The Lactating Sow

The Lactating Sow

M.W.A. Verstegen, P.J. Moughan and J.W. Schrama (editors)

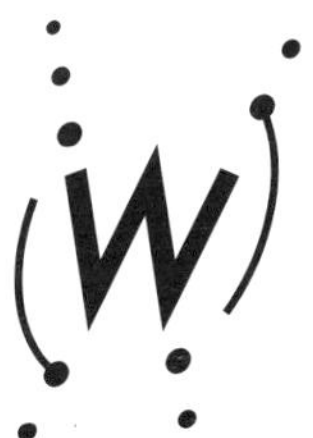

Wageningen Pers

**CIP-data Koninklijke Bibliotheek
Den Haag**

**ISBN 90-74134-43-2 hardbound
NUGI 835**

**Subject headings:
Milk production
Lactation
Pig**

First published, 1998

**Cover design:
Voorheen De Toekomst**

**Layout:
H. Kunst**

Printed in The Netherlands

List of authors

Prof. dr. L. **Babinszky**, head of the Department of Animal Nutrition and director of the Institute of Animal Physiology and Nutrition, Pannon University of Agriculture, Kaposvár, Hungary

Prof. dr. F. **Blecha**, professor of Immunophysiology, Department of Anatomy and Physiology, College of Veterinary Medicine, Kansas State University, Manhattan, USA

Dr. R.D. **Boyd**, director of Nutrition for the Pig Improvement Company USA, Franklin, USA

Prof. dr. P.H. **Brooks**, professor of Animal Production in the Seale-Hayne Faculty of Agriculture, Food and Land Use, University of Plymouth, England

Ms. J. **Burke** B.sc., postgraduate researcher at the Seale-Hayne Faculty of Agriculture, Food and Land Use, University of Plymouth, England

Dr. A.J. **Darragh**, research scientist at the Milk and Health Research Centre, Institute of Food, Nutrition and Human Health, Massey University, Palmerston North, New Zealand

Dr. G. **Dong**, scientist at the Southwest Agricultural University, Chongqing, Peoples Republic of China

Dr. J.-Y. **Dourmad**, director of research at INRA, Station de Recherches Porcines, St-Gilles, France

Dr. M. **Etienne**, director of research at INRA, Station de Recherches Porcines, St-Gilles, France

Dr. H. **Everts**, associate professor in Animal Nutrition at the Department of Large Animal Medicine and Nutrition, Faculty of Veterinary Medicine, Utrecht University, The Netherlands

Dr. ir. L.A. den **Hartog**, director of the Research Institute for Pig Husbandry, Rosmalen, The Netherlands

Dr. ir. B. **Kemp**, associate professor in Animal Reproduction at the Department of Animal Science, Wageningen Agricultural University, The Netherlands

Dr. R.S. **Kensinger**, associate professor of Animal Nutrition and Physiology at the Department of Dairy and Animal Science, Pennsylvania State University, Pennsylvania, USA

Dr. R.H. **King**, research scientist at the Victorian Institute of Animal Science, Werribee, Australia

Dr. D.D.S. **Mackenzie**, associate professor in Animal Science at the Institute for Food, Nutrition and Human Health, Massey University, Palmerston North, New Zealand

Dr. ir. C.A. **Makkink**, editor Animal Nutrition, De Molenaar, Leeuwarden, The Netherlands

Prof. dr. P.J. **Moughan**, head of the Institute of Food, Nutrition and Human Health, Massey University, Palmerston North, New Zealand

Dr. J. **Noblet**, director of research at INRA, Station de Recherches Porcines, St-Gilles, France

Ir. C.M.C. van der **Peet Schwering**, researcher in animal nutrition at the Research Institute for Pig Husbandry, Rosmalen, The Netherlands

Dr. J.E. **Pettigrew**, Pettigrew Consulting International, LLC, Louisiana, Missouri, USA and professor emeritus of the University of Minnesota, USA

Dr. J.R. **Pluske**, senior research scientist at the Monogastric Research Centre, Institute of Food, Nutrition and Human Health, Massey University, Palmerston North, New Zealand

Dr. D.K. **Revell**, lecturer in Animal Science at the Institute for Food, Nutrition and Human Health, Massey University, Palmerston North, New Zealand

Dr. ir. J.W. **Schrama**, head of the energy metabolism unit of the Wageningen Institute of Animal Science, Wageningen Agricultural University, The Netherlands

Dr. ir. J.W.G.M. **Swinkels**, senior researcher in Animal Welfare and Housing at the Research Institute for Pig Husbandry, Rosmalen, The Netherlands

Prof. dr. ir. M.W.A. **Verstegen**, professor of Animal Nutrition at Wageningen Institute of Animal Science, Wageningen Agricultural University, Animal Nutrition Group, The Netherlands

Prof. dr. C.T. **Whittemore**, professor of Agriculture & Rural Economy at the Institute of Ecology & Resource Management, University of Edinburgh, Scotland

Dr. I.H. **Williams**, senior lecturer in Animal Science at the Faculty of Agriculture, University of Western Australia, Nedlands, Australia

Contents

Introduction

World pig production has changed dramatically over the last three decades. Human population growth and an increase in the standard of living have considerably increased the demand for meat.

Animal production and pig production in particular have adapted to this demand through an increase in pig numbers. Other developments in animal agriculture have led to pigs which produce meat at a much higher efficiency and, moreover, the composition of the animals has changed towards more lean meat and less fat. Progress in animal, veterinary and the biological sciences (genetics, nutrition, reproductive physiology, husbandry) have led to the development of pigs with a high rate of gain in lean tissue and a low fat content. These modern animals are generally farmed under intensive production conditions.

Thus the modern lean type of pig has a much higher body lean content and less fat than the pig of several decades ago.

The piglets used for meat production are produced by sows which also have a reduced body fatness. Moreover in addition to this genetic selection for lean pigs, sows have been selected for producing a higher number of piglets per sow per year and higher litter weight. This has resulted in farms which wean up to 25 piglets per sow per year, when using the modern lean meat type of animal.

There is increasing awareness of a possible conflict between two aims, that of a lean type of animal and that of high reproductive performance. The biology of the lactating sow is increasingly studied with regard to these two aspects. In spite of this and compared to texts on the growing pig comprehensive textbooks on aspects of the lactating sow are not common.

The present book is focused on the sow. It aims to give an up-date on recent developments in research on biological aspects and on quantitative parameters about metabolism and production in the lactating sow. The seventeen chapters have been written by authors from several countries and leading international institutions.

The book brings together the various disciplines and it is aimed at students and scientists in animal, veterinary and biological sciences. It also aims to provide pig specialists with background and basic data on the lactating sow. This information can be used to develop nutritional, housing and management strategies for efficient pig production.

Wageningen and Palmerston North,
15 May 1998

Martin Verstegen
Paul Moughan
Johan Schrama

1 The Composition of Colostrum and Milk

A.J. Darragh and P.J. Moughan

1.1 Introduction

It is a long held belief that the milk of a given species is adapted to the nutrition of the young of that species (Oftedal, 1984). Indeed, the gross nutrient composition of milk is frequently used as the basis for developing an optimal diet for the neonate. This is readily seen in the manufacture of infant formulas for human infants where the gross chemical composition of breast milk is used as the 'gold' standard. Likewise, the gross composition of sow's milk is usually regarded as a suitable starting point when formulating milk-replacer diets for piglets. There is some debate, however, as to whether it is appropriate to use sow's milk composition in this manner (Hartmann *et al.*, 1984a).

Implicit in the assumption that milk is ideally suited to meet the neonate's nutrient requirements is an acceptance that the well-being of the neonate has been the primary selective force in the evolution of milk composition (Jenness & Sloan, 1970). It is also possible, however, that a dual selection process has occurred, whereby a compromise has been achieved between the neonate's nutrient requirements and those of the dam. The result would be a milk composition that, although meeting the minimum nutrient requirements of the neonate without depriving the dam of essential nutrients, is not necessarily optimal for the neonate. Closer scrutiny of this concept by Dewey *et al.* (1996), with regard to the human infant's protein requirements, has revealed that it is unlikely that there has been much evolutionary pressure to limit protein secretion in human milk. A similar study of the relationship between the piglet's needs and the composition of sow's milk has not been made. It is interesting to reflect upon the apparent compatibility between the amino acid profile of milk and the demands of a developing metabolic capacity in the newborn. Hartmann *et al.* (1984b) noted that human milk contains only small quantities of tyrosine and phenylalanine which match the limited capacity of the infant's relatively immature liver to metabolise these amino acids. The high level of cysteine in human milk, compared to other milks such as bovine milk (Jenness & Sloan, 1970) may also be uniquely suited to infant metabolism as the enzyme cystathionase, which converts methionine to cysteine, is absent in the premature infant's liver, and is thought to have limited capacity in the liver of the term infant (Gaull *et al.* 1972, Zlotkin *et al.* 1981, Zlotkin and Anderson, 1982). Also it would appear, that for humans at least, the metabolism of the lactating mother is able to buffer external factors to a considerable extent (Lönnerdal 1986, Finley 1986), and thus provide milk to the infant that is of consistent composition. It is reasonable to assume that this would also apply to the sow.

Thus, when determining an intake of nutrients that will optimise the growth and development of piglets, it is necessary to first consider the composition of sow's milk. This leads to an appreciation of the significance of this biological fluid, and the impact that it has on the piglet both in the provision of nutrients, and the maintenance of health and well-being.

1.2 Composition of sow's colostrum and milk

More than 130 years ago, von Gohren (1865) investigated the composition of sow's milk. Since then, many different aspects of sow's milk composition and milk production have been studied and reported in numerous publications (Braude *et al.*, 1947; Perrin, 1955; Bowland, 1966; Aumaitre & Seve, 1978; Pond & Houpt, 1978; Hartmann *et al.*, 1984a; Klobasa, *et al.*, 1987; Cranwell & Moughan, 1989; Hartmann & Holmes, 1989; Atwood & Hartmann, 1992; King *et al.*, 1993a; Wu & Knabe, 1994; Csapó *et al.* 1996).

The composition of sow's milk is in a constant state of change throughout lactation (Klobasa *et al.*, 1987; Csapó *et al.*, 1996), most markedly in the first few hours prior to, and immediately after parturition. Following a gradual accumulation of pre-colostrum in the mammary glands of the sow during gestation (Kensinger *et al.*, 1982), parturition results in appearance of the first-milk or colostrum (Hartmann & Holmes, 1989). Dramatic changes in milk composition occur during the first 2-3 days postpartum (Klobasa *et al.*, 1987). After the first week, the milk having passed through a transition stage can be regarded as being relatively stable or mature, although some changes will still occur right up to and beyond weaning (Klobasa *et al.*, 1987; Csapó *et al.*, 1996). The transition from colostrum to 'mature' milk is characterised by a substantial decrease in total solids and protein. Simultaneously, there is an increase in the concentration of lactose and fat. The ash content is lower in sow's colostrum compared to mature milk, which is the opposite to that found in many other species (Perrin, 1955). The extent of these changes in composition is outlined in Table 1.1.

The composition of sow's colostrum and milk is variable due to the following factors: variation between sows (Perrin, 1955); breed differences (Fahmy, 1972; Zou *et al.*, 1992); differing dietary regimens (King *et al.*, 1993b; Noblet & Etienne, 1986; Jackson *et al.*, 1995; Midgal 1991; Göransson 1990; Miller *et al.*, 1994); differences in body condition (Klaver *et al.* 1981); and varying disease status (Gooneratne *et al.*, 1982). Moreover, compositional data can be influenced by the techniques used to collect milk samples (Atwood & Hartmann, 1992), and the methods used for storage and chemical analysis. Therefore, to present a single set of compositional data as is the case here, albeit averaged across several sources of information, may be misleading, and care should be exercised when interpreting and applying such data.

Table 1.1. The major components of sow's colostrum and milk (g/100 g milk)

Component	Colostrum[1]	Mature Milk[2]	Reference[3]
Total Solids	24.8	18.7	b, c, d, e
Protein[4]	15.1	5.5	a, c, d, e, f
Non-protein Nitrogen	0.3	0.3	d, e
Lactose	3.4	5.3	a, b, c, e, f
Fat	5.9	7.6	a, b, c, d, e, f
Ash	0.7	0.9	c, d

[1] Taken immediately postpartum.
[2] Classified as milk samples collected between 14 and 21 days postpartum.
[3] a: Cranwell & Moughan (1989); b: Jenness & Sloan (1970); c: Oftedal (1984); d: Csapó *et al.* (1996); e: Klobasa *et al.* (1987); f: Atwood & Hartmann (1993).
[4] Total Protein as determined by N X 6.38.

Proteins and amino acids
Initially, the piglet is dependent upon an adequate intake of colostral proteins to obtain both humoral and surface protection against microbial infections. After approximately 24-36 hours, when the piglet can no longer obtain passive immunity by macromolecular absorption (Westrom *et al.* 1984), the role of proteins in the milk switches to that of primarily providing the amino acids essential for tissue maintenance and growth, although a degree of immune protection continues through the presence of specific whey proteins.

The proteins present in colostrum and milk can be grouped as two types: caseins and whey proteins. The caseins are made up of several subtypes (Jenness 1985), while the whey fraction consists of blood serum albumin, α-lactalbumin, β-lactoglobulin, immunoglobulin G (IgG), immunoglobulin A (IgA), immunoglobulin M (IgM), lactoferrin, and other minor proteins. The proportions of casein and whey proteins in sow's colostrum and milk are presented in Table 1.2.

The caseins are viewed predominantly as a source of dietary essential amino acids. In their synopsis of sow lactation, Hartmann & Holmes (1989) discussed the role of casein in sow's milk describing the prevalence of different casein subtypes and their functions. Casein is a carrier of calcium (Jenness & Sloan, 1970; Kitts & Yuan, 1992) and may help in the absorption of calcium in the neonate (Lee *et al.*, 1983; Sato *et al.*, 1986). Kappa-casein has been shown to stimulate the growth of *Bifidobacterium infantis* in human infants (Azuma *et al.*, 1984). It is possible that porcine κ-casein may also promote the growth of favourable bacteria in the gut of suckled piglets.

Table 1.2. The protein content of sow's colostrum and mature milk

	Colostrum[1]	Mature Milk[2]	References[3]
Total Protein[4] (g/100 g milk)	15.14	5.47	a, b, c, d, e
Casein (g/100 g milk)	1.48	2.74	c, d
Whey (g/100 g milk)	14.75	2.22	c, d
Serum albumin (mg/ml milk)	15.79	4.61	d
IgG[5] (mg/ml milk)	95.6	0.9	d
IgA[6] (mg/ml milk)	21.2	5.3	d
IgM[7] (mg/ml milk)	9.1	1.4	d
Lactoferrin ((g/ml milk)	1200	<100	f

[1] Taken immediately postpartum.
[2] Classified as milk samples collected between 14 and 21 days postpartum.
[3] a: Cranwell & Moughan (1989); b: Oftedal (1984); c: Csapó *et al.*, (1996); d: Klobasa *et al.* (1987); e: Atwood & Hartmann (1993); f: Elliot *et al.* (1984).
[4] Total Protein as determined by N X 6.38.
[5] Immunoglobulin G
[6] Immunoglobluin A
[7] Immunoglobulin M

Although casein serves a primary function of providing the neonate with a source of amino acids, some of the peptides arising during digestion of the casein proteins (Migliore-Samour & Jolles, 1988) are now recognised as being biologically active. For example, bovine β-casomorphin (Brantl *et al.*, 1979), human β-casomorphin (Brantl, 1984), and peptides from bovine α-casein are all thought to have immunomodulatory effects in the newborn (Migliore-Samour & Jolles, 1988). Although not, as yet, specifically identified in sow's milk, it would seem reasonable to assume that digestion of porcine caseins could also provide biologically active peptides to the piglet's gut.

Whey proteins make up approximately 90% of the total protein in colostrum at parturition, but account for less than 60% of total protein from day 5 postpartum onwards (Klobasa *et al.* 1987). Of the whey proteins found in early colostrum, over 90% can be attributed to the three major immunoglobulins which are essential for transferring passive immunity to the newborn piglet (Hartmann *et al.*, 1989). Immunoglobulin G (IgG) predominates in early colostrum (76% of total immunoglobulins), and is absorbed directly into the piglet's blood circulation (Pond & Houpt, 1978). Following a rapid decline in IgG concentrations during the first 24 hours after parturition (Figure 1.1), immunoglobulin A (IgA) emerges as the major immunoglobulin, accounting for more than 70% of total immunoglobulins from day 14 of lactation onwards. This shift in the concentrations of each immunoglobulin reflects the changing needs of the piglet, as absorption of whole proteins gives way to the maintenance of localised immune protection within the gut.

Once the secretion of mature milk has been established, albumin, β-lactoglobulin and α-lactalbumin account for the majority of the whey proteins. Previous studies with bovine and human whey proteins have found that serum albumin, β-lactoglobulin and α-lactalbumin are all highly digestible (Jakobsson *et al.*, 1982; Britton & Koldovsky, 1987). Alpha-lactalbumin, in particular, has an excellent nutritive value (Forsum, 1973), with a high content of lysine and cysteine and a particularly high tryptophan content (Heine *et al.*, 1991). In a recent study (Rutherfurd & Moughan, 1998) true ileal amino acid digestibility coefficients were determined for young growing pigs given a range of bovine milk-based proteins. High coefficients ranging from 0.83 for serine in casein to 1.0 for methionine in whey protein were determined. Rather than having a biological role within the gut, albumin, β-lactoglobulin and α-lactalbumin, together with the casein proteins, appear to serve to provide the piglet with essential amino acids.

There are a number of minor proteins in sow's milk which have been the subject of review (Hartmann & Holmes, 1989; Cranwell & Moughan, 1989). Lactoferrin, lysozyme, transferrin, vitamin B_{12}-binding protein and the bifidus factor have all been found in sow's milk (Gyorgy *et al.*, 1954; Schulze & Muller, 1980; Trugo & Newport, 1983; Elliot *et al.*, 1984; Jenness, 1986), and are thought to play a role

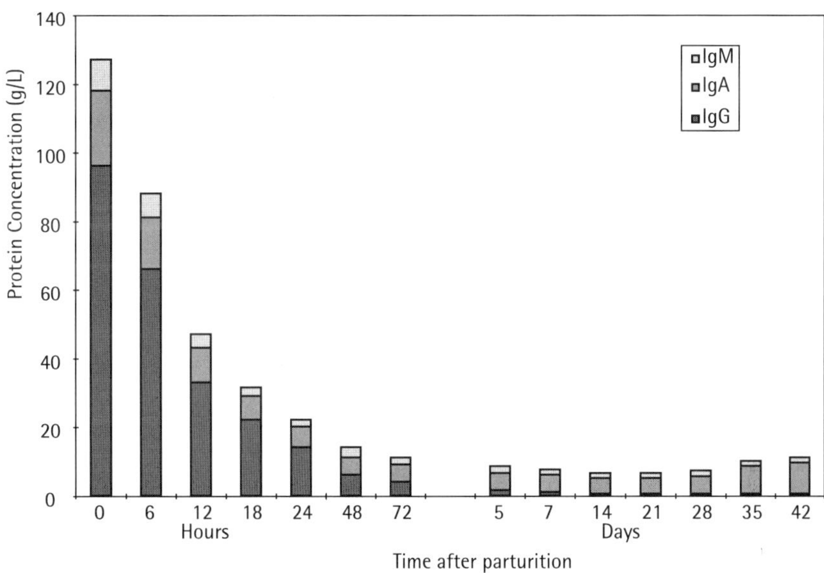

Figure 1.1. Changes in the concentration of immunoglobulins in sow's milk during a 42 day lactation (modified from Klobasa et al. 1987)

in protecting the piglet against disease. Lactoperoxidase, an enzyme found in bovine milk, has not, as yet, been identified in sow's milk (Jenness, 1986). Sow's milk contains several digestive enzymes, including lipase, α-amylase, esterase, protease and alkaline phosphatase, which are thought to assist digestion in the newborn (Hartmann & Holmes, 1989). In contrast, a protease inhibitor, found in sow's colostrum but rapidly declining to very low levels in milk secreted after the first few days of lactation (Westrom *et al.*, 1982), aids in the transfer of intact immunoglobulins into the blood of the newborn piglet (Westrom *et al.*, 1985).

The gross amino acid composition of sow's colostrum and milk are given in Table 1.3. Changes in the milk amino acid pattern during lactation reflect a change in the relative distribution of milk proteins with different amino acid patterns. The ratio of casein to whey, particularly immunoglobulins and α-lactalbumin, increases during the course of lactation. Whey proteins have generally lower concentra-

Table 1.3. The amino acid composition of sow's colostrum and milk (g/100g amino acid and, in brackets, as proportions of lysine = 100)

Amino Acid	Colostrum[1]		Mature Milk		References[3]
Lysine	6.5	(100)	7.5	(100)	a, b, c, d
Methionine	1.8	(28)	1.7	(23)	a, b, c, d
Cysteine	2.2	(34)	1.5	(20)	a, b, c, d
Histidine	2.3	(35)	2.4	(32)	a, b, c, d
Phenylalanine	4.5	(69)	3.9	(52)	a, b, c, d
Tyrosine	4.4	(68)	4.2	(56)	a, b, c, d
Threonine	5.5	(85)	3.9	(52)	a, b, c, d
Isoleucine	3.0	(46)	3.8	(51)	a, b, c, d
Leucine	9.8	(151)	8.8	(117)	a, b, c, d
Valine	5.5	(85)	4.7	(63)	a, b, c, d
Tryptophan	1.6	(25)	1.4	(19)	a, b, d
Arginine	5.4	(83)	5.2	(69)	a, b, c
Proline	9.2	(142)	11.3	(151)	b, c
Glycine	3.3	(51)	2.8	(37)	b, c
Glutamic Acid	17.4	(268)	21.6	(288)	b, c
Aspartic Acid	7.8	(120)	7.9	(105)	b, c
Serine	6.3	(97)	5.2	(69)	b, c
Alanine	4.4	(68)	3.2	(43)	b, c

[1] Taken immediately postpartum.

[2] Classified as milk samples collected between 14 and 21 days postpartum.

[3] a: Cranwell & Moughan (1989); b: Csapó *et al.*, (1996); c: Davis *et al.*, (1994); d: ARC (1981).

tions of glutamic acid, proline and methionine, and are richer in cysteine, glycine and threonine compared to the casein proteins (Heine *et al.*, 1991). These differences in amino acid composition between whey and casein proteins, are consistent with the different amino acid compositions found for colostrum and milk.

The gross amino acid compositions of sow's colostrum and milk as presented in Table 1.3, do not, however, provide a clear indication of the amounts of amino acids nutritionally available to the piglet. Immunoglobulins, being glycoproteins, are not readily hydrolysed in the gastrointestinal tract of the piglet (Hartmann *et al.*, 1984a), which aids in their role as providers of passive immunity at the gut mucosal level. Studies in human infants have shown that 79% of colostral IgA (Ogra *et al.*, 1977), and between 10 and 35% of the IgA in mature human milk (Prentice *et al.*, 1987; Davidson & Lönnerdal, 1987) can be identified in the faeces of infants.

Resistance of specific milk proteins to digestion, and subsequent failure to provide amino acids for absorption implies that the gross amino acid composition of milk will reflect neither the profile of amino acids absorbed by the neonate nor the neonate's amino acid requirements. This profile, which represents the nutritionally available amino acid composition, can only be obtained by determining digestibility coefficients for the individual amino acids in milk, and then using them to correct the gross amino acid composition. Such an approach has recently been used to determine the available amino acid composition of human milk (Darragh & Moughan, 1998) and some important compositional differences have been recorded (Table 1.4).

It can be argued that the absorbed amino acid composition of sow's milk is not a satisfactory basis for estimating the piglet's amino acid requirements for growth and development. Several studies, reviewed by Pluske *et al.* (1995), have shown that suckled piglets normally grow at less than their potential growth rate from birth to three weeks of age. The issue arises as to what constitutes a nutrient requirement. From a commercial point of view maximum growth rate is desirable, but this may not be the optimum in nature. Rather, the aim may be to achieve a subtle and dynamic balance between rapid growth, successful development, maximal resistance to disease and environmental changes, and adequate behavioural development. Further, it may be that the composition of milk reflects an evolutionary compromise between the nutritional needs of the dam and those of the offspring (Koletzko, 1997), though it is informative to note that the amino acid composition of sow's milk is very similar to that of piglet tissue (ARC, 1981) and that the protein in sow's milk is very efficiently utilised by piglets. The amino acid composition of sow's milk is likely to be a useful guide to the optimal balance of amino acids required by the young pig. Where the objective is to maximise piglet body growth rate, the absolute amounts of amino acids normally ingested by sucking piglets are seemingly too low. The absorbed amino acid profile of sow's milk should be used as a basis for an optimal dietary amino acid balance.

Table 1.4. Gross and absorbed amino acid composition of human milk[1] (mg/100 ml; mean ±SEM) (from Darragh, 1995)

Amino Acid	Gross[2]	Absorbed[3]
Aspartic Acid	102 ± 2.4	97 ± 2.3
Threonine	52 ± 1.6	44 ± 1.4
Proline	95 ± 2.3	87 ± 2.2
Valine	58 ± 1.4	52 ± 1.3
Isoleucine	57 ± 1.0	56 ± 1.0
Leucine	104 ± 1.8	103 ± 1.8
Phenylalanine	43 ± 1.9	39 ± 1.8
Histidine	26 ± 0.6	25 ± 0.6
Lysine	70 ± 1.5	68 ± 1.5
Methionine	16 ± 0.4	16 ± 0.4

[1] Mean values of samples taken from women in their 10th-14th weeks of lactation.
[2] Gross composition uncorrected for digestibility of individual amino acids.
[3] Absorbed composition calculated by correcting the gross amino acid composition with digestibility coefficients determined for the individual amino acids in human milk using the three-week-old piglet as a model animal for the three-month-old human infant.

Carbohydrates
Lactose is the major carbohydrate in sow's milk (Hartmann & Holmes, 1989), and is secreted into the lumen of the alveolus, along with other milk constituents such as the proteins, and some minerals, by exocytosis of the Golgi vesicles at the apical membrane of the epithelial cell. Lactose is also the primary osmotic constituent of milk (Jenness, 1985), and it is thought that the formation of lactose is a major determinant of milk yield (Hartmann & Holmes, 1989; See Chapter 5 by MacKenzie and Revell). The lactose concentration in milk nearly doubles during the first 1-2 weeks of lactation (see Table 1.1) and, thereafter, slowly decreases (Klobasa *et al.*, 1987), corresponding to a dramatic increase in milk volume reaching a peak flow at around 21 days (Oftedal, 1984), followed by a gradual decrease in milk volume as lactation proceeds. Intermediates of lactose synthesis, together with the ATP breakdown products ADP, AMP, cAMP, and the monosaccharides galactose and fructose also appear in sow's milk (Atwood & Hartmann, 1995). The quantities of these metabolites in sow's milk are given in Table 1.5.

During digestion, lactose is hydrolysed to yield glucose and galactose. These monosaccharides are readily absorbed into the piglet's blood, and are either metabolised directly, or used to replenish stores of liver and muscle glycogen (Hartmann *et al.*, 1989). Lactose is thought to improve the absorption of calcium

Table 1.5. Concentrations of selected metabolites in sow's milk[1] (Modified from Atwood & Hartmann, 1995)

Metabolite	Concentration (µmol/ml milk)
Glucose	0.67
G-6-P	0.06
G-1-P	0.02
UDPglc	0.30
UDPgal	0.64
Lactose	162
UDP	0.11
UMP	1.87
P_1	14
ATP	<0.0005
ADP	0.05
AMP	0.22
cAMP	0.02
Galactose	0.20
Fructose	0.23

[1] Milk collected from sows between days 5-11 of lactation.

in the newborn (Gaull *et al.* 1982), although this may be related to the presence of α-lactalbumin. Alpha-lactalbumin is part of the enzyme, lactose synthetase, which is responsible for lactose synthesis in the mammary gland (Blanc, 1981), and has been found to bind calcium in a 1:1 molar ratio (Lönnerdal & Glazier, 1985). It is possible that this calcium-binding property of α-lactalbumin may facilitate the absorption of calcium in the neonate.

Fat

Milk fat mainly comprises triglycerides, together with lesser amounts of di- and mono-glycerides, phospholipids, glycolipids, cholesterol, cholesterol ester, fat-soluble vitamins, and free fatty acids (Jenness, 1985), and the quantities of these components appearing in sow's colostrum and milk have been reviewed in detail (Hartmann & Holmes, 1989).

Unlike other nutrients in milk, the fat content can be substantially influenced by factors such as breed (Zou *et al.*, 1992), sow condition (Klaver *et al.*, 1981), and dietary regimen (Migdal, 1991; Göransson,1990; King *et al.*, 1993b; Jackson *et al.*, 1995). Furthermore, the method of milk collection can have a significant effect on the determined fat content of a milk sample (Atwood & Hartmann, 1992). Due to the number of factors that can influence the fat content of sow's colostrum and milk, the data reported here should be interpreted as merely indicative. Changes in the percentage of fat in sow's colostrum and milk observed in studies by Jackson *et al.* (1995), and Csapó *et al.*, (1996), are shown in Figures 1.2 and 1.3, respectively. Comparison of the two figures illustrates the degree of variability in fat content that can exist. In both studies, however, milk fat content was highest between 48-72 hours postpartum followed by a decrease as lactation progressed.

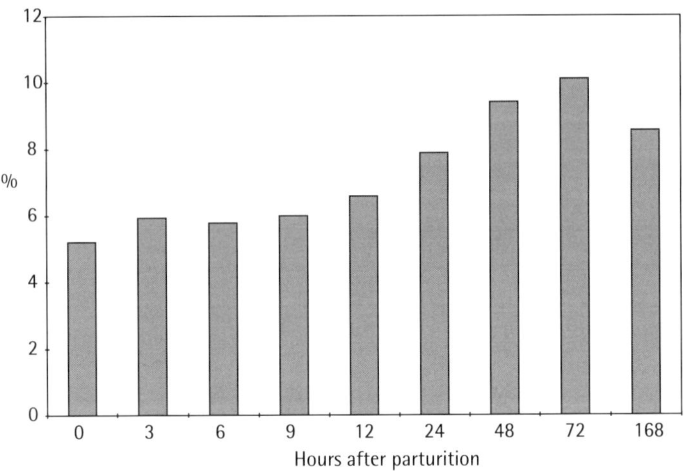

Figure 1.2. Changes in the concentration of fat in sow colostrum and milk (Adapted from Jackson et al., 1995)

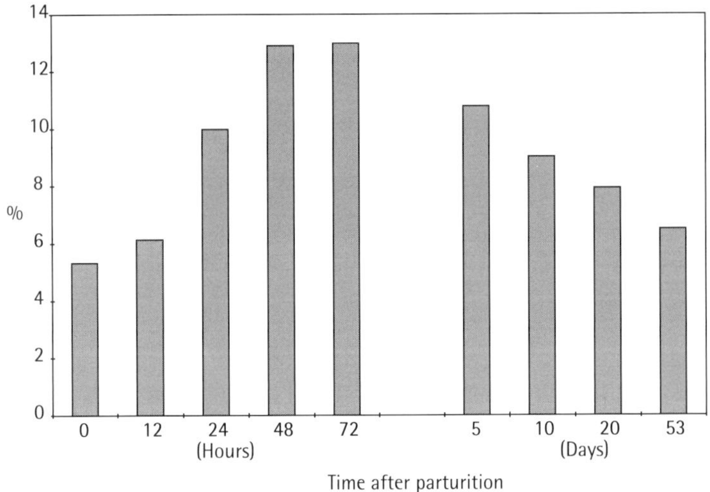

Figure 1.3. Changes in the concentration of fat in sow colostrum and milk (Adapted from Csapó et al., 1996)

A wide range of types of fatty acids has been found in the colostrum and milk of sows (Table 1.6). Colostrum appears to be devoid of short chain fatty acids, being dominated instead by oleic and palmitic acids, followed by linoleic acid. The proportions of fatty acids change continuously during lactation, consistent with changes in the fatty acid composition of blood triglycerides (Witter *et al.*, 1970), which are influenced by the type of fat in the sow's diet (Hartmann & Holmes, 1989). Hartmann & Holmes (1989) reviewed a collection of studies that showed there was a significant effect of diet on the fatty acid composition of sow's milk. An increase in oleic acid occurred when beef tallow was used, whereas the percentage of linoleic acid increased when corn oil was added to the diet. They concluded that well-fed, lactating sows utilise fatty acids of dietary origin for the synthesis of milk fats. Sows in a negative energy balance, however, such

Table 1.6. Fatty acids (%[1]) in the fat of sow's colostrum[2] and milk[3] (from Csapó et al., 1996)

Fatty Acid	Colostrum	Mature Milk
Butyric Acid (4:0)[4]	0	0.08
Caproic Acid (6:0)	0	0.09
Caprylic Acid (8:0)	0	0.03
Capric Acid (10:0)	0	0.01
Lauric Acid (12:0)	0	0.02
Myristic Acid (14:0)	3.2	3.71
Myristoleic Acid (14:1)	0.01	0
Pentadecanoic Acid (15:0)	0.03	0.01
Pentadecenoic Acid (15:1)	0.01	0
Palmitic Acid (16:0)	33.3	37
Palmitoleic Acid (16:1)	5.47	9.1
Heptadecanoic Acid (17:0)	0.08	0.09
Heptadecenoic Acid (17:1)	0.13	0.14
Stearic Acid (18:0)	6.31	6.02
Oleic Acid (18:1)	37.5	33
Linoleic Acid (18:2)	12.7	8.9
Linolenic Acid (18:3)	0.74	1.14
Arachidic Acid (20:4)	0.42	0.51
Behenic Acid (22:0)	0.01	0.01
Eicosatric Acid (20:3)/Erucic Acid (22:1)	0.11	0.13

[1] Relative percentages of the fatty acid methyl esters.

[2] Taken immediately postpartum.

[3] Classified as milk samples collected between 14 and 21 days postpartum.

[4] Values in parentheses indicate length of carbon chain and degree of saturation.

as would occur immediately post-partum, produced milk with increased levels of C_{18} fatty acids and a lower content of C_{14} and C_{16} fatty acids. This may, in part, explain why Csapó *et al.*, (1996) could not detect the shorter chain fatty acids in sow's colostrum.

Hormones and growth factors
Milk contains numerous hormones, growth-promoting factors and other compounds that may have regulatory roles, the physiological functions of which are only poorly understood (Cranwell & Moughan, 1989). Prolactin (Mulloy & Malven, 1979), oestrone (Farmer *et al.*, 1987), prostaglandin-like substances (Maffeo *et al.*, 1987), insulin, neurotensin, bombesin (Westrom *et al.*, 1987), and thyroid hormones (Slebodzinki *et al.*, 1986) have all been identified in sow's milk. Epidermal growth factor (Jaeger *et al.*, 1987) and insulin-like growth factor (Simmen *et al.*, 1988) have also been detected in sow's colostrum and milk. These compounds may have a range of specific physiological functions in the piglet, including being important in maturation of the digestive system (James *et al.*, 1987), and the induction and modulation of hormones and peptides secreted by the gut (Lucas, 1986).

Vitamins and Minerals
The quantity of vitamins found in sow's colostrum and milk, which will have originated from both the diet and from maternal stores (Pond & Houpt, 1978), can be influenced by a number of factors including seasonal changes, liver stores, and the maternal diet (Hartmann & Holmes, 1989). In Table 1.7, the concentrations of vitamins in colostrum and mature milk are presented. Vitamins A, D, E, and K_3 are all present in higher concentrations in colostrum compared to later secretions. The content of vitamin C, however, increases as lactation proceeded. On the contrary, Hidiroglou & Batra (1995) found that the vitamin C content of colostrum was more than twice that of subsequently produced milk. It is generally assumed that pigs can synthesise vitamin C, and do not require dietary supplementation. Thus it would appear that the piglet can obtain all the vitamin C it requires from either colostrum and milk, both of which appear to be rich sources of vitamin C, or by *de novo* synthesis. There have been reported cases of rickets (a disorder related to vitamin D deficiency) in piglets in the past, due to a lack of vitamin D in the milk (Hartmann & Holmes, 1989). This may be a reflection of the change of habitat that intensive pig production systems enforce on the sow and her piglets, as a primary source of vitamin D would normally be obtained from the conversion of the vitamin D precursor, 7-dehydrocholesterol by the ultraviolet component of sunlight.

Changes in the concentrations of various minerals as milk progresses from a colostral to mature secretion are shown in Table 1.7. In general, the mineral content of sow's milk increases as lactation progresses, with the exception of sodium and magnesium, both of which have lower concentrations in mature milk compared to colostrum. The concentration of calcium more than doubles from 0-21 days, while the phosphorus content of sow's milk also increases but less markedly than calcium, resulting in calcium to phosphorus ratios of 0.7:1 and 1.4:1 for colostrum and milk, respectively. The recommended calcium to phosphorus ratio for optimal growth in the piglet is between 1.1 to 1.5:1 (Pond & Houpt, 1978).

Table 1.7. Concentration of vitamins and minerals in sow's colostrum[1] and mature milk[2]

Nutrient	Colostrum	Mature Milk	References[3]
Vitamins *((g/100 ml milk)*			
Vitamin A	169	96	a, b
Vitamin D	1.58	0.95	a, b
Vitamin E	390	266	a, b
Vitamin C	7.2	8.42	a, b
Vitamin K_3	9.68	9.37	a, b
Vitamin B_{12}	–[4]	0.15	a
Thiamine	–	0.07	a
Riboflavin	–	0.28	a
Nicotinic Acid	–	0.74	a
Pantothenic Acid	–	0.46	a
Folic Acid	–	0.39	a
Biotin	–	1.4	a
Minerals *(mg/100 g milk)*			
Calcium	68.6	162.8	b, c
Phosphorus	101.7	118.3	b, c
Potassium	11.0	58.7	b, c
Sodium	68.5	39.3	b, c
Magnesium	7.9	9.0	b, c
Iron	0.2	0.2	b, c
Zinc	1.6	0.7	b, c
Sulphur	–	3.6	c
Copper	0.4	0.2	b, c

[1] Taken immediately postpartum.

[2] Classified as milk samples collected between 14 and 21 days postpartum.

[3] a: Cranwell & Moughan (1989); b: Csapó *et al.*, (1996); c: Park *et al.*, (1994).

[4] Not determined.

Both the iron and copper concentrations in sow's milk are considerably lower than for any of the other minerals, and iron deficiency can manifest itself in piglets that are intensively reared indoors (Pond & Houpt, 1978). This may suggest that sow's milk is naturally deficient in iron. More likely, however, it is the result of limited body stores of iron in both the sow and piglet, and an inability to access soil, which would, in the wild state, provide a ready supply of dietary iron. That sow's milk is deficient in iron is not so much a matter of evolutionary failure, rather it is indicative of the rearing systems adopted commercially. It would be wrong to conclude from this that sow's milk is not an appropriate form of nutrition for the piglet.

Cells

A variety of cells are secreted in milk and are thought to provide protection against infection in both the mammary gland and the digestive tract of the piglet (Reiter, 1978). Counts of different cell types, expressed as a percentage of the total cell count, in sow's colostrum and milk, are presented in Table 1.8. Neutrophils and lymphocytes constitute the majority of cells in colostrum, but decline in number as lactation proceeds. Epithelial cells, assumed to originate from abrasion of the lining of the mammary gland (Hartmann & Holmes, 1989), increase in later milk secretions.

Table 1.8. Differential cell counts[1] in sow's colostrum[2] and mature milk[3] (from Wuryastuti et al., 1993)

Cell Type	Colostrum	Milk
Neutrophils[4]	64	40.7
Macrophages	5.6	15.5
Lymphocytes	26.5	19.2
Eosinophils	0.7	0.4
Epithelial Cells	1.4	23.6

[1] Expressed as a percentage of total cell count.
[2] Taken immediately postpartum.
[3] Classified as milk samples collected between 14 and 21 days postpartum.
[4] Polymorphonuclear cells.

1.3 Summary

Milk, a natural secretion with a complex and tailored chemical composition and physical structure, must surely be regarded as more than merely a food. Subtle physiological roles of milk components are being increasingly discovered and described, and a view is emerging of a biologically active material of key importance in the regulation of overall development in the neonate. Milk is a relatively uncontaminated fluid. It supplies the sucking piglet with a frequent semi-continuous source of food, water, immune protection and biological regulatory factors. The nursing of offspring by the dam also involves key behavioural and social elements which need to be considered from social and ethical as well as production related perspectives.

In order to design production systems for rearing healthy, functional pigs the unique properties and composition of milk must be completely understood. At present our understanding is less than complete.

1.4 References

Agricultural Research Council, 1981. The nutrient requirements of pigs. Commonwealth Agricultural Bureaux, Slough.

Atwood, C.S. & P.E. Hartmann, 1992. Collection of fore and hind milk from the sow and the changes in milk composition during suckling. J. Dairy Res. 59:287-298

Atwood, C.S. & P.E. Hartmann, 1993. The concentration of fat, protein and lactose in sows' colostrum from sucked and unsucked glands during lactogenesis II. Aust. J. Agric. Res. 44:1457-65

Atwood, C.S. & P.E. Hartmann, 1995. Assessment of mammary gland metabolism in the sow. I. Development of methods for the measurement of cellular metabolites in milk and colostrum. J. Dairy Res. 62:189-206

Aumaitre, A. & B. Seve, 1978. Nutritional importance of colostrum in the piglet. Ann. Rech. Vet. 9:181-192

Azuma, N., K. Yamauchi & T. Mitsuoka, 1984. Bifidus growth-promoting activity of a glycomacropeptide derived from human κ-casein. Agric. Biol. Chem. 48:2159-2162

Blanc, B., 1981. Biochemical aspects of human milk - comparison with bovine milk. Wrld Rev. Nutr. Diet. 36:1-89

Bowland, J.P., 1966. Swine in Biomedical Research. Editors, L.K. Bustad, R.O. McClellan & M.P. Burns. Pacific Northwest Laboratory, Washington. 97-107

Brantl, V., 1984. Novel opioid peptides derived from human β-casein: Human β-casomorphins. Europ. J. Pharm. 106:213-214

Brantl, V., H. Teschemacher, A. Henschen & F. Lattspeich, 1979. Novel opioid peptides derived from casein (β-casomorphins). Hoppe-Seyler's Z. Physiol. Chem. 360:1211-1216

Braude, R., M.E. Coates, K.M. Henry, S.K. Son, S.J. Rowland, S.Y. Thomson & D.M. Walker, 1947. A study of the composition of sow's milk. Brit. J. Nutr 1:64-77

Britton, J.R. & O. Koldovsky, 1987. Luminal digestion of human milk proteins in suckling and weanling rats. Nutr. Res. 7:1041-1049

Cranwell, P.D. & P.J. Moughan, 1989. Biological limitations imposed by the digestive system to the growth performance of weaned pigs. In: Manipulating Pig Production II. Proceedings of the Australasian Pig Science Association, Editors, J.L. Barnett & D.P. Hennessy, Australasian Pig Science Association, Werribee. 140-159

Csapó J., T.G. Martin, Z.S. Csapó-Kiss & Z. Házas, 1996. Proteins, fats, vitamin and mineral concentrations in porcine colostrum and milk from parturition to 60 days. Int. Dairy J. 6:881-902

Darragh, A.J., 1995. The Amino Acid Composition of Human Milk - Towards Determining the Amino Acid Requirements of the Human Infant. PhD Thesis, Massey University, Palmerston North, New Zealand.

Darragh, A.J. & P.J. Moughan, 1998. The amino acid composition of human milk corrected for amino acid digestibility. Brit. J. Nut. (in press)

Davidson, L.A. & B. Lönnerdal, 1987. Persistence of human milk proteins in the breast-fed infant. Acta Paediatr. Scand. 76:733-740

Davis, T.A, H.V. Nguyen, R. Garcia-Bravo, M.L. Fiorotto, E.M. Jackson & P.J. Reeds, 1994. Amino acid composition of the milk of some mammalian species changes with stage of lactation. Brit. J. Nutr 72:845-853

Dewey, K.G., G. Beaton, C. Fjeld, B. Lönnerdal & P. Reeds, 1996. Protein requirements of infants and children. Euro. J. Clin. Nut 50:S119-S150

Elliot, J.I, B.Senft, G. Erhardt & D. Fraser, 1984. Isolation of lactoferrin and its concentration in sows' colostrum and milk during a 21-day lacation. J. Anim. Sc 59:1080-1084

Fahmy, M.H., 1972. Comparative study of colostrum and milk composition of seven breeds of swine. Can. J. Anim. Sci. 52:621-627

Farmer, C., S.K. Houtz & D.R. Hagen, 1987. Estrone concentration in sow milk during and after parturition. J. Anim. Sci. 64:1086-1089

Finley, D.A., 1986. Effects of vegetarian diets upon the composition of human milk. In: Human Lactation 2: Maternal and Environmental Factors. Editors, M. Hamosh & A.S. Goldman. Plenum Press, New York. 89-92

Forsum, E., 1973. Nutritional evaluation of whey protein concentrates and their fractions. J. Dairy Sci. 57:665-670

Gaull, G.E., R.G. Jensen, D.K. Rassin & M.H. Malloy, 1982. Advances in Perinatal Medicine. Volume 2. Editors, A. Milunsky, E.A. Friedman & L. Gluck. Plenum Publishing Corporation, New York. 47-120

Gaull, G., J.A. Sturman & N.C.R. Raiha, 1972. Development of mammalian sulphur metabolism: Absence of cystathionase in human fetal tissues. Pediatr. Res. 6: 538-547.

Gooneratne, A.D., P.E. Hartmann & H.M. Nottage, 1982. The initiation of lactation in sows and the mastitis-metritis-agalactia syndrome. Anim. Reprod. Sci. 5:135-140

Göransson, L., 1990. The effect of late pregnancy feed allowance on the composition of the sow's colostrum and milk (sic). Acta Vet. Scand. 31:109-115

Gyorgy, P., R. Kuhn, C.S. Rose & F. Zilliken, 1954. Bifidus factor. II. Its occurrence in milk from different species and its other natural products. Arch. Biochem. 48:202-207

Hartmann, P.E. & M.A. Holmes, 1989. Sow lactation. In: Manipulating Pig Production II. Proceedings of the Australasian Pig Science Association, Editors, J.L. Barnett & D.P. Hennessy, Australasian Pig Science Association, Werribee. 72-97

Hartmann, P.E., P.H. Bird & M.A. Holmes, 1989. The influence of lactation on piglet survival. In: Manipulating Pig Production II. Proceedings of the Australasian Pig Science Association, Editors, J.L. Barnett & D.P. Hennessy, Australasian Pig Science Association, Werribee. 101-134

Hartmann, P.E., I. McCauley, A.D. Gooneratne & J.L Whitely, 1984a. Inadequacies of sow lactation: survival of the fittest. In: Physiological Strategies in Lactation. Symposia of the Zoological Society of London, Volume 51. Editors, M. Peaker. R. G. Vernon & C.H. Knight, Academic Press, London. 301-326

Hartmann, P.E., S. Rattigan, C.G. Prosser, L. Saint & P.G. Arthur, 1984b. Human lactation: back to nature. In: Physiological Strategies in Lactation. Symposia of the Zoological Society of London, Volume 51. Editors, M. Peaker. R. G. Vernon & C.H. Knight, Academic Press, London. 337-368

Heine, W.E., P.D. Klein & R.J. Reeds, 1991. The importance of α-lactalbumin in infant nutrition. J. Nutr. 121:227-283

Hidiroglou, M. & T.R. Batra, 1995. Concentrations of vitamin C in milk of sows and in plasma of piglets. Can. J. Anim. Sci. 75:275-277

Jackson, J.R., W.L. Hurley, R.A. Easter, A.H. Jensen & J. Odle, 1995. Effects of induced or delayed parturition and supplemental dietary fat on colostrum and milk composition in sows. J. Anim. Sci. 73:1906-1913

Jaeger, L.A., C.H. Lamar, G.D. Bottoms & T.R. Cline, 1987. Growth-stimulating substances in porcine milk. Am. J. Vet. Res. 48:1531-1533

Jakobsson, I., T. Lindberg 7 B. Benediktsson, 1982. In vitro digestion of cow's milk protein by duodenal juice from infants with various gastrointestinal disorders. J. Pediatr. Gastroenterol. Nutr. 1:183-191

James, P.S., M.W. Smith, D.R. Tivey & T.J.G. Wilson, 1987. Epidermal growth factor selectively increases maltase and sucrase activities in neonatal piglet intestine. J. Physiol. 393:583-594

Jenness, R., 1985. Lactation. Editors, B. L. Larson & R.R. Anderson. Iowa State University Press, Iowa. 164-167

Jenness, R., 1986. Inter-species comparison of milk proteins. Developments in Dairy Chemistry, Volume 1. Applied Science, London. 87-114

Jenness, R. & R.E. Sloan, 1970. The composition of milks of various species: A review. Dairy Sci. Abstr. 32:599-612

Kensinger, R.S., R.J. Collier, F.W. Bazer, C.A. Ducsay & H.N. Becker. 1982. Nucleic acid, metabolic and histological changes in gilt mammary tissue during pregnancy and lactogenesis. J. Anim. Sci. 54:1297-1308

King, R.H., C.J. Rayner & M. Kerr, 1993a. A note on the amino acid composition of sow's milk. Anim. Prod. 57:500-502

King, R.H., M.S. Toner, H. Dove, C.S. Atwood & W.G. Brown, 1993b. The response of first-litter sows to dietary protein level during lactation. J. Anim. Sci. 71:2457-2463

Kitts, D.D. & Y.V. Yuan, 1992. Caseinophosphopeptides and calcium bioavailability. Trends Food Sci. and Tech. 3:31-35

Klaver, J., G.J.M. van Kempen, P.G.B. de Lange, M.W.A. Verstegen & H. Boer, 1981. Milk composition and daily yield of different milk components as affected by sow condition and lactation/feeding regimen. J. Anim. Sci. 52:1091-1097

Klobasa, F., E. Werhahn & J.E. Butler, 1987. Composition of sow milk during lactation. J. Anim. Sci. 64:1458-1466

Koletzko, B., 1997. Can infant formula be made more similar to human milk? In: Proceedings of the 16th International Congress of Nutrition: From Nutrition Science to Nutrition Practice for Better Global Health. Montreal, Canada. Abstract S4.4

Lee, C.S., I. McCauley & P.E. Hartmann, 1983. Light and electron microscopy of cells in pig colostrum, milk and involution secretion. Acta. Anat. 116:126-135

Lönnerdal, B., 1986. Effect of maternal nutrition on human lactation. In: Human Lactation 2: Maternal and Environmental Factors. Editors, M. Hamosh & A.S. Goldman. Plenum Press, New York. 301-323

Lönnerdal, B. & C. Glazier, 1985. Calcium binding by α-lactalbumin in human milk. J. Nutr. 115:1209-1216

Lucas, A., 1986. Breastfeeding and gut hormones. In: The Breastfed Infant - a model for performance. Editors, L.J. Filer & S.J. Fomon, Ross Laboratories, Ohio. 73-83

Maffeo, G, M. Damasio, R. Balabio & W. Jochle, 1987. Detection of prostaglandin-like substances in sows' milk. Zuchthygiene 22:209-214

Midgal, W., 1991. Chemical composition of colostrum and milk in sows fed diets supplemented with animal fat. Wrld Rev. Anim. Prod. 26:11-15

Migliore-Samour, D. & P, Jolles, 1988. Casein, a prohormone with an immunomodulating role for the newborn? Exp. 44:188-193

Miller, M.B., T.G. Hartsock, B. Erez, L. Douglass & B. Alston-Mills, 1994. Effect of dietary calcium concentrations during gestation and lactation in the sow on milk composition and litter growth. J. Anim. Sci. 72:1315-1319
Mulloy, A.L. & P.V. Malven, 1979. Relationships between concentrations of porcine prolactin in blood serum and milk of lactating sows. J. Anim. Sci. 48:876-881
Noblet, J. & M. Etienne, 1986. Effect of energy level in lactating sows on yield and composition of milk and nutrient balance of piglets. J. Anim. Sci. 63:1888-1896
Oftedal, O.T., 1984. Milk composition, milk yield and energy output at peak lactation: A comparative review. In: Physiological Strategies in Lactation. Symposia of the Zoological Society of London, Volume 51. Editors, M. Peaker. R.G. Vernon & C.H. Knight, Academic Press, London. 33-85
Ogra, S.S., D. Weintraub & P.L. Ogra, 1977. Immunologic aspects of human colostrum and milk. III. Fate and absorption of cellular and soluble components in the gastrointestinal tract of the newborn. J. Immunol. 119:245-248
Park, Y.W., M. Kandeh, K.B. Chin, W.G. Pond & L.D. Young, 1994. Concentrations of inorganic elements in milk of sows selected for high and low serum cholesterol. J. Anim. Sci. 72:1399-1402
Perrin, D.R., 1955. The chemical composition of the colostrum and milk of the sow. J. Dairy Res. 22:103-107
Pluske, J.R., I.H. Williams & F.X. Aherne, 1995. Nutrition of the Neonatal Pig. In: The neonatal pig: Development and Survival. Editor, M.A. Varley, CAB International, Oxon, 187-235
Pond, W.G. & K.A. Houpt, 1978. The biology of the pig. Cornell University Press, New York. 226-335
Prentice, A., G. Ewing, S.B. Roberts, A. Lucas, A. MacCarthy, L.M.A. Jarjou & R.G. Whitehead, 1987. The nutritional role of breast-milk IgA and lactoferrin. Acta Pediatr. Scand. 76:592-598
Reiter, B., 1978. Review of the progress of dairy science: Antimicrobial systems in milk. J. Dairy Res. 45:131-147
Rutherfurd, S.M. & P.J. Moughan, 1998. The digestible amino acid composition of several milk proteins - application of a new bioassay. J. Dairy Sci. (In press).
Sato, R., R. Noguchi & H. Naito, 1986. Casein phosphopeptide (CCP) enhances calcium absorption from the ligated segment of rat small intestine. J. Nutr. Sci. Vitaminology 32:67-76
Schulze, F. & G. Muller, 1980. Lysozyme in sow's milk and its importance for bacterial colonisation of the gastrointestinal tract of the unweaned piglet. Arch. Exp. Vetmed. 34:317-324
Simmen, F.A., R.C.M. Simmen & G. Reinhardt, 1988. Maternal and neonatal somatomedin C/insulin-like growth factor-1 (IGF-1) and IGF binding proteins during early lactation in the pig. Develop. Bio. 130:16-27
Slebodzinski, A.B., J, Nowak, H. Gaweka & A. Sechman, 1986. Thyroid hormones and insulin in milk: A comparative study. Endocr. Exp. 20:247-255
Trugo, N.M.F. & M.H. Newport, 1983. Resistance of vitamin B_{12}-binding protein in sow's milk to proteolysis *in vivo*. In: Proceedings of the 6th International Congress of Food Science and Technology. Editors, J.V. McLoughlin & B.M. McKenna, Boole Press, Dublin. 77-78
von Gohren, T., 1865. Analyse der schweinemilch. Landwirtsch. Versuchsstation Baden 7:351
Westrom, B.R., R. Ekman, L. Svendsen, J. Svendsen & B.W. Karlsson, 1987. Levels of immunoreactive insulin, neurotensin, and bombesin in porcine colostrum and milk. J. Pediatr. Gastroeneterol. Nutr. 6:460-465

Westrom, B.R, B.G. Ohlsson., J. Svendsen, C. Tagesson & B.W. Karlsson, 1985. Intestinal transmission of macromoelcules (BSA and FITC-labelled dextrans) in the neonatal pig: Enhancing effect of colostrum, proteins and proteinase inhibitors. Biol. Neonate 47:359-366
Westrom, B.R., J. Svendsen & B.W. Karlsson, 1982. Protease inhibitor levels in porcine mammary secretions. Biol. Neonate 42:185-194
Westrom, B.R., J. Svendsen, B.G. Ohlsson, C. Tagesson & B.W. Karlsson, 1984. Intestinal transmission of macromoelcules (BSA and FITC-labelled dextrans) in the neonatal pig: Influence of age of piglet and molecular weight of markers. Biol. Neonate 46:20-26
Witter, R.C. & J.A.F. Rook, 1970. The influence of the amount and nature of dietary fat on milk fat composition in the sow. Brit. J. Nutr. 24:749-760
Wu, G. & D.A. Knabe, 1994. Free and protein-bound amino acids in sow's colostrum and milk. J. Nutr. 124:415-424
Wuryastuti, H., H.D. Stowe, R.W. Bull & E.R. Miller, 1993. Effects of vitamin E and selenium on immune responses of peripheral blood, colostrum, and milk leukocytes of sows. J. Anim. Sci. 71:2464-2472
Zlotkin, S.H. & G.H. Anderson, 1982. The development of cystathionase activity during the first year of life. Pediatr. Res. 16: 65-68.
Zlotkin, S.H., M.H. Bryan & G.H. Anderson, 1981. Cysteine supplementation to cysteine-free intravenous feeding regimens in newborn infants. Am. J. Clin. Nutr. 34: 914-923.
Zou, S., D.G. McLaren & W.L. Hurley, 1992. Pig colostrum and milk composition: comparisons between Chinese Meishan and US breeds. Livest. Prod. Sci. 30:115-127

2 Immunological aspects: comparison with other species

Frank Blecha

2.1 Introduction

Porcine immunology is grounded in the same fundamentals and principles as all studies of immunity, regardless of species. However, there are some traits and characteristics that are unique to the porcine immune system and some that, although shared by other ungulates, are totally different from humans or rodents. Because of the agricultural importance of pigs and because pigs are increasingly being used for human health needs, such as animal models for human diseases and sources of tissues and organs for xenotransplantation, it is necessary to thoroughly understand the immune response in this species. Consequently, over the last five years there have been several excellent reviews on porcine immunology in general (Gaskins and Kelley, 1995; Lunney, 1994) and also on specific segments of the porcine immune response (Blecha, 1997; Chitko-McKown and Blecha, 1992; Tumbleson and Schook, 1996; Vandenbroeck and Billiau, 1997). This chapter will review the acquisition of passive immunity in the pig and discuss the cells and mediators that comprise nonspecific and specific aspects of active immunity in pigs. Throughout the chapter and summarized at the end, particular attention will be given to those aspects of immunity that are unique to the pig.

2.2 Passive immunity

Immune cells and immunological responses can be detected early in gestation in the foetal pig. For example, by 28 days of gestation lymphoid cells are detected in the thymic region, liver, and peripheral blood; lymphocytes expressing characteristic T and B cell markers are present by the sixth week of gestation. If immunized *in utero*, antigen-specific antibody responses are detectable at 55 days of gestation; and, as early as 5 weeks before birth, umbilical-cord blood lymphocytes respond to mitogenic stimulation (Nielsen, 1987; Tlaskalova-Hogenova, *et al.*, 1994; Trebichavsky, *et al.*, 1996). However, because of the epitheliochorial placentation in the pig, where six tissues separate the maternal and fetal circulations (Brambell, 1969), the foetal pig is well protected from external antigenic stimulation. Consequently, under normal conditions, immune responses are not elicited in the foetal pig. Thus, at birth the neonatal pig, like equine and ruminant newborns, differs from other mammalian neonates in being immunologically naive and is critically dependent on acquiring immune protection passively from the sow. This passive immunity is conferred primarily by the ingestion and absorption of colostral immunoglobulins. However, colostral leukocytes and other factors also are passively transferred from the sow to the pig and may contribute to the initial immune protection of the neonatal pig.

2.2.1 Immunoglobulins

The neonatal pig is born virtually agammaglobulinanemic and is dependent on ingestion and absorption of colostral immunoglobulins for passive antibody immunity. High concentrations of immunoglobulins (Ig) G, M, and A are present in the first colostral samples taken after parturition, with IgG comprising about 75 % of the total (Table 2.1). However, Ig concentrations and isotype profiles change rapidly during lactation. Over a 6-week lactation, concentrations of IgG, IgM and IgA can decrease 100-, 6-, and 4-fold, respectively, with much of the decrease occurring during the first 24 hours (Klobasa and Butler, 1987). This rapid reduction in colostral Ig emphasizes the importance of the newborn pig ingesting sufficient quantities of Ig-rich colostrum during the first few hours of life, when they can be efficiently absorbed. At 24 hours after birth, serum Ig values are similar to those of the sow (Holland, 1990) and by 48 hours of life 'gut closure' has effectively occurred in the newborn pig with the cessation of intestinal absorption of Ig. By day 3 of lactation, IgA is the prominent isotype in lacteal secretions and constitutes over 50 % of total lacteal Ig at the end of the first week of lactation.

As lactation proceeds, IgA becomes the predominant isotype in milk, which is a consequence of local synthesis and secretion by the mammary gland (Bourne, *et al.*, 1978) Immunoglobulin A is relatively resistant to degradation by digestive

Table 2.1. Concentrations of lacteal immunoglobulins (mg/ml) during lactation in the sow

Day of Lactation	IgG	IgM	IgA
0[1]	95.6	9.1	21.2
0.5	32.1	4.2	10.1
1	14.2	2.7	6.3
3	3.5	2.3	5.5
7	1.5	1.8	4.8
14	1.0	1.5	4.8
21	0.9	1.5	5.3
42	0.8	1.8	9.4

[1] Day 0 lactation samples were taken immediately after birth. Values are means (n=25). Adapted from Klobasa and Butler, 1987.

enzymes, and is effective in neutralizing viruses, inhibiting the attachment of bacteria to enterocytes, and opsonizing or coating bacteria, which facilitates bacterial destruction (Tizard, 1996). Thus, a vigorously nursing newborn pig is provided good immune protection by the colostral and milk immunoglobulins that it ingests. However, the half-life of maternal Ig in newborn pigs is only a matter of a few days to weeks: IgA = 2 - 3 days, IgM = 2.5 - 3 days, and IgG = 6.5 - 22.5 days (Curtis and Bourne, 1973). In addition, it is important to remember that the maternal Ig that the neonate receives are specific for antigens that the sow has encountered and, thus, are a reflection of the immunization history and pathogen exposure of the dam. Consequently, older sows may provide more protective Ig, both in quantity and quality, to the young pig. This is illustrated in Figure 2.1 where older sows, which have been through more lactations and presumably have experienced more exposure to several antigens, have higher relative concentrations of milk IgA and colostral IgG than sows in their first lactations.

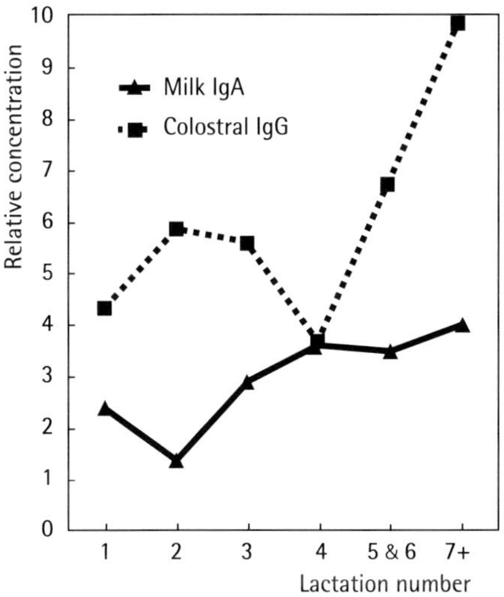

Figure 2.1. Relative concentrations of milk IgA (day 42 of lactation) and colostral IgG for sows of different parity. Relative concentration = mg ml^{-1} of Ig / mg ml^{-1} of albumin. Adapted from Klobasa and Butler, 1987

2.2.2 Leukocytes

Discussions about the acquisition of passive immunity in neonates, generally, only consider the absorption of colostral immunoglobulins. However, colostrum contains many leukocytes, including neutrophils, macrophages, and lymphocytes, at concentrations that are comparable to those in peripheral blood (Le Jan, 1996; Riedel-Caspari and Schmidt, 1990). Studies in neonatal pigs have established that colostral leukocytes are absorbed intracellularly in the upper small intestine, enter the lymphatic vessels, and are transported to the mesenteric lymph nodes (Tuboly, *et al.*, 1988; Williams, 1993). Within two hours of ingesting colostral leukocytes, maternal cells can be detected in the neonate's blood and by 24 hours they can be found in gastrointestinal tissues, lymph nodes, liver, spleen, and lung (Williams, 1993). Some degree of selectivity appears to be involved in colostral leukocyte absorption, in that cells from the neonatal pig's own mother are absorbed and travel to tissue sites better than cells from a sow other than the pig's mother (Tuboly, *et al.*, 1988). In addition, blood lymphocytes or heat-treated colostral lymphocytes are not absorbed (Tuboly, *et al.*, 1988).

Clearly, significant numbers of lymphoid cells are contained in colostrum and are absorbed by the neonatal pig. However, are these maternal leukocytes functional in the pig and do they contribute to disease defence capabilities of the neonate? Colostral leukocytes that were fed to neonatal pigs and then isolated and stimulated with T- and B-lymphocyte mitogens, showed significant proliferative responses, implying that they may contribute to cellular immunity in the neonate (Williams, 1993). Similarly, an extensive series of well-controlled studies by Riedel-Caspari and colleagues (Riedel-Caspari, *et al.*, 1991; Riedel-Caspari and Schmidt, 1991a; Riedel-Caspari and Schmidt, 1991b; Riedel-Caspari and Schmidt, 1991c) has shown that colostral leukocytes are functional in neonatal calves and exhibit enhanced lymphocyte blastogenic responses, higher concentrations of antibodies against *Escherichia coli,* and increased lysozyme activity, when compared to neonates fed cell-depleted colostrum. Importantly, neonates that were orally infected with enteropathogenic *E. coli,* shed less bacteria in their faeces and cleared the bacteria early when they were fed pooled colostrum that had been supplemented with colostral leukocytes compared to calves fed cell-depleted pooled colostrum (Riedel-Caspari, 1993). Calves that received the colostral leukocytes also had higher concentrations of *E. coli*-specific IgA and IgM antibodies. Thus, although the number of studies that have investigated the involvement of colostral leukocytes in the acquisition of neonatal passive immunity is limited, it is clear that they contribute to the initial immune capabilities and disease defence mechanisms of the newborn.

2.2.3 Other factors

In addition to immunoglobulins and leukocytes, colostrum contains many other substances which may contribute to passive immunity in the neonate. Growth factors, such as epidermal growth factor (EGF) and insulin-like growth factor-I (IGF-I) are present in lacteal secretions and contribute to neonatal gastrointestinal development (Donovan, *et al.*, 1994; Houle, *et al.*, 1997; Odle, *et al.*, 1996;). However, because recent findings have shown that IGF-I is a potent regulator of immune responses (Arkins, *et al.*, 1993; Kelley, *et al.*, 1992; Liu, *et al.*, 1997), it is likely that colostral IGF-I also influences immune responses in the neonate. Similarly, several cytokines including interleukin-1β (IL-1β), IL-6, tumor necrosis factor-α (TNF-α), and interferon-γ (IFN-γ) have been detected in colostrum (Munoz, *et al.*, 1990; Bocci, *et al.*, 1991; Bocci, *et al.*, 1993). It has been suggested that these colostral cytokines exert an immunostimulatory role particularly on the oropharyngeal-associated lymphoid tissue (Bocci, *et al.*, 1991). Finally, a novel proline-rich cytokine called colostrinine has been isolated from sheep and human colostrum and has been shown to induce the synthesis of IFN-γ, IFN-β, and TNF-α (Blach-Olszewska and Janusz, 1997; Inglot, *et al.*, 1996; Piasecki, *et al.*, 1997). Whether this novel cytokine, or any of the other colostral factors are important mediators of passive immunity in pigs has not been established. However, the presence of these growth factors and cytokines in colostrum suggests that they may be involved in immune regulatory signals.

2.3 Active immunity

In contrast to passive immunity, where immune cells and mediators are obtained either by transfer from the mother to the offspring or are administered artificially, active immunity encompasses all of the immune cells and mediators that are endogenous to the animal. Although the foetal pig can respond immunologically to many stimuli, active immune responses are generally low at birth in the neonatal pig (Blecha and Charley, 1990; Gaskins and Kelley, 1995) and require several weeks to attain adult capabilities. Active immune responses can be divided into two categories: innate (nonspecific) immunity and adaptive (specific) immunity.

2.3.1 Innate immune responses

Innate immune responses are nonspecific. Cellular mediators of innate immunity do not require prior exposure to the pathogen to effectively engage and neutralize it. The advantage of innate immune responses is that they can be rapidly mobilized and quickly limit the pathogen to the site of invasion. Phagocytic cells, such as neutrophils and macrophages, and cytolytic natural killer cells are the primary cells that confer nonspecific immunity in the pig.

Neutrophils

Polymorphonuclear granulocytes or neutrophils are one of the first lines of defence against infections; they are the first leukocytes to arrive at sites of inflammation and are well-equipped to sequester and eliminate pathogens. Like all leukocytes, these granule-rich cells originate in the bone marrow from pluripotent stem cells, and, under the influence of various cytokines, differentiate and mature into neutrophils. Neutrophils have several potent antimicrobial defence mechanisms, including both oxidative and nonoxidative killing processes.

When neutrophils engage and phagocytose pathogens, their oxygen consumption increases dramatically. This respiratory burst is initiated by the activation of a plasma membrane-bound enzyme complex called reduced nicotinamide-adenine dinucleotide phosphate (NADPH) oxidase (Rotrosen, 1992). This multicompent enzyme catalyzes the reduction of molecular oxygen to superoxide anion using NADPH as an electron donor. In a reaction, catalysed by superoxide dismutase, superoxide anion rapidly dismutates to hydrogen peroxide, which is converted to hypochlorite in a reaction catalyzed by myeloperoxidase. These and other reactive oxygen intermediates are important and potent components of the neutrophil's antimicrobial defences within the phagosomes of the cell. However, these toxic oxidants also are very destructive to surrounding tissue when released extracellularly, and thus, their generation and inactivation is tightly regulated.

At least five proteins comprise the NADPH phagocyte oxidase (phox) complex: two proteins ($gp91^{phox}$ and $p22^{phox}$) comprise the membrane flavocytochrome b_{558}, and three proteins ($p47^{phox}$, $p67^{phox}$, and a GTP binding protein, $p21^{Rac}$) are cytosolic proteins (Quinn, 1995). Activation and assembly of the NADPH oxidase complex is not fully elucidated; however, it is clear that multiple protein-protein interactions occur among the components, which are regulated by several signalling intermediates. Recently, an endogenous porcine peptide has been shown to be a potent regulator of the phagocyte NADPH oxidase (Shi, *et al.*, 1996). This proline-arginine (PR)-rich peptide, PR-39, is contained in porcine neutrophils (Shi, *et al.*, 1994) and was discovered and isolated on the basis of its antibacterial properties (Agerberth, *et al.*, 1991). This peptide has several activities, including, wound-healing properties (Gallo, *et al.*, 1996) neutrophil chemoattractant activity (Huang, *et al.*, 1997), and, through binding to $p47^{phox}$, PR-39 is also a potent inhibitor of the NADPH oxidase (Shi, *et al.*, 1996). The paradoxical finding of an antibacterial peptide also possessing NADPH oxidase inhibitory activity is intriguing and suggests a mechanism for interaction between oxidative and nonoxidative defence mechanisms in porcine neutrophils.

In addition to oxygen-dependent killing mechanisms, neutrophils and other phagocytes have potent nonoxidative defence mechanisms, including enzymes such as lysozyme, proteinase, phospholipases, and granule-associated antibacterial peptides (Elsbach and Weiss, 1992). Antibacterial peptides are an ancient and fundamental defence mechanism that virtually all organisms in the plant and animal kingdoms use (Broekaert, *et al.*, 1995; Lehrer, *et al.*, 1991). These natural antibiotics are produced by a diverse array of cells and are often found in leukocytes (Ganz and Lehrer, 1997). In pigs, all of the neutrophil antibacterial peptides discovered to date belong to the cathelicidin family (Table 2.2).

Cathelicidins share a highly conserved prepro-sequence followed by structurally variable mature peptide sequences. These peptides are called cathelicidins because their pro-sequences share identity to cathelin, a 96 amino-acid peptide originally isolated from porcine neutrophils (Zanetti, *et al.*, 1995). Cathelicidins are synthesized by bone marrow progenitors and stored in neutrophil granules. Three

Table 2.2. Porcine cathelicidins

Peptide	MW (Da)	Comments	References
PR-39	4,720	Proline-arginine-rich peptide with multiple functions, including, antibacterial activities primarily against Gram-negative bacteria, involvement in wound repair, NADPH oxidase inhibition, and neutrophil chemotaxis	Agerberth *et al.*, 1991; Gallo *et al.*, 1994; Shi *et al.*, 1996; Huang *et al.*, 1997; Zhang *et al.*, 1997
Protegrins	~2,000	Five known isoforms with four cysteines forming two intra-chain disulphide bonds; potent broad-spectrum activity against bacteria, fungi, and viruses	Kokryakov *et al.*, 1993
Prophenins	8,683	Two known congeners rich in proline and phenylalanine; peptides contain six nearly perfectly repeated decamers; mainly active against Gram-negative bacteria	Harwig *et al.*, 1995
PMAP-23 PMAP-36 PMAP-37	2963 2525 4365	All three porcine myeloid antimicrobial peptides (PMAP) have been deduced from bone marrow cDNAs; synthetic peptides are active against Gram-positive and -negative bacteria	Zanetti *et al.*, 1994 Storici *et al.*, 1994 Tossi *et al.*, 1995

cathelicidins have been isolated from porcine neutrophils: PR-39, protegrin, and prophenin (Agerberth, *et al.*, 1991; Harwig, *et al.*, 1995; Kokryakov, *et al.*, 1993). In addition, three porcine myeloid antimicrobial peptides (PMAP), which have not been isolated, are characterized as cathelicidins based on their cDNA-predicted gene products (Storici, *et al.*, 1994; Tossi, *et al.*, 1995; Zanetti, *et al.*, 1994). The initial discovery of porcine neutrophil antibacterial peptides only took place a few years ago; however, because these peptides offer the possibility of devising new and perhaps more effective antimicrobial defence strategies, information about their regulation and control will accumulate rapidly.

Macrophages

As the name implies, macrophages are large phagocytic leukocytes. These cells, which differentiate from myeloid progenitors in the bone marrow to circulating blood monocytes and then tissue macrophages, are widely distributed in the body (Carrasco, *et al.*, 1995; Chitko-McKown and Blecha, 1992; Hu, *et al.*, 1996). They are important mediators of host defence and tissue repair and, through secretion of several cytokines and presentation of antigen, are central to the regulation of immune responses. Although macrophages populate many tissue sites, they are not a homogeneous cell population and their functions and activities may vary widely between tissue sites and even within the same tissue compartment (Bullido, *et al.*, 1997; Khanna, *et al.*, 1996; Kielian, *et al.*, 1995; Scamurra, *et al.*, 1996).

The porcine lung contains at least three macrophage populations: alveolar, intravascular, and interstitial. Porcine alveolar and intravascular macrophages have been extensively studied (Charley, 1982; Staub, 1989). Lavage fluid from the lungs of newborn pigs contains few macrophages; however, within a few days of birth, they appear inside the lung alveoli and adult values are attained by 2 weeks of age (Rothlein, *et al.*, 1981). Similarly, differentiated intravascular macrophages are rare in newborn pigs and appear in discrete stages of differentiation by 3 to 7 days of age (Winkler, 1989). In contrast to humans and rats, pulmonary intravascular macrophages play a major role in the clearance of blood-borne bacteria and particulates in pigs (Staub, 1989). However, because of the difficulty of isolating pulmonary intravascular macrophages, few studies have evaluated the immunological functions of these cells (Chitko-McKown and Blecha, 1992). Although it appears that porcine intravascular macrophages may have lower phagocytic activity than alveolar macrophages, they may be more efficient at killing ingested bacteria (Chitko-McKown, *et al.*, 1991). In addition, porcine intravascular macrophages appear to be more spontaneously cytolytic than alveolar macrophages. Thus, although macrophages often are considered as a homogenous entity, it is apparent that the potency and function of these cells in distinct tissue compartments are different, and additional study is needed to fully understand their role in host defence.

Natural killer cells
Non-T, non-B cells of lymphocytic lineage that can spontaneously kill tumour or virus-infected cells are called natural killer (NK) cells. Phenotypic characterization of immune cells is based on the expression of cluster of differentiation (CD) antigens on the cell membrane. Recently, the phenotype of porcine NK cells was determined to be surface Ig^-, $CD2^+$, $CD3^-$, and $CD8^{lo}$, which is similar to human NK cells (Yang and Parkhouse, 1996). The porcine CD5 antigen also is an important discriminator of NK cells, in that they are $CD5^-$, as compared to MHC-restricted $CD8^+$ cytotoxic T cells, which are $CD5^+$ (Saalmüller, *et al.*, 1994).

Two characteristics come to mind when considering porcine NK cells. First, NK cell activity is virtually absent in newborn pigs and takes 2 to 3 weeks to develop. This developmental delay in NK cell activity has been observed regardless of the target cells used (see Blecha and Charley, 1990 for review). It should be noted, however, that Kovaru and colleagues have reported peripheral blood NK cell activity at 100 days of gestation in the fetal pig (Kovaru, *et al.*, 1994). This finding was attributed to the use of a permissible target cell (rat astrocytoma fused with porcine thymocyte surface determinants). The second characteristic that is peculiar to porcine NK cell activity is the length of the assay. Human and rodent NK cell assays usually entail incubating the effector NK cells with the target cells for 4 hours. Typically, porcine NK cell assays require an incubation period that is four to five times longer (Cepica and Derbyshire, 1984; Hennessy, *et al.*, 1990; Onizuka, *et al.*, 1987; Yang and Schultz, 1986). It is not known why porcine NK cells exhibit a delayed lysis; however, it does not appear to relate to delayed target cell recognition (Pinto and Ferguson, 1988). Finally, a novel antimicrobial peptide termed NK-lysin has been recently cloned, and is suggested to be a new effector molecule of porcine cytotoxic T cells and NK cells (Andersson, *et al.*, 1995; Andersson, *et al.*, 1996).

2.3.2 Adaptive immunity

Adaptive immune responses are learned and exhibit memory. That is, once the host has encountered the pathogen, long-lived memory cells are produced and upon re-encountering the pathogen, a rapid and robust immune response is generated. Many cells and mediators interact to generate a specific immune response; however, B and T lymphocytes are primary cellular mediators of adaptive immunity and cytokines coordinate their interaction.

B lymphocytes
Humoral immunity is mediated by antibodies produced by plasma cells which are end-stage differentiated B lymphocytes. Immunoglobulins or antibodies are the secreted form of the B-cell receptor that recognizes antigen. Over the last several years, Butler and colleagues at the University of Iowa have published many articles and reviews on immunoglobulin diversity in several species (Butler, 1995;

Butler, 1997; Butler and Brown, 1994; Sun and Butler, 1996). Their work shows that in pigs the constant regions for the heavy chains of IgM, IgE, and IgA are encoded by single genes. This is similar to the situation in mice and cattle, but differs from humans that have two genes that encode the heavy chain of IgA. Similarly, pigs, which have as many as nine genes for the constant region of the IgG heavy chain, differ from mice and humans, which have four. Pigs also differ from mice and humans, in that they do not have IgD, which is similarly absent in cattle, sheep, rabbits and chickens. Finally, the high degree of similarity among human and swine genes emphasizes the difficulty in predicting Ig gene structure, organization and sequence similarity on the basis of phylogeny (Butler, 1997).

T lymphocytes

Similar to other mammals, CD4 antigens are expressed on porcine T-helper lymphocytes, and CD8 antigens are expressed on cytotoxic T lymphocytes. However, based on the expression of CD4 and CD8 antigens, porcine T lymphocytes are divided into four subpopulations: $CD4^{+}CD8^{-}$, $CD4^{-}CD8^{+}$, $CD4^{+}CD8^{+}$ and $CD4^{-}CD8^{-}$. T lymphocytes are further categorized on the basis of their T-cell receptor chains as either $\alpha\beta$ or $\gamma\delta$. In humans and rodents, $\alpha\beta$ T lymphocytes are the most prominent subclass expressed on peripheral T lymphocytes and $\gamma\delta$ T lymphocytes, which are $CD4^{-}CD8^{-}$, are a minor subclass (Binns, 1994; Hirt, *et al.*, 1993; Thome, *et al.*, 1994). Similarly, dual positive CD4/CD8 T lymphocytes are rare in humans and rodents. However, both dual positive and dual negative CD4/CD8 populations, can comprise 40 to 60% of peripheral lymphocytes in pigs (Carr, *et al.*, 1994; Pescovitz, *et al.*, 1994; Yang and Parkhouse, 1996; Zuckermann and Gaskins, 1996; Zuckermann and Husmann, 1996). T-lymphocytes expressing $\gamma\delta$ T-cell receptors are numerous in young pigs (Yang and Parkhouse, 1996) and as the pig ages, $\alpha\beta$ T lymphocytes become prominent (Yang and Parkhouse, 1996; Zuckermann and Husmann, 1996). Because dual positive CD4/CD8 T lymphocytes exhibit properties of mature antigen-experienced cells, it is likely that this population includes memory T cells (Zuckermann and Husmann, 1996). Thus, porcine T-lymphocyte populations appear to be the most heterogenous of all mammalian species studied thus far and are particularly useful for studying T lymphocyte diversity.

Cytokines

Cytokines are the protein mediators of the immune system that orchestrate the complex events and interactions that are involved in the development and regulation of an immune response. Two recent texts have reviewed several topics relative to cytokines in domestic food animals, including pigs (Myers and Murtaugh, 1995; Schijns and Horzinek, 1997). Similarly, the molecular biology of porcine cytokines and chemokines (chemoattractants) and the *in vivo* application of cytokines in pigs have recently been reviewed (Blecha, 1997; Vandenbroeck and Billiau, 1997). Table 2.3 summarizes the current list of porcine cytokines and chemokines and brief comments relative to their cellular sources and targets, and primary biological effects.

Table 2.3. Porcine cytokines and chemokines: GenBank accession number, cellular source and target, and primary biological effect

Cytokine	Accession number	Primary cell sources	Primary cell targets	Primary effects	References
IFN-α	M28623 X57191	Macrophages monocytes (synthesis can occur in any cell)	Receptors are ubiquitous; therefore, most cells are targets	Inhibit viral replication, antiproliferative activity, increased expression of MHC class I antigens	Lefèvre and La Bonnardière, 1986; Lefèvre *et al.*, 1990c; 1990b; Yerle *et al.*, 1986
IFN-β	M86762 S41178	Fibroblasts (synthesis can occur in any cell)	Macrophages, NK cells	Same as IFN-α	Artursson *et al.*, 1992
IFN-γ	X53085 S63967	T lymphocytes, NK cells, trophoblast	Macrophages, NK cells endometrial epithelium	Macrophage activation, increased expression of MHC class I and class II antigens, viral protection of the conceptus	Dijkmans *et al.*, 1990; Vandenbroeck *et al.*, 1991; 1993b; 1994; Lefèvre *et al.*, 1990a
IFN-ω	X57192 X57193 X57194 X57195 X57196	Trophoblast	Endometrial epithelium	Maternal recognition of pregnancy by maintaining the function of the *corpus luteum*	Lefèvre *et al.*, 1990b; Mège *et al.*, 1991
IFN-δ	Z22706 Z22707 Z22708	Trophoblast	Endometrial epithelium	Transiently expressed by trophoblastic cells of pig conceptuses at implantation; may have a role in viral protection of the conceptus	Lefèvre and Boulay, 1993; Niu *et al.*, 1995; Lundgren and Langer, 1997
TNF-α	M29079 X54001 X57321 X54859	Macrophages	Hepatocytes, endothelial cells	Key mediator of inflammation, co-stimulant for lymphocyte proliferation	Pauli *et al.*, 1989; Drews *et al.*, 1990; Choi *et al.*, 1991; Kuhnert *et al.*, 1991

TNF-β	X54859	T lymphocytes	Tumour cells	Induces tumour apoptosis, activates neutrophils, macrophages, B cells	Kuhnert *et al.*, 1991
IL-1α	X52731 M86730	Macrophages, Langerhans cells, neutrophils, T and B lymphocytes, NK cells, endothelium, fibroblasts keratinocytes	T and B lymphocytes, NK cells, neutrophils, eosinophils dendritic cells, fibroblasts, endothelial cells, hepatocytes, monocytes	Co-stimulators of Th2 cells, induces acute-phase response	Maliszewski *et al.*, 1990; Huether *et al.*, 1993
IL-1β1 IL-1β2	X74568 M86725				Vandenbroeck *et al.*, 1993a Huether *et al.*, 1993
IL-1RA	L38849	Macrophages, monocytes	Cells expressing IL-1 receptors	IL-1 receptor antagoist	Yin and Murtaugh, 1996
IL-2	X58428 X56750	Th1 lymphocytes	T and B lymphocytes, NK cells macrophages	Activates T and B lymphocytes, NK cells	Goodall *et al.*, 1991; Lefèvre *et al.*, 1991
IL-4	X68330 L12991	Th2 lymphocytes	B and T lymphocytes, macrophages, endothelial cells, fibroblasts, mast cells	Stimulates B cell growth and differentiation; inhibits IL-1, IL-6 and TNF-α secretion	Bailey *et al.*, 1993; Zhou and Murtaugh, 1993
IL-6	M86722 M80258	Macrophages, T and B lymphocytes, bone marrow stromal cells, fibroblasts, keratinocytes, mesangial cells	T and B lymphoctyes, bone marrow stromal cells	Promotes IL-2 production and T lymphocyte differentiation; stimulates acute-phase response	Richards and Saklatvala, 1991; Mathialagan *et al.*, 1992; Scamurra *et al.*, 1996
IL-8	M99367 M86923 X61151	Macrophages, fibroblasts, lymphocytes, granulocytes, endothelial cells, hepatocytes keratinocytes	Neutrophils, basophils, lymphocytes	Chemoattractant for neutrophils, basophils, some T lymphocytes, activates neutrophils	Goodman *et al.*, 1992; Lin *et al.*, 1994; Sanjanwala, 1994
IL-10	L20001	Th2 ymphocytes, macrophages	Th1 and B lymphocytes, macrophages, NK cells, mast cells, thymocytes	Inhibits activation of Th1 cells and NK cells, suppresses macrophage function	Blancho *et al.*, 1995
IL-12	U08317 L35765	Macrophages	Th1 lymphocytes, NK cells	Stimulates Th1 lymphocyte secretion of IL-2 and IFN-γ, enhances T lymphocyte and NK cell proliferation	Foss and Murtaugh, 1995

IL-15	U58142	Lymphocytes	T lymphocytes, NK cells	Enhances proliferation of T lymphocytes and induces lymphokine activated killer cells	Canals, *et al.*, 1996
IL-18	U68701	Alveolar macrophages	Th1 lymphocytes, NK cells	Growth and differentiation factor for Th1 cells, induces IFN-γ production	Foss and Murtaugh, 1997
GM-CSF	D21074 U61139 U67175 U67318	T lymphocytes, macrophages, endothelial cells, fibroblasts	Haemopoietic stem cells, granulocyte/macrophage progenitors	Simulates proliferation of granulocyte, macrophage, and erythrocyte progenitors; activates macrophages, neutrophils and eosinophils	Inumaru and Takamatsu, 1995 Foss and Murtaugh, 1996 Gloster *et al.*, 1996; 1997
TGFβ1 TGFβ2 TGFβ3	M23703 X70142 X14150	Lymphocytes, monocytes, kidney, placenta, platelets, bone	Fibroblasts, osteoblasts, smooth muscle cells, Schwann cells, keratinocytes, haemopoietic progenitors, lymphocytes	Potent inhibitor of cell proliferation often inhibiting proliferation induced by other growth factors; increases cell density, fibrosis, and angiogenesis	Kondaiah *et al.*, 1988 Mulheron, 1992 Derynck *et al.*, 1988
AMCF-II	M99368	Alveolar macrophages	Neutrophils	Neutrophil chemotaxis	Goodman *et al.*, 1992
NAP-2	X77935	Platelets	Neutrophils	Neutrophil chemotaxis/activation	Power *et al.*, 1994
MCP-1	Z48479	Luteal cells	Monocytes/macrophages	Chemoattraction of monocytes/ macrophages towards the *corpus luteum* at the end of a nonfertile cycle	Hosang *et al.*, 1994a; 1994b Zach *et al.*, 1995

Abbreviations: AMCF-II, alveolar macrophage-derived chemotactic factor II; GM-CSF, granulocyte-macrophage colony-stimulating factor; IFN, interferon; IL, interleukin; IL-1RA, IL-1 receptor antagonist; MCP, monocyte chemoattractant protein; NAP-2, neutrophil-activating peptide-2; Th1, T helper type I; Th2, T helper type 2; TGF, transforming growth factor; TNF, tumour necrosis factor.

Table 2.4. Characteristics unique to porcine immunology or different from human and rodent immunology

Characteristic	Uniqueness	References
Dual Positive CD4/CD8 T cells	Pigs have an increased percentage of $CD4^+CD8^+$ T lymphocytes.	Pescovitz *et al.*, 1994; Zuckermann and Husmann, 1996
IFN-γ	In addition to T cells and NK cells, IFN-γ also is produced by trophoectoderm cells in pigs.	Lefèvre *et al.*, 1990a
IFN-δ	A type I interferon expressed by the pig trophoblast. Initially called short porcine type I IFN, now designated IFN-δ.	Lefèvre and Boulay, 1993; Niu *et al.*, 1995;Lundgren and Langer, 1997
IL-1 genes	Pigs have two IL-1β genes, IL-1β1 and IL-1β2.	Vandenbroeck and Billiau, 1997
[1]Lymph node structure and circulation	The lymph node cortex is located towards the centre and the medulla is at the periphery of the node; lymphocytes leave the node and enter the blood not lymph vessels.	Binns and Pabst, 1994; Tizard, 1996
[1]fMLP receptors	Porcine neutrophils do not express receptors for fMLP	Nelson *et al.*, 1979; Chenoweth, *et al.*, 1980
[1]IgD	Pigs do not have an IgD isotype.	Butler, 1997
[1]MHC class II	Major histocompatibility class II antigens are expressed on resting T lymphocytes.	Saalmuller, *et al.*, 1991 Davis *et al.*, 1987
[1]γδ T lymphocytes	Dual negative CD4/CD8 lymphocytes expressing the γδ T-cell receptor are a major subpopulation in peripheral blood of young pigs.	Yang and Parkhouse, 1996 Davis and Hamilton, 1997

[1] Not totally unique to pigs: elephants, hippopotamuses, rhinoceroses, and dolphins have a similar lymph node structure; bovine neutrophils also do not have formyl-methionyl-leucyl-phenylalanine (fMLP) receptors; IgD has only been reported in humans and mice; MHC class II antigens also are expressed on resting T lymphocytes of horses, dogs, and cats; γδ T-cells also are numerous in young ruminants.

2.4 Summary of comparisons of the porcine immune system with other species

Most aspects of porcine immunology are similar to those in other mammalian species. However, there are some important differences that are totally unique to the porcine immune system, and some, which may be similar in other ungulates, are certainly different from humans and rodents. For example, characteristics that are unique to porcine immunology include a high percentage of $CD4^{+}CD8^{+}$ peripheral lymphocytes (Pescovitz, *et al.*, 1994; Zuckermann and Husmann, 1996); IFN-δ, a novel type I interferon (Lefèvre and Boulay, 1993); the secretion of IFN-γ by trophoectoderm cells (Lefèvre, *et al.*, 1990b); and the existence of two distinct genes for IL-1β (Vandenbroeck and Billiau, 1997). These unique characteristics and characteristics that are different from human and rodent immunology are summarized in Table 2.4.

2.5 Concluding remarks

A complete understanding of the immune system of pigs is becoming increasingly important. From an agricultural standpoint, health management programmes must consider the unique aspects of porcine immunology to ensure effective preventive and therapeutic strategies. Vaccination and herd health programmes can only be optimized if the immunological capabilities and differences of pigs are considered. From a human health perspective, a thorough understanding of porcine immunology is necessary to allow valid interpretation of experimental findings when pigs are used as models for human disease. Furthermore, porcine immunology must be understood to facilitate the rational use of porcine tissues and organs in xenotransplantation. Thus, because of these two separate but equally important reasons for investigating the immune system of pigs, new information and advances in our understanding of porcine immunology will continue to receive high priority.

2.6 References

Agerberth, B.J., J.Y. Lee, T. Bergman, H.G. Boman, V. Mutt & H. Tornvall, 1991. Amino acid sequence of PR-39: isolation from pig intestine of a new member of the family of proline-arginine-rich antibacterial peptides. Eur. J. Biochem. 216, 623-629.

Andersson, M., H. Gunne, B. Agerberth, A. Boman, T. Bergman, R. Sillard, H. Jornvall, V. Mutt, B. Olsson, H. Wigzell, Å. Dagerlind, H.G. Boman & G.H. Gudmundsson, 1995. NK-lysin, a novel effector peptide of cytotoxic T and NK cells. Structure and cDNA cloning of the porcine form, induction by interleukin 2, antibacterial and antitumour activity. EMBO J. 14, 1615-1625.

Andersson, M., H. Gunne, B. Agerberth, A. Boman, T. Bergman, B. Olsson, Å. Dagerlind, H. Wigzell, H.G. Boman & G.H. Gudmundsson, 1996. NK-lysin, structure and function of a novel effector molecule of porcine T and NK cells. Vet. Immunol. Immunopath. 54, 123-126.

Arkins, S., R. Dantzer & K.W. Kelley, 1993. Somatolactogens, somatomedins, and immunity. J. Dairy Sci. 76, 2437-2450.

Artursson, K., A. Gobl, M. Lindersson, M. Johansson & G. Alm, 1992. Molecular cloning of a gene encoding porcine interferon-beta. GenBank, direct submission.

Bailey, M., A.C.F. Perry, P.W. Bland, C.R. Stokes & L. Hall, 1993. Nucleotide and deduced amino acid sequence of porcine interleukin-4 cDNA derived from lamina propria lymphocytes. Biochim. Biophys. Acta. 1171, 328-330.

Binns, R.M., 1994. The null/ΓδTCR+T cell family in the pig. Vet. Immunol. Immunopath. 43, 69-77.

Binns, R.M. & R. Pabst, 1994. Lymphoid tissue structure and lymphocyte trafficking in the pig. Vet. Immunol. Immunopathol. 43, 79-87.

Blach-Olszewska, Z. & M. Janusz, 1997. Stimulatory effect of ovine colostrinine (a proline-rich polypeptide) on interferons and tumor necrosis factor production by murine peritoneal cells. Arch. Immunol. Ther. Exp. (Warsz), 45, 43-47.

Blancho, G., P. Gianello, S. Germana, M. Baetscher, D.H. Sachs & C. LeGuern, 1995. Molecular identification of porcine interleukin 10: regulation of expression in a kidney allograft model. Proc. Natl. Acad. Sci. USA, 92, 2800-2804.

Blecha, F., 1998. Cytokine applications in pigs. In: Cytokines in Veterinary Medicine. V.E.C.J. Schijns and M.C. Horzinek, eds. CAB International, Wallingford, In press.

Blecha, F. & B. Charley, 1990. Rationale for using immunopotentiators in domestic food animals. In: Immunomodulation in Domestic Food Animals. F. Blecha and B. Charley, eds. Academic Press, Orlando, pp. 3-19.

Bocci, V., K. von Bremen, F. Corradeschi, E. Luzzi & L. Paulesu, 1991. What is the role of cytokines in human colostrum? J. Biol. Regul. Homeost. Agents, 5, 121-124.

Bocci, V., K. von Bremen, F. Corradeschi, F. Franchi, E. Luzzi & L. Paulesu, 1993. Presence of interferon-gamma and interleukin-6 in colostrum of normal women. Lymphokine Cytokine Res. 12, 21-24.

Bourne, F.J., T.J. Newby, P. Evans & K. Morgan, 1978. The immune requirements of the newborn pig and calf. Ann. Rech. Vét. 9, 239-244.

Brambell, F.W.R., 1969. The transmission of immunoglobulins from the mother to the foetal and newborn young. Proc. Nutr. Sci. 23, 35-41.

Broekaert, W.F., F.R. Terras, B.P. Cammue & R.W. Osborn, 1995. Plant defensins: novel antimicrobial peptides as components of the host defence system. Plant Physiol. 108, 1353-1358.

Bullido, R., M. Gomez del Moral, F. Alonso, A. Ezquerra, A. Zapata, C. Sanchez, E. Ortuno, B. Alvarez & J. Dominguez, 1997. Monoclonal antibodies specific for porcine monocytes/macrophages: macrophage heterogeneity in the pig evidenced by the expression of surface antigens. Tissue Antigens, 49, 403-413.

Butler, J.E., 1995. Antigen receptors, their immunomodulation and the immunoglobulin genes of cattle and swine. Livest. Prod. Sci., 42, 105-121.

Butler, J.E., 1997. Immunoglobulin gene organization and the mechanism of repertoire development. Scand. J. Immunol. 45, 455-462.

Butler, J.E. & W.R. Brown, 1994. The immunoglobulins and immunoglobulin genes of swine. Vet. Immunol. Immunopath. 43, 5-12.

Canals, A., D.R. Grimm, L.C. Gasbarre, J.K. Lunney & D.S. Zarlenga, 1996. Molecular cloning of cDNA encoding the porcine interleukin 15. GenBank, direct submission.

Carr, M.M., C.J. Howard, P. Sopp, J.M. Manser & K.R. Parsons, 1994. Expression on porcine gamma delta lymphocytes of a phylogenetically conserved surface antigen previously restricted in expression to reminant gamma delta T lymphocytes. Immunology, 81, 36-40.

Carrasco, L., M.J. Bautista, J. Martin de las Mulas, J.C. Gomez-Villamandos, A. Espinosa de los Monteros & M.A. Sierra, 1995. Description of a new population of fixed macrophages in the splenic cords of pigs. J. Anat. 187, 395-402.

Cepica, A. & J.B. Derbyshire, 1984. Antibody-dependent and spontaneous cell-mediated cytotoxicity against Transmissible Gastroenteritis virus infected cells by lymphocytes from sows, fetuses and neonatal piglets. Can. J. Comp. Med. 48, 258
Charley, B., 1982. Swine alveolar macrophages: description and functional analysis. Ann. Rech. Vét. 13, 1-9.
Chenoweth, D.E., T.A. Lane, J.G. Rowe & T.E. Hugli, 1980. Quantitative comparisons of neutrophil chemotaxis in four animal species. Clin. Immunol. Immunopathol. 15, 525-535.
Chitko-McKown, C.G. & F. Blecha, 1992. Pulmonary intravascular macrophages: a review of immune properties and functions. Ann. Rech. Vet. 23, 201-214.
Chitko-McKown, C.G., S.K. Chapes, R.E. Brown, R.M. Phillips, R.D. McKown & F. Blecha, 1991. Porcine alveolar and pulmonary intravascular macrophages: comparison of immune functions. J. Leuk. Biol. 50, 364-372.
Choi, C.S., T.W. Molitor, G.F. Lin & M.P. Murtaugh, 1991. Complete nucleotide sequence of a cDNA encoding porcine tumor necrosis factor-alpha. Anim. Biotechnol. 2, 97-105.
Curtis, J. & F.J. Bourne, 1973. Half-lives of immunoglobulins IgG, IgA, and IgM in the serum of new-born pigs. Immunol. 24, 147-155.
Davis, W.C., S. Marusic, H.A. Lewin, G.A. Splitter, L.E. Perryman, T.C. McGuire & J.R. Gorham, 1987. The development and analysis of species specific and cross reactive monoclonal antibodies to leukocyte differentiation antigens and antigens of the major histocompatibility complex for use in the study of the immune system in cattle and other species. Vet. Immunol. Immunopath. 15, 337-376.
Davis, W.C. & M.J. Hamilton, 1997. Unique characteristics of the immune system in ruminants and pigs. USDA Internet Virtual Conference, URL: http://www.nadc.ars.usda.gov/virtconf/subpost.posters.G00061m.html, 1-5.
Derynck, R., P.B. Lindquist, A. Lee, D. Wen, J. Tamm, J.L. Graycar, L. Rhee, A.J. Mason, D.A. Miller, R.J. Coffey, H.L. Moses & E.Y. Chen, 1988. A new type of transforming growth factor-beta, TGF-beta 3. EMBO J. 7, 3737-3743.
Dijkmans, R., K. Vandenbroeck, E. Beuken & A. Billiau, 1990. Sequence of the porcine interferon-gamma (IFN-Γ) gene. Nucleic Acids Res. 18, 4259.
Donovan, S.M., R.T. Zijlstra & J. Odle, 1994. Use of the piglet to study the role of growth factors in neonatal intestinal development. Endocr. Regul. 28, 153-162.
Drews, R.T., B.W. Coffee, A.K. Prestwood & R.A. McGraw, 1990. Gene sequence of porcine tumor necrosis factor alpha. Nucleic Acids Res. 18, 5564.
Elsbach, P. & J. Weiss, 1992. Oxygen-independent antimicrobial systems of phagocytes. In: Inflammation: Basic Principles and Clinical Correlates. J.I. Gallin, I.M. Goldstein and R. Snyderman, eds. Raven Press, Ltd. New York, pp. 603-636.
Foss, D.L. & M.P. Murtaugh, 1995. Cloning and characterization of porcine interleukin-12. GenBank, direct submission.
Foss, D.L. & M.P. Murtaugh, 1996. Cloning and expression of recombinant porcine granulocyte-macrophage colony-stimulating factor. GenBank, direct submission.
Foss, D.L. & M.P. Murtaugh, 1997. Cloning of porcine interferon-gamma inducing factor (interleukin 18). GenBank, direct submission.
Gallo, R.L., M. Ono, T. Povsic, C. Page, E. Eriksson, M. Klagsbrun & M. Bernfield, 1994. Syndecans, cell surface heparan sulfate proteoglycans, are induced by a proline-rich antimicrobial peptide from wounds. Proc. Natl. Acad. Sci. USA, 91, 11035-11039.
Ganz, T. & R.I. Lehrer, 1997. Antimicrobial peptides of leukocytes. Current Opinion in Hematology, 4, 53-59.
Gaskins, H.R. & K.W. Kelley, 1995. Immunology and neonatal mortality. In: The Neonatal Pig *Development and Survival.* M.A. Varley, ed. Cab International, Wallingford, pp. 39-55.

Gloster, S.E., R.M. Sandeman & A.D.G. Strom, 1996. Cloning of a cDNA and gene encoding porcine granulocyte-macrophage-colony stimulating factor (GM-CSF). GenBank, direct submission.

Gloster, S.E., R.M. Sandeman & A.D.G. Strom, 1997. Cloning of a cDNA and gene encoding porcine granulocyte-macrophage colony-stimulating factor (GM-CSF). GenBank, direct submission.

Goodall, J.C., D.C. Emery, M. Bailey, L.S. English & L. Hall, 1991. cDNA cloning of porcine interleukin 2 by polymerase chain reaction. Biochim. Biophys. Acta. 1089, 257-258.

Goodman, R.B., D.C. Foster, S.L. Mathewes, S.G. Osborn, J.L. Kuijper, J.W. Forstrom & T.R. Martin, 1992. Molecular cloning of porcine alveolar macrophage-derived neutrophil chemotactic factors I and II: identification of porcine IL-8 and another intercrine-I protein. Biochemistry, 31, 10483-10490.

Harwig, S.S.L., V.N. Kokryakov, K.M. Swiderek, G.M. Aleshina, C. Zhao & R.I. Lehrer, 1995. Prophenin-1, an exceptionally proline-rich antimicrobial peptide from porcine leukocytes. FEBS Letters, 362, 65-69.

Hennessy, K.J., F. Blecha, B.W. Fenwick, R.C. Thaler & J.L. Nelssen,1990. Human recombinant interleukin-2 augments porcine natural killer cell cytotoxicity in vivo. Ann. Rech. Vet. 21, 101-109.

Hirt, W., A. Saalmüller & M.J. Reddehase, 1993. Expression of gamma/delta T-cell receptors in porcine thymus. Immunobiology, 188, 70-81.

Holland, R.E., 1990. Some infectious causes of diarrhoea in young farm animals. Clin. Microbiol. Rev., 3, 345-375.

Hosang, K., I. Knoke, J. Klaudiny, F. Wempe, W. Wuttke & K.H. Scheit, 1994a. Porcine luteal cells express monocyte chemoattractant protein-1 (MCP-1): analysis by polymerase chain reaction and cDNA cloning. Biochem. Biophys. Res. Commun. 199, 962-968.

Hosang, K., I. Knoke, J. Klaudiny, F. Wempe, W. Wuttke & K.H. Scheit 1994b. Porcine luteal cells express monocyte chemoattractant-2 (MCP-2): analysis by cDNA cloning and Northern analysis. Biochem. Biophys. Res. Commun. 205, 148-153.

Houle, V.M., E.A. Schroeder, J. Odle & S.M. Donovan, 1997. Small intestinal disaccharidase activity and ileal villus height are increased in piglets consuming formula containing recombinant human insulin-like growth factor-I. Pediatr. Res. 42, 78-86.

Hu, S., C.C. Chao, K.V. Khanna, G. Gekker, P.K. Peterson & T.W. Molitor, 1996. Cytokine and free radical production by porcine microglia. Clin. Immunol. Immunopathol. 78, 93-96.

Huang, H.J., C.R. Ross & F. Blecha, 1997. Chemoattractant properties of PR-39, a neutrophil antibacterial peptide. J. Leuk. Biol. 61, 624-629.

Huether, M.J., G. Lin, D.M. Smith, M.P. Murtaugh & T.W. Molitor, 1993. Cloning, regulation and sequencing of mRNA encoding porcine interleukin-1J. Gene, 129, 285-289.

Inglot, A.D., M. Janusz & J. Lisowski, 1996. Colostrinine: a proline-rich polypeptide from ovine colostrum is a modest cytokine inducer in human leukocytes. Arch. Immunol. Ther. Exp. (Warsz), 44, 215-224.

Inumaru, S. & H. Takamatsu, 1995. cDNA cloning of porcine granulocyte-macrophage colony-stimulating factor. Immunol. Cell Biol. 73, 474-476.

Kelley, K.W., S. Arkins & Y.M. Li, 1992. Growth hormone, prolactin, and insulin-like growth factors: new jobs for old players. Brain Behav. Immun. 6, 317-326.

Khanna, K.V., C.S. Choi, G. Gekker, P.K. Peterson & T.W. Molitor, 1996. Differential infection of porcine alveolar macrophage subpopulations by nonopsonized *Mycobacterium bovis* involves CD14 receptors. J. Leuk. Biol. 60, 214-220.

Kielian, T.L., C.R. Ross, D.S. McVey, S.K. Chapes & F. Blecha, 1995. Lipopolysaccharide modulation of a CD14-like molecule on porcine alveolar macrophages. J. Leuk. Biol. 57, 581-586.

Klobasa, F. & J.E. Butler, 1987. Absolute and relative concentrations of immunoglobulins G, M, and A, and albumin in the lacteal secretion of sows of different lactation numbers. Am. J. Vet. Res. 48, 176-182.

Kokryakov, V.N., S.S.L. Harwig, E.A. Panyutich, A.A. Schevchenko, G.M. Aleshina, O.V. Shamova, H.A. Korneva & R.I. Lehrer, 1993. Protegrins: leukocyte antimicrobial peptides that combine features of corticostatic defensins and tachyplesins. FEBS Letters, 327, 231-236.

Kondaiah, P., E. Van Obberghen-Schilling, R.L. Ludwing, R. Dhar, M.B. Sporn & A.B. Roberts, 1988. cDNA cloning of porcine transforming growth factor-beta 1 mRNAs. Evidence for alternate splicing and polyadenylation. J. Biol. Chem. 263, 18313-18317.

Kovaru, H., F. Kovaru, R. Halouzka & H. Kozakova,1994. Pig development of natural killer cytotoxicity with modified C-6 glioma cell line as targets. Cell Biology International, 18, 531(Abstract).

Kuhnert, P., C. Wüthrich, E. Peterhans & U. Pauli, 1991. The porcine tumor necrosis factor-encoding genes: sequence and comparative analysis. Gene, 102, 171-178.

Le Jan, C., 1996. Cellular components of mammary secretions and neonatal immunity: a review. Vet. Res. 27, 403-417.

Lefèvre, F., 1991. Molecular cloning of porcine interleukin 2 cDNA by the polymerase chain reaction. GenBank, direct submission.

Lefèvre, F. & V. Boulay 1993. A novel and atypical type one interferon gene expressed by trophoblast during early pregnancy. J. Biol. Chem. 268, 19760-19768.

Lefèvre, F. & C. La Bonnardière, 1986. Molecular cloning and sequencing of a gene encoding biologically active porcine alpha-interferon. J. Interferon Res. 6, 349-360.

Lefèvre, F., F. Martinat-Botté, M. Guillomot, K. Zouari, B. Charley & C. La Bonnardière, 1990a. Interferon-gamma and protein are spontaneously expressed by the porcine trophectoderm early in gestation. Eur. J. Immunol. 20, 2485-2490.

Lefèvre, F., D. Mege, R. L'Haridon, S. Bernard, C. de Vaureix & C. La Bonnardière, 1990b. Contribution of molecular biology to the study of the porcine interferon system. Vet. Micro. 23, 245-257.

Lefèvre, F., R. Haridon, F. Borras-Curest & C. La Bonnardière, 1990c. Production, purification and biological properties of an *Escherichia coli*-derived recombinant porcine alpha interferon. J. Gen. Virol. 71, 1057-1063.

Lehrer, R.I., T. Ganz & M.E. Selsted, 1991. Defensins: endogenous antibiotic peptides of animal cells. Cell, 64, 229-230.

Lin, G., A.E. Pearson, R.W. Scamurra, Y. Zhou, M.J. Baarsch, D.J. Weiss & M.P. Murtaugh, 1994. Regulation of interleukin-8 expression in porcine alveolar macrophages by bacterial lipopolysaccharide. J. Biol. Chem. 269, 77-85.

Liu, Q., D. Schacher, C. Hurth, G.G. Freund, R. Dantzer & K.W. Kelley, 1997. Activation of phosphatidylinositol 3'-kinase by insulin-like growth factor-I rescues promyoloid cells from apoptosis and permits their differentiation into granulocytes. J. Immunol. 159, 829-837.

Lundgren, E. & J.A. Langer, 1997. Nomenclature of interferon receptors and interferon-delta. J. Interferon Cytokine Res. 17, 315-316.

Lunney, J.K., 1994. Special Issue: Porcine Immunology. Vet. Immunol. Immunopath. 43, 1-333.

Maliszewski, C.R., B.R. Renshaw, M.A. Schoenborn, J.F. Urban & P.E. Baker, 1990. Porcine IL-1 alpha cDNA nucloetide sequence. Nucleic Acids Res. 18, 4282.

Mathialagan, N., Bixby & M.R. Roberts, 1992. Expression of interleukin-6 in porcine, ovine, and bovine preimplantation conceptuses. Mol. Reprod. Dev. 32, 324-330.

Mege, D., F. Lefèvre & C. La Bonnardière, 1991. The porcine family of interferon-w: cloning, structural analysis, and functional studies of five related genes. J. of Interf. Res., 11, 341-350.

Mulheron, G.W., J.G. Mulheron, D. Danielpour & D.W. Schomberg, 1992. Porcine granulosa cells do not express transforming growth factor-beta 2 (TGF-beta 2) messenger ribonucleic acid: molecular basis for their inability to produce TGF-beta activity comparable to that of rat granulosa cells. Endocrinology, 131, 2609-2614.

Munoz, C., S. Endres, J. van der Meer, L. Schlesinger, M. Arevalo & C. Dinarello, 1990. Interleukin-1 beta in human colostrum. Res. Immunol. 141:6, 505-513.

Myers, M.J. & M.P. Murtaugh, 1995. Cytokines in Animal Health and Disease. Marcel Dekker, Inc. New York, 465 pages.

Nelson, R.D., S.K. Ackerman, V.D. Fiegel, M.P. Bauman & S.D. Douglas, 1979. Cytotaxin receptors of neutrophils: evidence that F-methionyl peptides and pepstatin share a common receptor. Infect. Immun. 26, 996-999.

Nielsen, J. 1987. Mitogenic reactivity of mononuclear cells isolated from thymus, spleen and umbilical cord blood of pig foetuses. Vet. Immunol. Immunopath. 16, 123-138.

Niu, P.D., F. Lefèvre, D. Mege & C. La Bonnardière, 1995. Atypical porcine type I interferon. Biochemical and biological characterization of the recombinant protein expressed in insect cells. Eur. J. Biochem. 230, 200-206.

Odle, J., R.T. Zijlstra & S.M. Donovan, 1996. Intestinal effects of milkborne growth factors in neonates of agricultural importance. J. Anim. Sci. 74, 2509-2522.

Onizuka, N., Y. Maede, T. Ohsugi & S. Namioka, 1987. Nonspecific cell-mediated cytotoxicity of peripheral blood lymphocytes derived from suckling piglets. Jpn. J. Vet. Res. 35, 41-48.

Pauli, U., B. Beutler & E. Peterhans, 1989. Porcine tumor necrosis factor alpha: cloning with the polymerase chain reaction and determinatin of the nucleotide sequence. Gene, 81, 185-191.

Pescovitz, M.D., A.G. Sakopoulos, J.A. Gaddy, R.J. Husmann & F.A. Zuckermann, 1994. Porcine peripheral blood $CD4^+/CD8^+$ dual expressing T-cells. Vet. Immunol. Immunopath. 43, 53-62.

Piasecki, E., A.D. Inglot, M. Winiarska, K. Krukowska, M. Janusz & J. Lisowski, 1997. Coincidence between spontaneous release of interferon and tumor necrosis factor by colostral leukocytes and the production of a colostrinine by human mammary gland after normal delivery. Arch. Immunol. Ther. Exp. (Warsz), 45, 109-117.

Pinto, A. & F. Ferguson, 1988. Characteristics of Yorkshire swine natural killer cells. Vet. Immunol. Immunopath. 20, 15-29.

Power, C.A., A.E.I. Proudfoot, E. Magnenat, K.B. Bacon & T.N.C. Wells, 1994. Molecular cloning and characterization of a neutrophil chemotactic protein from porcine platelets. Eur. J. Biochem. 221, 713-719.

Quinn, M.T., 1995. Low-molecular-weight GTP-binding proteins and leukocyte signal transduction. J. Leuk. Biol. 58, 263-276.

Richards, C.D. & J. Saklatvala, 1991. Molecular cloning and sequence of porcine interleukin 6 cDNA and expression of mRNA in synovial fibroblasts in vitro. Cytokine, 3, 269-276.

Riedel-Caspari, G., 1993. The influence of colostral leukocytes on the course of an experimental *Escherichia coli* infection and serum antibodies in neonatal calves. Vet. Immunol. Immunopath. 35, 275-288.

Riedel-Caspari, G. & F.W. Schmidt, 1990. Review article: colostral leukocytes and their significance for the immune system of newborns. DTW Dtsch Tierarztl Wochenschr, 4, 180-186.

Riedel-Caspari, G. & F.W. Schmidt, 1991a. The influence of colostral leukocytes on the immune system of the neonatal calf. I. Effects on lymphocyte responses. DTW Dtsch Tierarztl Wochenschr, 98, 102-107.

Riedel-Caspari, G. & F.W. Schmidt, 1991b. The influence of colostral leukocytes on the immune system of the neonatal calf. II. Effects on passive and active immunization. DTW Dtsch Tierarztl Wochenschr, 98, 190-194.

Riedel-Caspari, G. & F.W. Schmidt 1991c. The influence of colostral leukocytes on the immune system of the neonatal calf. III. Effects on phagocytosis. DTW Dtsch Tierarztl Wochenschr, 98, 330-334.

Riedel-Caspari, G., F.W. Schmidt & J. Marquardt, 1991. The influence of colostral leukocytes on the immune system of the neonatal calf. IV. Effects on bactericidity, complement and interferon; synopsis. DTW Dtsch Tierarztl Wochenschr, 98, 395-398.

Rothlein, R., R. Gallily & Y.B. Kim, 1981. Development of alveolar macrophages in specific pathogen-free and germ-free Minnesota miniature swine. J. Reticuloendoth. Soc. 30, 483-495.

Rotrosen, D., 1992. The respiratory burst oxidase. In: Inflammation: Basic Principles and Clinical Correlates. J.I. Gallin, I.M. Goldstein and R. Snyderman, eds. Raven Press, Ltd. New York, pp. 589-601.

Saalmüller, A., E. Weiland & M.J. Reddehase, 1991. Resting porcine T lymphocytes expressing class II major histocompatibility antigen. Immunobiology, 183, 102-114.

Saalmüller, A., W. Hirt, S. Maurer & E. Weiland, 1994. Discrimination between two subsets of porcine $CD8^{+}$ cytolytic T lymphocytes by the expression of CD5 antigen. Immunology, 81, 578-583.

Sanjanwala, M. 1994. Cloning and sequencing of cDNA encoding porcine IL 8 protein. GenBank, direct submission.

Scamurra, R., C. Arriaga, L. Sprunger, M.J. Baarsch & M.P. Murtaugh, 1996. Regulation of interleukin-6 expression in porcine immune cells. J. Interferon Cytokine Res. 16, 289-296.

Schijns, V.E.C.J. & M.C. Horzinek, 1997. Cytokines in Veterinary Medicine. CAB International, Wallingford, In press.

Shi, J., C.R. Ross, M.M. Chengappa & F. Blecha, 1994. Identification of a proline-arginine-rich antibacterial peptide from neutrophils that is analogous to PR-39, an antibacterial peptide from the small intestine. J. Leuk. Biol. 56, 807-811.

Shi, J., C.R. Ross, T.L. Leto & F. Blecha, 1996. PR-39, a proline-rich antibacterial peptide that inhibits phagocyte NADPH oxidase activity by binding to Src homology 3 domains of $p47^{phox}$. Proc. Natl. Acad. Sci. USA, 93, 6014-6018.

Staub, N.C., 1989. The Pulmonary Intravascular Macrophage. Futura, Mount Kisco, pp. 1-180.

Storici, P., M. Scocchi, A. Tossi, R. Gennaro & M. Zanetti, 1994. Chemical synthesis and biological activity of a novel antibacterial peptide deduced from a pig myeloid cDNA. FEBS Letters, 337, 303-307.

Sun, J. & J.E. Butler 1996., Molecular characterization of VDJ transcripts from a newborn piglet. Immunology, 88, 331-339.

Thome, M., W. Hirt, E. Pfaff, M.J. Reddehase & A. Saalmüller, 1994. Porcine T-cell receptors: molecular and biochemical characterization. Vet. Immunol. Immunopath. 43:103, 13-18.

Tizard, I.R., 1996. Veterinary Immunology: An Introduction. W.B. Sanders Company, Philadelphia, 531 pages.

Tlaskalova-Hogenova, H., L. Mandel, I. Trebichavsky, F. Kováoù, R. Barot & J. Sterzl, 1994. Development of immune responses in early pig ontogeny. Vet. Immunol. Immunopath. 43, 135-142.

Tossi, A., M. Scocchi, M. Zanetti, P. Storici & R. Gennaro, 1995. PMAP-37, a novel antibacterial peptide from pig myeloid cells. cDNA cloning, chemical synthesis and activity. Eur. J. Biochem. 228, 941-946.

Trebichavsky, I., H. Tlaskalová, B. Cukrowska, I. Splíchal, J. Sinkora, Z. Oeháková, M. Sinkora, R. Pospisil, F. Kovaru, B. Charley, R. Binns & A. White, 1996. Early ontogeny of immune cells and their functions in the fetal pig. Vet. Immunol. Immunopath. 54, 75-81.

Tuboly, S., S. Bernath, R. Glavits & I. Medveczky, 1988. Intestinal absorption of colostral lymphoid cells in newborn piglets. Vet. Immunol. Immunopath. 21, 75-85.

Tumbleson, M.E. & L.B. Schook, 1996. Advances in Swine in Biomedical Research. Plenum Press, New York 422 pages.

Vandenbroeck, K. & A. Billiau, 1997. Recent progress in the molecular characterization of porcine lymphokines, monokines and chemokines. In: Cytokines in Veterinary Medicine. V.E.C.J. Schijns and M.C. Horzinek, eds. CAB International, Wallingford, In press.

Vandenbroeck, K., R. Dijkmans, A. Van Aerschot & A. Billiau, 1991. Engineering by PCR-based exon amplification and ligation of the genomic porcine interferon-gamma DNA for expression in *Eschericia coli*. Biochem. Biophys. Res. Commun. 180, 1408-1415.

Vandenbroeck, K., P. Fiten, E. Beuken, E. Martens, A. Jannsen, J. Van Damme, G. Opdenakker & A. Billiau, 1993a. Gene sequence, cDNA construction, expression in *Escherichia coli* and genetically approached purification of porcine interleukin-1J. Eur. J. Biochem. 217, 45-52.

Vandenbroeck, K., E. Martens, S. d'Andrea & A. Billiau, 1993b. Refolding and single step purification of porcine interferon-, from *Escherichia coli* inclusion bodies. Conditions for reconstitution of dimeric IFN-γ. Eur. J. Biochem. 215, 481-486.

Vandenbroeck, K., L. Willems, A. Billiau, G. Opdenakker & R. Huybrechts, 1994. Glycoform heterogeneity of porcine interferon-γ expressed in Sf9 cells. Lymphokine and Cytokine Res., 13, 253-258.

Williams, P.P., 1993. Immunomodulating effects of intestinal absorbed maternal colostral leukocytes by neonatal pigs. Can. J. Vet. Res. 57, 1-8.

Winkler, G.C., 1989. Developmental Biology in the Pig. In: The Pulmonary Intravascular Macrophage. N.C. Staub, ed. Futura, Mount Kisco, pp. 1-22.

Yang, H. & R.M.E. Parkhouse, 1996. Phenotypic classification of porcine lymphocyte sub-populations in blood and lymphoid tissues. Immunology, 89, 76-83.

Yang, W.C. & R.D. Schultz, 1986. Ontogeny of natural killer cell activity and antibody dependent cell mediated cytotoxicity in pigs. Dev. Comp. Immunol. 10, 405-418.

Yerle, M., J. Gellin, G. Echard, F. Lefèvre & M. Gillois, 1986. Chromosomal localization of leukocyte interferon gene in the pig *(Sus scrofa domestica* L.) by in situ hybridization. Cytogenet Cell Genet, 42, 129-132.

Yin, J. & M.P. Murtaugh, 1996. Characterization of IRAP in morphine treated pig. GenBank, direct submission.

Zach, O.R., H.C. Bauer, K. Richter, G. Webersinke & H. Bauer, 1995. Sequence of the porcine full-length cDNA encoding ribosomal protein rpS12. Gene, 159, 277-278.

Zanetti, M., R. Gennaro & D. Romeo, 1995. Cathelicidins: a novel protein family with a common proregion and a variable C-terminal antimicrobial domain. FEBS Letters, 374, 1-5.

Zanetti, M., P. Storici, A. Tossi, M. Scocchi & R. Gennaro, 1994. Molecular cloning and chemical synthesis of a novel antibacterial peptide derived from pig myeloid cells. J. Biol. Chem. 269, 7855-7858.

Zhang, G., C.R. Ross, S.S. Dritz, J.C. Nietfeld & F. Blecha, 1997. Salmonella infection increases porcine antibacterial peptide concentrations in serum. Clinical & Diagnostic Laboratory Immunology, In press.

Zhou, Y. & M.P. Murtaugh, 1993. Regulation of interleukin-4 expression in porcine T lymphocytes. GenBank, direct submission.

Zuckermann, F.A. & H.R. Gaskins, 1996. Distribution of porcine CD4/CD8 double-positive T lymphocytes in mucosa-associated lymphoid tissues. Immunology, 87, 493-499.

Zuckermann, F.A. & R.J. Husmann, 1996. Functional and phenotypic analysis of porcine peripheral blood CD4/CD8 double-positive T cells. Immunology, 87, 500-512.

3 Factors influencing the utilisation of colostrum and milk

J.R. Pluske and G.Z. Dong

3.1 Introduction

Increasing efficiencies and associated reduced production costs are continually required to maintain pig production levels and enhance profitability. One of the greatest opportunities for increasing production and profitability is exploitation of the rapid growth potential of the young pig. In a large commercial herd in Australia, Tritton *et al.* (1993) recorded pre-weaning growth rates of 215 g/day in litter sizes of 9-10 piglets. However, if piglets are artificially reared from birth, they are capable of growing at at least twice the rate than if they are suckled by the sow during lactation (Hodge, 1974; Williams, 1976). This disparity between what is observed commercially and what is attainable will have a large impact on profitability. For example, B.P. Mullan (personal communication) simulated the effect of an increase in pre-weaning piglet growth rate from 200 to 250 g/day using a computerized pig growth simulation model (AUSPIG; Black *et al.*, 1986), and reported that slaughter weight increased by over 5 kg and net revenue per sow almost doubled.

In this respect, the widespread adoption of management practices such as segregated early weaning (weaning at 10-17 days of age) and multi-site production have, to some extent, circumvented this inequality by exploiting the rapid growth potential of the young pig in the post-weaning period. The system of pig production in some countries, however, does not lend itself to such strategies, and hence more 'traditional' weaning ages (22-26 days) are still used.

This chapter describes the interplay between the production of milk by the sow and the utilisation of milk by the piglet. A brief description of the composition of colostrum and milk is provided, although the reader is referred to the chapter by Darragh and Moughan (1998) in this text for a complete account. Emphasis is placed on the biological utilisation of milk by piglets, and biologically optimum production versus that found in practice. Attention is also paid to the interaction between the sow and the piglet around the time of, and including, milk letdown, as evidence is now mounting that the piglet itself has a significant bearing on sow milk production. Finally, reference is made to milk-borne growth factors present in sow's milk and their biological activities, and the chapter closes with a discussion of supplementary feeding as a means of increasing piglet growth rate during lactation and, in turn, increasing overall production and profitability.

3.2 Milk as a food for the piglet

Secretory activity by the sow during lactation (i.e. the production of colostrum and milk) is associated with the final phase of the reproductive cycle. Colostrum and milk provide the sole nutrient supply early in life, and are complex secretions possessing unique properties and compounds, many of which have yet to be identified and their functions discovered. To date, for example, close to 90 oligosaccharides in human milk have been isolated and their structures confirmed. However, more than 900 structural permutations of oligosaccharides are possible based on the moieties of the molecule (Newburg, 1997). Similar scenarios are therefore likely in sow's mammary secretions. With this in mind, Hartmann & Holmes (1989) have outlined the following major properties of sow's colostrum and milk: -

1. They provide the young pig with a source of nourishment ideally adapted to its digestive and metabolic requirements;
2. They provide the young pig with protection against microbes through the intake of immunoglobulins contained in both colostrum and milk;
3. They suppress inflammatory reactions in the gastrointestinal tract of the piglet;
4. They supplement the digestive enzymes of the young pig;
5. They may exercise a degree of control over metabolism;
6. They may modulate the endocrine system;
7. They may contain biologically active compounds that have the potential to influence the behaviour of the young pig; and
8. They have the potential to stimulate cell division and differentiation in the small intestine due to the presence of specialized compounds (e.g. polyamines), hormones and growth factors (see Koldovsky, 1996; Odle *et al.*, 1996; Xu, 1996).

A discussion of each of these points is outside the confines of this particular chapter. For further information the reader is directed to the reviews of Hartmann & Holmes (1989), Moughan *et al.* (1992), and Pluske *et al.* (1995a). However, as remarked upon by Pluske *et al.* (1995a), it is worth considering, purely from an evolutionary perspective, that the unique properties and composition of colostrum and milk are likely to have developed to enhance the chances of survival of the neonatal piglet and, ultimately, continuation of the species. In this context, attempts to change milk composition and the milk production of sows to meet commercial expectations for piglet growth rate may be complex.

With respect to milk composition, most recent interest has focused on points 7 and 8 (above), with Xu (1996) summarizing some of the biologically active substances present in a range of mammalian milks (Table 3.1). In the young pig, attention has focused predominately on the effects of bioactive polypeptides contained in colostrum and milk, such as epidermal growth factor (EGF) and the insulin-like growth factors (IGF-I and IGF-II), on intestinal growth and development. A common feature of their biological action is the interaction with cell surface receptors (Morgan *et al.*, 1996), which in turn may have an effect on the way in which the young pig can digest and absorb the milk it consumes from the sow. The biological functions of some of these components are discussed later in this chapter.

3.2.1 Colostrum and milk composition

The gross compositions of colostrum and milk have been described on many occasions (see Darragh & Moughan, 1998, for a complete account of the composition of sow's mammary secretions in lactation). Nevertheless, and for the purposes of this chapter, it is worth reiterating that colostrum and milk not only supply the piglet with energy and essential amino acids, but also contain specific proteins and peptides, nucleotides, essential fatty acids, minerals, trace elements, vitamins, enzymes and carbohydrates, such as oligosaccharides. Colostrum has a high concentration of total solids and protein but lower levels of lactose and fat (Table 3.2). The high concentration of immunoglobulins found

Table 3.1. Some of the biologically-active substances found in milk and their possible effects on neonatal gastrointestinal development (adapted from Xu, 1996)

Milk-borne substance	Possible biological effects
Hormones	
insulin	Modulating intestinal enzyme activity and epithelial cell migration
cortisol	Stimulating gut enzyme maturation, gut closure and pancreatic growth
thyroxine	Stimulating gut maturation
Growth factors	
epidermal growth factor (EGF)	Trophic effects on GI tract
transforming growth factor (TGF)	Trophic effects on GI tract
nerve growth factor (NGF)	Trophic effects on sympathetic nerve cells
insulin-like growth factors I and II (IGF-I, IGF-II)	Trophic effects on GI tract, liver, pancreas
Others	
opioid peptides	Enhancing mother and young bond, inducing sleep
bombesin	Trophic effects on intestine, stimulating gastrin secretion
lactoferrin	Trophic effect on lymphocytes & intestinal crypt cells
neurotensin	Trophic effects on the intestine

Table 3.2. The main components of colostrum and milk of sows and their relative contribution to gross energy (from Fowler and Gill, 1989)

	Fresh sample		% of total gross energy
	g/kg	kJ/kg	
Colostrum (3 hours after farrowing)			
Total crude protein	175	4148	56.5
Total immunoglobulins	96		
Pre-albumin + albumin	47		
Casein	32		
Total lipids	67	2653	36.1
Lactose	32	544	7.4
Total Energy		7345	100.0
Milk (day 7 of lactation)			
Total crude protein	56	1327	21.5
Total immunoglobulins	20		
Pre-albumin + albumin	13		
Casein	23		
Total lipids	101	4000	65.0
Lactose	49	833	13.5
Total Energy		6160	100.0

Compiled from Bourne (1969), Elsley (1971), and Atwood and Hartmann (1992).

in colostrum coincides with the period of time following parturition when the newborn piglet can absorb these macromolecules across the gut and into the circulation. A decline in total solids and protein (mainly immunoglobulins) and a simultaneous rise in fat and lactose distinguish the transition from colostrum to milk during the first two to three days postpartum. It is clear from Table 3.2 that in milk, the greatest energy source quantitatively for the sucking pig is the fat component. Yet, as will be explained further on, it is the imbalance between protein and energy in sow's milk that has the greatest influence on piglet growth and body composition.

3.2.2 Additional factors in sow's milk

As mentioned above, sow's milk contains a host of metabolites and biologically-active substances that perform specific functions in the piglet, many of which we are just beginning to appreciate. This is important because by isolating and understanding the biological functions of these substances, new opportunities for enhancing growth of the young pig may be possible. For example, Comber &

Hartmann (1993) discovered the presence of creatine phosphate in sow's milk, whilst Kennaugh & Hartmann (1995) measured concentrations of total creatine in sow's colostrum and milk some 400% higher than those found in either human or cow's milk. Although the piglet's requirement for creatine is unknown, creatine is crucial for the development of skeletal muscle and brain function. The higher concentration in sow's secretions compared to those of other mammals may be related to the enormous growth rate of the neonatal piglet compared to the human infant and calf, which take 25 and 9 times longer, respectively, to double their birthweight (Kennaugh & Hartmann, 1995). During this period of rapid muscle growth it is possible that the piglet is unable to synthesize sufficient creatine to meet its creatine demand, hence the high concentration of this compound in sow's colostrum and milk. Using this knowledge, it may then be possible to design, for example, milk replacement formulas enriched in this compound to assist piglet growth.

3.3 Biological utilisation of milk

How the sucking piglet digests, absorbs and metabolizes colostrum and milk provided by the sow can only be appreciated by understanding how the gastrointestinal tract develops and functions. There are many excellent reviews in the field of porcine digestive physiology, the most recent being by Cranwell (1995), and it is not our intention to repeat this information here. Nevertheless, it is worth reiterating that the gastrointestinal tract of the young pig has evolved so as to utilize the mammary secretions of the sow to the fullest extent. For example, chymosin (or rennin) is the most important milk-clotting protease secreted by the gastric mucosa. Pig chymosin has very weak general proteolytic activity but has a milk-clotting activity significantly greater than pig pepsin A. The properties of chymosin have evolved to match the requirements of the newborn pig, acting specifically against the κ-casein fraction of milk protein to clot milk without further proteolytic activity against peptide bonds. The weak, general proteolytic activity of pig chymosin, therefore, allows peptides, growth factors and immunoglobulins present in colostrum and milk to pass undegraded into the duodenum (see Cranwell, 1995).

3.3.1 Energy and amino acid utilisation in relation to sow's milk composition

If we are to develop methods and technologies aimed at enhancing piglet growth rate during lactation, not only is a thorough understanding of porcine digestive physiology a prerequisite, but also how these processes influence the nutrient requirements of the young pig must be known. More than 20 years ago, Williams (1976) conducted a comprehensive study of the nutrient requirements of piglets for protein (amino acids) and energy during the first three weeks of life. Cow's milk protein was fed to piglets from 1.8 to 6.4 kg bodyweight at two levels of energy intake (3.2 and 5.2 MJ GE/day) or approximately 2.5 and 4.0 times maintenance, respectively (Figure 3.1). The response of nitrogen retention to nitrogen intake was similar at both levels of energy intake, which suggests that nitrogen (protein/amino acids) requirements are linearly related to energy intake. Calculating from the lower level of energy intake, the piglets required 12.0 g cow's milk protein per MJ DE assuming the apparent digestibility of milk energy to be 0.96.This value can be adjusted for both digestibility and quality of protein so that the requirement becomes 10.0 g of 'ideal' protein/MJ of DE. Taking the calculation a stage further and assuming that amino acids in milk are fully available after absorption, then the piglet's tissue requirement for lysine was 0.7 g/MJ of DE.

The piglets in this study (Williams, 1976) were representative of the genotypes in Australia at that time but they do not represent the fast-growing genotypes used today. As Campbell and Taverner (1988) have shown, genotypes have changed substantially over the last 20 years. Modern strains are capable of much higher rates of protein deposition, they retain proportionally more water in the fat-free empty body and they have higher maintenance requirements than conventional strains of twenty years ago. However, and as Williams (1995) argued, most if not all of these changes can be explained by the simple assumption that modern genotypes differ from traditional ones only in their mature body size. It follows that if comparisons are made at the same proportion of mature body size (similar degree of physiological maturity) then differences between genotypes disappear. If this

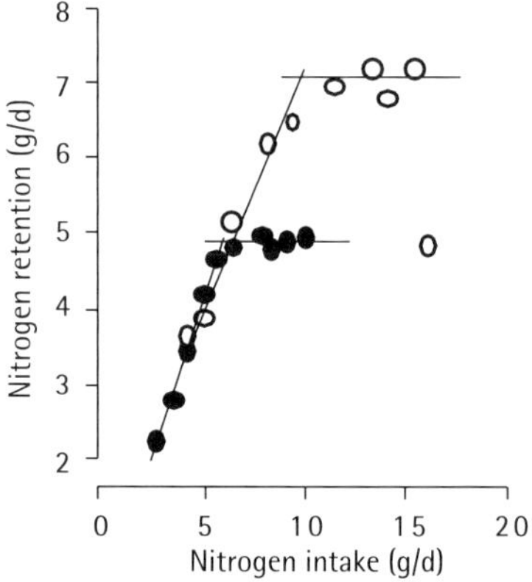

Figure 3.1. Two-phase response of nitrogen retention (NR) to nitrogen intake (NI) for piglets given low (3.2 MJ GE/day)(●) or high (5.2 MJ GE/day) (○) energy intakes from 1.8 to 6.4 kg liveweight.Maximum NR was 7.03 g for the high-energy piglets and 4.86 g for the low-energy piglets.When NI was limiting NR, the relationship was described by NR = 0.83NI - 0.17 for the low energy and NR = 0.72NI + 0.33 for the high energy intakes (from Williams, 1976).

simple explanation is correct it follows that the nutrient requirements of these modern genotypes, expressed relative to each other, should be the same as that of the older genotypes. For example, the amount of ideal protein per MJ of DE should be the same for a large or small genotype but the absolute amounts of either energy or protein needed will be different; they will increase for the bigger genotype. With respect to the sucking piglet, Auldist & King (personal communication) re-examined the protein (amino acid) requirements of baby pigs but used a modern genotype, very different to that used by Williams (1976). Their estimate of the lysine requirement for piglets between 2 and 7 kg liveweight fed cow's milk was 0.74 g available lysine/MJ of DE and, in keeping with the hypothesis described above, suggests there has been little change in requirements despite substantial genetic changes.

3.4 Is sow's milk optimum for maximizing piglet growth?

The sucking piglet generally grows at 180 to 240 g/day between birth and weaning at three to four weeks of age. When this is calculated as a percentage of body weight, the growth rate of the young pig is unequalled by most other domestic species. For example, Harrell *et al.* (1993) reported that a growth rate of 300 g/day for a 5.0 kg pig equated to a 6% increase in body weight per day. During the first week of post-natal life the energy contained in a piglet increases by a factor of between four and five (Okai *et al.*, 1977). This rapid deposition of body tissue is effected by a level of consumption of metabolizable energy equivalent to about four times the pig's estimated requirement for maintenance (Fowler and Gill, 1989).

Despite this impressive rate of growth, a large number of experiments conducted with artificially-reared piglets weaned shortly after birth have demonstrated that when pigs are healthy and fed ad libitum, provision of liquid milk diets generally increases growth rate in comparison to sucking piglets farmed under commercial conditions. The fastest growth rates reported were by Hodge (1974), who fed reconstituted cows' milk (20% dry matter) to pigs ad libitum and found they gained 576 g/day from 10-30 days of age, and 832 g/day from 30-50 days of age. It would appear that the growth potential of the young pig can only be fully realized when it is removed from the sow at birth, or very soon after, and is offered a liquid diet.

There are two major reasons why piglets sucking the sow are restricted in their rate of growth. Firstly, the amount of milk produced by the sow limits the growth of the piglet. Harrell *et al.* (1993) calculated that milk production becomes limiting to the sucking piglet at around 8-10 days of age and that the difference between need and supply progressively increases as lactation proceeds (Figure 3.2). These authors estimated that, by day 21 of lactation, the sow needs to produce in excess of 18 kg/day of milk in order to supply piglets with enough energy to grow at rates comparable to artificially-reared piglets of the same age. Such a rate of milk production exceeds that of even the highest-producing sows in many herds. Apart from small increases in production that may be expected with indirect genetic selection for milk yield, the disparity in growth rate between what is achievable when pigs are raised artificially and the growth rates observed commercially during lactation, will remain a concern for researchers interested in maximizing piglet growth.

Secondly, the potential for lean tissue growth in the baby pig is most likely restricted by the composition of sow's milk per se. The piglet at birth is the most cold-sensitive ungulate because it is small in body size and has a large surface area to body weight ratio relative to other farm animals (Herpin & Le Dividich, 1995). Unlike the wild pig, the piglet born under conventional commercial conditions has a sparse pelage accounting for at most 15% of thermal insulation (Mount, 1968). In addition, the newborn piglet has very low amounts of body lipid (1-2% of total body weight; Mellor & Cockburn, 1986) and thus the glycogen stored in its liver and the protein in its skeletal muscle represent the main energy stores that can be used to maintain body temperature. These energy stores are small which means that unless the piglet has frequent access to large amounts of dietary energy it will rapidly succumb to cold and become hypothermic and die. The low capacity to conserve heat is reflected in the observation that each 1°C decrease below the lower critical temperature is associated with a 1.46 kJ/kg$^{0.75}$/hour increase in heat production, which is about threefold higher than that in a 35 kg pig (Herpin & Le Dividich, 1995).

Sow's milk seems well designed for the survival of piglets because it is high in fat and it is delivered at frequent intervals (approximately once each hour) by the sow. It is not only rich in fat but it is also low in protein and, because of this

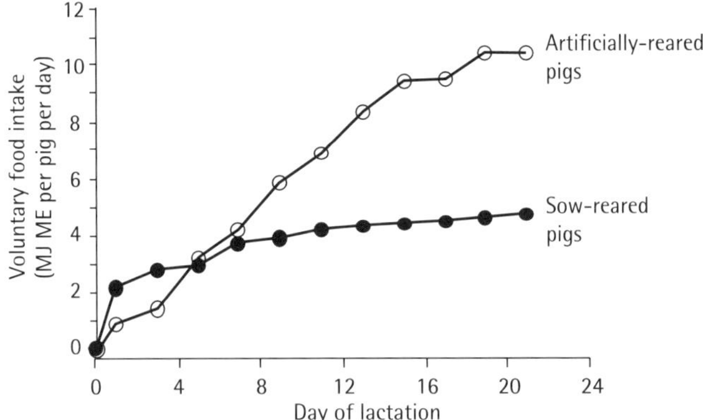

Figure 3.2. Voluntary food intakes (MJ ME/pig/day) of pigs either suckled by the sow (●——●) or fed milk replacer (○——○) following weaning at 2-3 days of age (from Harrell et al., 1993)

relatively low protein to energy ratio (9.2 to 10.4 g/MJ GE), the deposition of fat is favoured. Much of this fat is deposited subcutaneously and can serve both as an energy store and as an insulation layer. Sow's milk, therefore, appears to be designed primarily to promote the deposition of fat in the piglet rather than support lean tissue gain, and this seems to be the case for at least the first three weeks of life (Pluske *et al.*, 1995a). Apart from encouraging survival by building the energy stores of the piglet, low-protein diets may also be an advantage in certain disease states. This is certainly the case when piglets become dehydrated as a result of diarrhoea caused directly by microorganisms or indirectly by indigestible nutrients reaching the large intestine. In these circumstances, high-protein diets can be lethal because excess protein is deaminated to urea, a diuretic, which will dehydrate an animal further (Pluske *et al.*, 1995a).

3.4.1 How deficient in protein is sow's milk?

In the same study described previously, Williams (1976) removed piglets from the sow at two days of age and raised them from 1.8 to 6.4 kg liveweight on liquid milk diets in an attempt to mimic the sow. He offered diets which ranged in dietary protein concentration from 113 to 460 g crude protein/kg dietary dry matter at two levels of energy intake (1.3 or 2.1 MJ GE/kg$^{0.75}$/day). At the end of the experiment when the piglets weighed 6.4 kg liveweight (6.0 kg empty bodyweight) they were slaughtered and, together with some of their sow-suckled counterparts, body composition was measured (Figure 3.3). At either energy intake an increase in dietary protein reduced body fat of the artificially-reared piglets and minimum body fat was induced with a diet containing a little over 300 g cow's milk protein/kg dry matter. Body fat content of the sow-suckled pigs (153 g/kg) indicated that they had consumed a diet with approximately 200 g protein/kg dry matter, much lower than that needed to promote minimum body fat and maximum lean gain (Williams, 1976). Although fat deposition probably aids the survival of piglets reared outdoors, it is doubtful whether the piglet needs to deposit such a high ratio of fat so early in life if it is raised in modern commercial facilities where the physical and microbiological environment can be more closely controlled. Perhaps more important is whether early deposition of fat has adverse effects on subsequent growth and development. For example, if lean growth is restricted early in postnatal life does this reduce the potential for lean growth at a later stage? Does fat deposited in early life have long-term effects on fat deposition or food intake? These questions are outside the scope of this review, but are clearly questions warranting further investigation.

In view of the preceding discussion, an obvious question that may be asked is whether the protein concentration of sow's milk can be altered to achieve a higher protein to energy ratio. Discussion of this topic is also outside the scope of this review, but the reader is directed towards the review of Williams (1995) for a discussion on attempts to modify the nutrient profile of sow's milk.

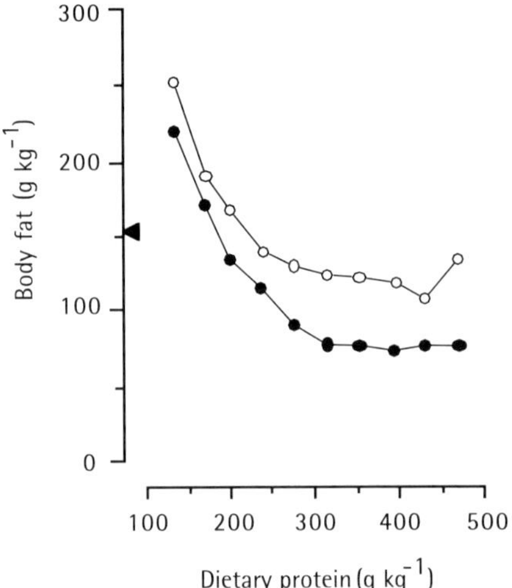

Figure 3.3. The effect of dietary protein on the body fat content of piglets reared artificially on either 1.3 (●——●) or 2.1 (○——○) MJ GE/kg live weight$^{0.75}$/day from 1.8 to 6.4 kg liveweight. The amount of body fat contained in sow-suckled piglets killed at 6.4 kg live weight is represented by (◄), and corresponds to a protein content in sow's milk of ≈200 g/kg (from Williams, 1976)

3.5 Biological efficiency of piglet utilisation of sow's milk

Although sow's milk may be protein deficient relative to energy, there is little doubt that the protein it does contain is used with high efficiency. Interestingly, few studies have been conducted to quantify the efficiency of nutrient utilisation of sow's milk in the very young pig, presumably because of the technical difficulties associated with harvesting the large amount of milk required to feed young pigs at *ad libitum* levels of intake. Unpublished results from a study conducted nearly 40 years ago (Livingstone *et al.*, 1959; cited by Lucas and Lodge, 1961), where pigs were weaned at two days of age and offered 1000 ml of sow's milk daily, showed apparent digestibility coefficients for crude protein and ether extract ranging between 0.97 and 0.99 for piglets aged up to 27 days of age (Table 3.3). Moughan *et al.* (1992) summarized several data sets and reported that the apparent digestibility of nitrogen in dried butter, milk powder or skim milk powder fed to young piglets as the major or sole source of nitrogen in semi-synthetic diets ranged from 86 to 98%. Using the three-week-old piglet as a model for the human infant, Darragh & Moughan (1995) reported mean true digestibilities of total nitrogen and amino acid nitrogen of 88% and 95%, respectively, when piglets were fed human milk. Lipids in cow's whole milk were reported to have an apparent digestibility of 98% (Braude & Newport, 1973).

Table 3.3. Apparent digestibility in the piglet of several components of sow's milk (from Livingstone et al., 1959; cited by Lucas & Lodge, 1961)

Component	Coefficient of digestibility	
	10-16 days of age	17-26 days of age
Dry matter	0.97	0.98
Crude protein	0.97	0.98
Ether extract	0.99	0.98
Ash	0.91	0.94
Calcium	0.89	0.92
Phosphorus	0.95	0.98

Noblet & Etienne (1987) used gaseous exchange methodology and comparative slaughter to determine the efficiency of utilisation of sow's milk and, as anticipated, found high levels of efficiency (Table 3.4). Gross energy was retained in the piglet body with an efficiency of between 52 and 55% depending upon the technique used for measurement. These values are very similar to those reported by Hodge (1974) in piglets fed reconstituted cow's whole milk between 10 and 30 days of age (52 to 57%). Nitrogen was retained in the empty body with an efficiency of 88%, although Williams (1995) commented that consideration of endogenous losses and nitrogen digestibility would result in a biological value nearing 1.0. These data concur with those of Livingstone *et al.* (1959), and provide compelling evidence that the young pig has a gastrointestinal tract capable of very efficient digestion and absorption of nutrients. In this respect, it is of little surprise that the young pig can grow at double its rate when removed from the sow early in its life.

3.5.1 Efficiency of piglet gain

Milk dry matter is converted to piglet gain with an efficiency ratio of about 0.75 to 0.80:1 (Lucas & Lodge, 1961), or about 3.8 g milk per gram of liveweight gain. Results from a number of studies conducted worldwide suggest that this conversion ratio is relatively stable despite wide fluctuations in nutrient intake by the sow and subsequent nutrient delivery to the piglet. Nevertheless, this ratio was established many years ago, and may now differ given the changes that have occurred over the last three decades in nutrition, genetics, litter size, milk production and environmental conditions. Revell *et al.* (1995) and Pluske *et al.* (1998) have recently calculated efficiencies with which piglets convert milk to body gain, and observed differences in this ratio dependent, essentially, upon the metabolic state of the sow during lactation. In the study described by Revell *et al.* (1995), piglets had a mean efficiency ratio of 5.2 g milk to 1 g of body gain when milk production was estimated between days four and six of lactation, and

Table 3.4. Energy, nitrogen and fat balance of sucking piglets between birth and weaning at 22 days of age (n = 20; results correspond to a litter and are expressed per piglet per day) (from Noblet & Etienne, 1987)

	Mean
Bodyweight at birth, kg	1.39
Bodyweight gain, g	195
Nitrogen intake from milk, g	5.43
Nitrogen retained[1], g	4.78
Efficiency of N retention, %	88.0
Fat intake from milk, g	53.5
Fat retained[1], g	28.7
Efficiency of fat retention, %	53.6
Energy intake as milk, kJ	3628
Retained energy RQ, kJ[2]	1908
Retained energy ST, kJ[1]	1984
RQ[2]	0.84
Efficiency of milk energy retention by RQ, %	52.5
Efficiency of milk energy retention by ST, %	54.7

[1] As measured by the Comparative Slaughter technique (ST); [2] Respiratory Quotient: retained energy estimated as difference between metabolizable energy intake as milk (milk energy x 0.95) and heat production (Brouwer, 1965).

a ratio of 3.7:1 in late lactation (days 25 to 27). However, the ratio was dependent upon both the level of sow body fatness at parturition and the level of crude protein in the lactation diet fed to the first-litter sows. Pluske *et al.* (1998) established an experimental model whereby primiparous sows were either made *grossly catabolic* (restrictedly fed), *slightly catabolic* (*ad libitum*-fed), or *anabolic* (superalimented via a gastric cannula) by the end of a 28-day lactation (see Pluske *et al.*, 1995b). Then, at two stages during lactation (*mid*, days 10-15, and late, days 21-25), milk production was estimated.

In mid lactation, and for restrictedly fed, *ad libitum*-fed and superalimented sows respectively, piglets required 4.2, 3.8 and 3.8 g milk per g body gain. In late lactation, and for restrictedly-fed, *ad libitum*-fed and superalimented sows respectively, piglets required 4.1, 3.9 and 3.9 g milk per g body gain. This occurred in the absence of statistically significant differences in both sow milk production

Table 3.5 Mean (± SE) milk yield, piglet growth rates, and milk composition determined at two different stages of lactation in primiparous sows which were restrictedly-fed (Restrict), ad libitum-fed (Ad libitum), or superalimented (Super) (from Pluske et al.*, 1998)*

	Treatment		
Item	Restrict	Ad libitum	Super
Mid lactation (d 10-15)			
Milk yield, kg/d	8.9 ± .65	9.2 ± .51	9.8 ± .57
Piglet growth, g/d[1]	248 ± 21.8	280 ± 16.9	290 ± 19.2
Milk composition, %			
Protein	5.2 ± .13	5.1 ± .13	5.1 ± .15
Fat	7.9 ± .92	7.4 ± .22	7.8 ± .23
Lactose	5.6 ± .11	5.5 ± .07	5.3 ± .16
Total Solids[2]	19.6	18.9	19.1
Late lactation (d 21-25)			
Milk yield, g/kg	7.3 ± .53	8.8 ± .46	8.3 ± .61
Piglet growth, g/d[1]	210 ± 17.9	269 ± 15.6	206 ± 20.3
Milk composition, %			
Protein	5.2 ± .16	5.2 ± .18	5.1 ± .15
Fat	7.1 ± .37	6.8 ± .43	7.6 ± .24
Lactose	5.3 ± .11	5.6 ± .06	5.3 ± .18
Total solids[2]	18.5	18.5	18.9

[1] Pig growth rate as determined within each milk production estimation period (adjusted for litter size at the start of each milk production estimation period).
[2] Assumes an ash concentration of 8.8 g/kg (Elliott *et al.*, 1971).

(although milk yield of restrictedly-fed sows was numerically lower than that of *ad libitum*-fed or superalimented sows) and milk composition (Table 3.5). Similarly, piglets sucking restrictedly-fed sows were about 1 kg lighter at weaning, but again this difference was not statistically significant (Pluske *et al.*, 1998). Nevertheless, the lower milk conversion efficiency of pigs sucking restrictedly-fed sows may be most simply explained by piglet body maintenance representing a greater proportion of intake. Another possibility, and most likely acting in concert with an increased maintenance requirement, is that a greater proportion of milk substrates was coming from maternal reserves in restrictedly-fed sows than from the diet. This may have caused subtle changes in milk composition, particularly the protein: energy ratio, which probably decreases in situations of severe catabolism in sows during lactation (I.H. Williams, personal communication). This may have occurred despite our observation that milk composition remained stable during lactation and did not vary with sow feeding treatment.

3.6 The role of piglets in determining milk production and milk intake

We have focused our discussion until now on the composition of sow's milk and the amount of milk produced by the sow as key determinants of piglet growth during lactation. While it has been known for some time that milk yield increases as a function of litter size (Elsley, 1971; King *et al.*, 1989; Auldist *et al.*, 1994; Toner *et al.*, 1995), and that milk intake per piglet increases with decreasing litter size because of larger glands (Auldist *et al.*, 1995), we are now beginning to understand that the size (weight) of the piglet along with sucking vigour (or intensity) play a major role in the amount of milk produced by the sow, and hence consumed by the piglet. These observations stem from the work 35 years ago by Hartman *et al.* (1962) who documented a positive, linear relationship between birth weight and milk intake of the young pig. Since then, a number of workers (e.g., Fraser & Morley Jones, 1975; Hemsworth *et al.*, 1976) have confirmed this relationship.

But how might litter size influence sow milk production? The effect of litter size on suckling frequency was examined by Auldist *et al.* (1994). Litters of 6, 8, 10, 12 or 14 piglets were established by fostering within 36 h post-partum. Auldist *et al.* (1994) reported a shorter suckling interval (i.e., period of time between successful sucklings) in early (day 10) compared to late (d 24) lactation (48.2 vs. 52.2 min, $P < 0.05$) commensurate with a longer period of milk ejection (14.6 vs. 12.8 seconds, $P < 0.05$).The period that milk is withdrawn from each teat is less in late lactation as opposed to early lactation because there are fewer sucklings and milk letdown is shorter (Auldist & King, 1995). Despite this though, measured sow milk production was similar, suggesting that the larger pigs in late lactation have a greater sucking strength and were able to extract more milk from each gland.

Support for this notion comes from the work of Hoy and Puppe (1992), who observed that growth rate from birth to weaning was higher in piglets sucking from the anterior teats compared to their littermates sucking either medial or posterior teats. Pluske and Williams (1996) also made this observation, and confirmed the likely mechanism of action by finding a strong, negative relationship between milk intake and teat number (Figure 3.4). Collectively, these data provide clear evidence that heavier piglets in a litter, which are also likely to be more active during udder massage and letdown, are more efficient at draining their teats than the lighter, less active piglets, and may therefore stimulate greater milk flow.

3.6.1 Piglet size (weight) and milk consumption

Numerous authors (e.g. van der Steen & de Groot, 1992; Head and Williams, 1995; King *et al.*, 1997) have reported very large differences in milk production dependent upon the weight, and hence sucking vigour, of piglets at birth. The

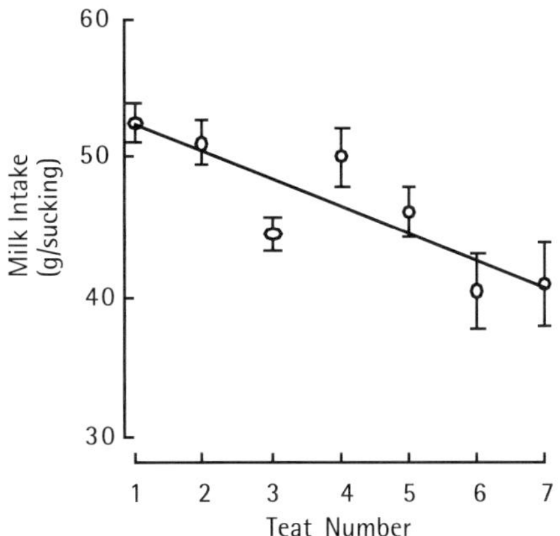

Figure 3.4. The relationship between average milk intake of piglets prior to split weaning (y-axis) and teat order (x-axis), with teats numbered one to seven from the anterior to the posterior end of the udder ($y = -1.929x + 54.214$; $R^2 = 0.757$; $P < 0.001$) (from Pluske & Williams, 1996)

work described by van der Steen & de Groot (1992) clearly elucidated the relationship between piglet weight, sucking demand, and milk intake. This experiment used both Chinese Meishan and Large White x Landrace sows and piglets, and involved transferring piglets within 24-48 hours of birth to establish litters of approximately half Chinese Meishan piglets and half Large White x Landrace piglets. The heavier Large White x Landrace piglets consumed similar amounts of milk and grew at similar rates irrespective offrom which sow genotype they suckled. However, Chinese Meishan piglets failed to consume as much milk as piglets born to Large White x Landrace sows despite being given the opportunity to do so from the potentially high milk-producing Large White x Landrace sows (Table 3.6). Further evidence that piglet milk demand has a direct bearing on sow milk yield is provided by the fact that heavy Chinese Meishan piglets and light Large White x Landrace piglets, which were similar in weight at birth, had comparable pre-weaning growth rates (van der Steen & de Groot, 1992).

Furthermore, King *et al.* (1997) found an increase in milk production of 26% during the first week of lactation when two-week-old piglets were fostered on to newly farrowed sows.Conversely, fostering newborn piglets on to sows already into their third week of lactation reduced subsequent milk production in that week by 22%. These data lend support to the general hypothesis that it is the piglet that primarily determines sow milk yield during early lactation but, as lactation proceeds, it is the supply of substrates needed for milk synthesis, controlled primarily by sow food intake but also by mobilisation of body reserves, that determines milk production towards the end of a 28-day lactation (Auldist

Table 3.6. Pre-weaning performance of piglets born to Chinese Meishan and Large White x Landrace sows and cross-fostered within 48 hours of birth to create litters of equal size but with the same number of piglets from each sow genotype (from van der Steen & de Groot, 1992)

Sows:	Chinese Meishan		Large White x Landrace	
Piglets:	Chinese Meishan	Large White x Landrace	Chinese Meishan	Large White x Landrace
Birth weight, kg	0.89	1.38	0.89	1.38
Lactation growth rate, g/day	164	191	154	205
Average milk intake, g/day	684	852	612	924
g milk : g body gain	4.17	4.46	3.97	4.51

& King, 1995). Alternatively, and as demonstrated recently by Pluske *et al.* (1998) where first-litter sows given 38% more energy via a gastric cannula than *ad libitum*-fed sows throughout a 28-day lactation did not produce more milk nor grow their piglets any faster, the ceiling to milk production may represent nothing more than a shortage of milk secretory cells.

Why may piglet size (weight) influence sow milk production and piglet milk intake? Algers & Jensen (1991) showed that the duration and intensity of stimulation given to a teat influenced the production of milk from that teat during the first few days of life. Fraser (1984) suggested that a larger pig may massage the teat more vigorously before ejection and achieve a greater blood flow to the teat. This, in turn, may cause more oxytocin to reach the udder resulting in greater contraction of the alveolar myoepithelial cells and hence greater milk flow. Alternatively, and assuming that heavier pigs are more efficient at draining teats, reduced levels of the feedback inhibitor of lactation (Hartmann *et al.*, 1995; Wilde *et al.*, 1995) would reside in the cistern after milk letdown. This would reduce the deleterious effects of this autocrine inhibitor on subsequent milk production.

3.6.2 The role of hormones in milk production and piglet milk consumption

The secretion of other lactogenic hormones such as prolactin has also been implicated (Algers *et al.*, 1991). In this regard, a series of experiments by Spencer and colleagues (see Spencer, 1986) found that immunization of lambs and goats against somatostatin, or somatotropin (growth hormone) release inhibiting factor (SRIF), increased growth rate and improved the efficiency of feed utilisation. Subsequent studies by Sun *et al.* (1990a, b) and Westbrook and colleagues

(Westbrook *et al.*, 1993, 1994) where ewes were passively immunized against somatostatin during gestation have confirmed these data. Sun *et al.* (1990b) reported an 11.3% increase in ewe milk yield when ewes were immunized against somatostatin during gestation. Westbrook *et al.* (1993) reported a 20-30% increase in milk intake in the first six weeks postpartum by lambs that were born to ewes immunized against somatostatin during gestation, an effect thought to be mediated by increased appetite (Westbrook *et al.*, 1994).

This work was extended to investigate the effect of immunization against somatostatin in pregnant primiparous sows on litter performance to weaning at 28 days of age (reported by McCauley *et al.*, 1995). Piglets sucking from first-litter sows immunized against somatostatin were found to be 20% heavier at weaning than their counterparts sucking from sows not immunized against somatostatin (8.9 compared with 7.6 kg, $P < 0.05$). There was no difference in birthweight between piglets born to both groups of sows, but differences in piglet liveweight were evident from day seven to weaning. Reasons for this marked increase in weaning weight are unknown, but piglets sucking from sows immunized against somatostatin consumed more milk and/or converted the milk more efficiently to body gain. It is recognised that somatostatin has a regulatory effect on gut hormone secretion (Spencer, 1986) and influences gut motility (Barry *et al.*, 1985), factors which most likely caused the improvement in digestion of dry feeds in crossbred lambs observed by Sun *et al.* (1990a). However, and given that the true digestibility of sow's milk approaches 100% regardless (Williams, 1995), it is unlikely that any increase in the digestibility of sow's milk caused by the transfer of somatostatin from the milk of the sow to the piglet is sufficient to account for the large difference in weaning weight between the groups of piglets. Nevertheless, the retention time of digesta in sheep immunized against somatostatin is increased (Barry *et al.*, 1985), so a subtle change in transit time may have allowed greater digestion and absorption of nutrients in the small intestine, and hence greater growth. An interesting result in this respect is that reported by Bird *et al.* (1990), who estimated that 30% of all lactose consumed by piglets is not hydrolyzed and enters the large intestine. If this is indeed true, then only a small reduction in transit time would be required to change lactose digestibility and effect an increase in piglet growth. Alternatively, immunization against somatostatin may have somehow altered the protein to energy ratio of sow's milk, although Westbrook *et al.* (1993, 1994) reported no differences in the protein and energy concentrations of milk when ewes were immunized against somatostatin during pregnancy. In summary, the increase in piglet weaning weight in response to immunization against somatostatin in sows is an interesting finding, and raises the possibility that hormonal and (or) neural factors may also be involved in the piglet's drive to consume milk and (or) utilize its digestive breakdown products.

3.7 Effects of substances and growth factors present in sow's colostrum and milk

Stimulatory effects of colostrum and milk on growth and development of the intestine in neonates has long been recognized (e.g. Widdowson & Crabb, 1976; Widdowson *et al.*, 1976), and the putative role of milk-borne growth factors in mediating this development has been the subject of considerable investigation (see Odle *et al.*, 1996; Xu, 1996; Burrin, 1997, for recent reviews). However, it is only relatively recently that we have been able to quantify with a reasonable degree of confidence the concentrations of milk-borne growth factors present in porcine colostrum and milk. These growth factors comprise a variety of proteins and peptides capable of stimulating cell growth and (or) expression of differentiated function in the intestinal tract. In the young pig, most attention to date has been centred upon epidermal growth factor, insulin, and the insulin-like growth factors, IGF-I and IGF-II (Odle *et al.*, 1996).

3.7.1 Insulin-like growth factors

As this area of research has evolved, an underlying hypothesis has been that milk-borne growth factors in mammalian secretions such as colostrum and milk, and in particular IGF-I and IGF-II, have a functional role in the growth and development of neonates. However, it seems that the amount of IGF-I received by the pig has a large bearing on the subsequent response. Using a pharmacological dose of recombinant human IGF-I (rhIGF-I) (3.5 mg/kg body weight) given to pigs from birth until four days of age, Burrin *et al.* (1996) showed increases in intestinal weight, protein and DNA content, and also increased villous height (Table 3.7). Small intestinal length and crypt depth were not altered. The quantity of rhIGF-I supplied to neonatal piglets was in excess of that normally ingested by piglets in both colostrum (≈ 100 µg/kg body weight) and milk (≈ 5 µg/kg body weight), bringing into question the biological relevance of IGF-I under normal conditions of suckling. Other studies in young pigs (Xu *et al.*, 1994; Houle *et al.*, 1995) and calves (Baumrucker *et al.*, 1994) have demonstrated that more physiological oral doses of IGF-I have elicited measurable increases in villous height and crypt cell proliferation but no demonstrable increases in intestinal mass or length. In addition, Houle *et al.* (1996) observed that oral administration of IGF-I (500 µg/L fed on an *ad libitum* basis) increased small intestinal lactase activity when caesarean-derived piglets were killed at 14 days of age, suggesting an influence of IGF-I on enterocyte maturation and disaccharidase activity. This, in turn, may have an impact on the efficiency with which the young pig can digest disaccharides.

Another important question regarding the possible function of milk-borne IGF-I is whether it survives luminal digestion and is absorbed into the peripheral circulation in a biologically-active form. There is significant absorption of intact macromolecules during the perinatal period, a function that is critical for acquisition of immunoglobulins (Lecce *et al.*, 1964). It is possible, therefore, that ingested polypeptide growth factors can also be absorbed intact across the small intestine into the general circulation and exert systemic effects, for example on organ development and muscle growth. However, a recent study in young pigs by Donovan *et al.* (1997) found that although as much as 30% of an orally administered dose of ^{125}I-labelled IGF-I was recovered in the intestinal mucosa, there was very limited absorption into the circulation. On the other hand, Xu & Wang (1996) reported significant absorption of IGF-I in both newborn and three-day-old piglets, whilst Xu *et al.* (1994) described heavier pancreas weights and increased pancreatic DNA content when newborn pigs were fed IGF-I and IGF-II.

Table 3.7. Changes in mucosal growth and morphology of the small intestine in neonatal piglets fed a milk replacer or milk replacer plus added rhIGF-I which provided 3.5 mg/kg bodyweight/day for four days after birth (from Burrin et al., 1996)

	Treatment		Pooled SD	P-value
	Milk replacer	Milk replacer + rhIGF-I		
Weight, g/kg BW[1]				
jejunum	13.7	17.5	2.6	0.013
ileum	15.6	20.0	2.3	0.003
Length, cm/kg BW				
jejunum	158	149	18	0.369
ileum	157	151	18	0.497
DNA, mg/kg BW				
jejunum	66	108	27	0.010
ileum	64	91	12	0.001
Protein, mg/kg BW				
jejunum	1,597	2,332	405	0.004
ileum	1,769	2,167	382	0.041
Villous height, µm				
jejunum	472	822	151	0.001
ileum	702	944	189	0.029
Crypt depth, µm				
jejunum	117	118	32	0.935
ileum	107	111	20	0.690

[1] BW: bodyweight.

Recently, we have observed significant differences in spleen, liver and thymus weights when piglets were fed bovine-derived milk products enriched with IGF-I during a 28-day lactation (Pluske *et al.*, unpublished data). These data support the work of Xu & Wang (1996) who reported that absorption of IGF-I occurred after gut closure in the young pig. These data also concur with those reported by Dunshea & Walton (1995) for artificially-reared pigs infused with an analogue of IGF-I. The physiological significance of these findings is yet to be determined, but clearly this is an exciting area of research. Opportunities for exogenous supplementation of, for example, milk replacers with gut-protected growth factors, may assist gut growth and development which, in turn, may increase the efficiency of piglet growth and enhance animal health.

3.8 Increasing piglet growth using milk supplements

To supplement waning sow milk production during lactation, producers (especially those weaning piglets greater than 25 days old) often provide piglets with a 'creep' or 'starter' diet. The idea is that piglets will choose to eat a dry 'creep' feed to complement their decreased intake of milk, and hence will be heavier at weaning. Evidence to support the notion that creep feeding increases weaning weight, however, is equivocal, and the published data suggest that the intake of creep food is generally small and extremely variable (Pluske *et al.*, 1995a).

Supplementation during lactation with liquid milk diets, however, offers the potential to provide a major boost to piglet growth rate during lactation, and hence to increase weaning weight. In spite of the considerable amount of work conducted in the 1960's and 1970's related to milk feeding of the young piglet, very few studies have quantified the response to feeding milk supplements to entire litters. Reale (1987) offered cow's whole milk to piglets from 10.00 h each day, adding fresh milk every two hours until 23.00 h, from day 7 to day 28 of lactation. Growth was stimulated by 151 g/day (70%) in the fourth week of lactation and, from days 7 to 28, by 87 g/day, an amount that increased piglet weaning weight by 1.8 kg in comparison to 'creep-fed' controls. As suggested by Williams (1995), and as is seen commercially, it is worth reflecting on why piglets continue sucking the sow when a more ample supply of nutrients is available nearby. Obviously, the sow provides both nutritive and non-nutritive needs to her offspring, an imprinting that would appear impossible to manipulate.

In another study of 171 litters over a three-year period, Azain *et al.* (1996) offered a commercial milk replacer (150 g/L dry matter) to litters on an *ad libitum* basis from within 24 hours of parturition to weaning at 21 days of age. Average pig weight was 16.4% higher (5.5 compared with 6.4 kg, $P < 0.001$) at weaning for litters receiving the milk replacer compared to those not receiving a supplement. The advantage in weaning weight conferred by provision of the milk replacer was most evident in warmer months, where intake was fourfold greater than in the cooler months and compensated for decreased sow milk production. Piglets converted milk replacer to body weight gain with an efficiency similar to that of sow's milk, the ratio being 0.85 to 1 (i.e. g milk replacer dry matter to g body gain) in the cooler months and 1.18 to 1 in the warmer months (Azain *et al.*, 1996). So, provided piglets drink the milk replacer offered and the regimen is economic, then supplementary milk feeding offers a practical way to increase piglet growth during weaning, especially during the warmer months when sow food intake, and hence sow milk production, is decreased.

3.9 Conclusion

In this chapter we have attempted to address some of the major issues related to the consumption and utilisation of colostrum and milk by sucking piglets. Colostrum and milk are associated with the final phase of the reproductive cycle of the sow and, it may be argued, their composition and production are designed to abet the survival of the neonatal piglet and to allow the sow to reproduce. This would appear to be in conflict with the aspirations of commercial pig production where piglets are expected to grow at the fastest rate possible. It is little wonder, therefore, that the composition of sow's colostrum and milk is extremely resilient to nutritional and environmental influences and that, despite the best efforts of researchers and practitioners, piglet growth rates during lactation still remain, at best, half of what can be achieved under artificial rearing. Exciting advances have been made in our understanding of how piglet size and behaviour influence the frequency and duration of suckling, and hence the amount of milk consumed. The question remains whether these stimuli can be manipulated in a practical fashion to effect increases in piglet gain. Current interest has focused on the physiological functions of the many substances, hormones and growth factors (such as IGF-I and IGF-II) present in colostrum and milk, and exciting opportunities exist for their incorporation into supplements. However, evidence of a response in overall digestive and absorptive capacity and increased weight gain to milk-borne growth factors remains elusive. The provision of milk replacers to piglets during lactation to augment diminishing sow milk supply offers a practical means of increasing the efficiency of piglet growth and profitability. Finally, the piglet is extremely efficient at digesting the milk it consumes, which is testimony to a gastrointestinal tract that is superbly adapted to handling milk protein (amino acids), fats, and lactose. Having said this, and while it is evident that current rates of growth fall well short of biological potential, the challenge to researchers and producers in the future is to devise nutritional regimens within the current systems of farm management to fulfil this goal.

3.10 References

Algers, B. & P. Jensen, 1991. Teat stimulation and milk production in early lactation of sows. Can. J. Anim. Sci. 71, 51-60.
Algers, B., A. Madej, S. Rojanasthien & K. Uvnas-Moberg, 1991. Quantitative relationships between suckling-induced teat stimulation and release of prolactin, gastrin, somatostatin, insulin, glucagon and vasoactive intestinal polypeptide in sows. Vet. Res. Commun. 35, 395-407.
Atwood, C.S. & P.E. Hartmann, 1992. Collection of fore and hind milk from the sow and the changes in milk composition during suckling. J. Dairy Res. 59, 287-298.
Auldist, D.E., D. Carlson, L. Morrish, C. Wakeford & R.H. King, 1995. Effect of increased suckling frequency on mammary development and milk yield of sows. In: Manipulating Pig Production V (eds D.P. Hennessy & P.D. Cranwell), p. 137. Australasian Pig Science Association, Werribee, Victoria, Australia.
Auldist, D.E. & R.H. King, 1995. Piglet's role in determining milk production in the sow. In: Manipulating Pig Production V (eds D.P. Hennessy & P.D. Cranwell), pp. 114-118. Australasian Pig Science Association, Werribee, Victoria, Australia.
Auldist, D.E., L. Morrish, M. Thompson & R.H. King, 1994. Response of sows to varying litter size. Proc. Nutr. Soc. Aust. 18: 175.
Azain, M.J., T. Tomkins, J.S. Sowinski, R.A. Arentson & D.E. Jewell, 1996. Effect of supplemental pig milk replacer on litter performance: seasonal variation in response. J. Anim. Sci. 74, 2195-2202.
Barry, T.N., G.J. Faichney & C. Redekopp, 1985. Gastro-intestinal tract function in sheep infused with somatostatin. Aust. J. Biol. Sci. 38, 393-403.
Baumrucker, C.R., D.L. Hadsell & J.W. Blum, 1994. Effects of dietary insulin-like growth factor-1 on growth and insulin-like growth factor receptors in neonatal calf intestine. J. Anim. Sci. 72, 428-433.
Bird, P.H., A. Di Rosso & P.E. Hartmann, 1990. Galactose and glucose changes in the blood after ingestion of either lactose or galactose plus glucose by piglets with diarrhoea. Proc. Nutr. Soc. Aust. 15, 50.
Black, J.L., R.G. Campbell, I.H. Williams, K.J. James & G.T. Davies, 1986. Simulation of energy and amino acid utilisation in the pig. Res. Dev. Agric. 3, 121-145.
Bourne, F.J., 1969. Studies on colostral and milk whey proteins in the sow. 1. The transition of mammary secretions from colostrum to milk with natural sucking. Anim. Prod. 11, 337-343.
Braude, R. & M.J. Newport, 1973. Artificial rearing of pigs. 4. The replacement of buttermilk in a whole-milk diet by either beef tallow, coconut oil or soyabean oil. Br. J. Nutr. 29, 447-455.
Brouwer, E., 1965. Report of sub-committee on constants and factors. In Energy Metabolism (ed K.L. Blaxter), pp. 441-443. European Association of Animal Production No. 11. Academic Press, London, UK.
Burrin, D.G., 1997. Is milk-borne insulin-like growth factor-1 essential for neonatal development? J. Nutr. 127, 975S-979S.
Burrin, D.G., T.J. Wester, T.A. Davis, S. Amick & J.P. Heath, 1996. Orally administered IGF-I increases intestinal mucosal growth in formula-fed neonatal pigs. Am. J. Physiol. 270, R1085-R1091.
Campbell, R.G. & M.R. Taverner, 1988. Genotype and sex effects on the relationship between energy intake and protein deposition in growing pigs. J. Anim. Sci. 66, 676-686.
Comber, M.F. & P.E. Hartmann, 1993. In: Manipulating Pig Production IV (ed E.S. Batterham), p. 263. Australasian Pig Science Association, Werribee, Victoria, Australia.

Cranwell, P.D., 1995. Development of the neonatal gut and enzyme systems. In: The Neonatal Pig: Development and Survival (ed M.A. Varley), pp. 99-154. CAB International, Wallingford, Oxon, U.K.
Darragh, A.J. & P.J. Moughan, 1995. The digestibility of amino acids in human milk. In: Manipulating Pig Production V (eds D.P. Hennessy & P.D. Cranwell), p. 132. Australasian Pig Science Association, Werribee, Victoria, Australia.
Darragh, A.J. & P.J. Moughan, 1998. Composition of sow's colostrum and milk. In: The Lactating Sow (eds. M.W.A. Verstegen, P.J. Moughan & J. Schrama), pp. 1-19. Wageningen Pers, Wageningen, The Netherlands.
Donovan, S.M., J.C-J. Chao, R.T. Zijlstra & J. Odle, 1997. Orally administered iodinated recombinant human insulin-like growth factor-1 (IGF-I) is poorly absorbed by the neonatal piglet. J. Pediatr. Gastroenterol. Nutr. (In press).
Dunshea, F.R. & P.E. Walton, 1995. Potential of exogenous metabolic modifiers for the pig industry. In: Manipulating Pig Production V (eds. D.P. Hennessy & P.D. Cranwell), pp. 42-51. Australasian Pig Science Association, Werribee, Victoria, Australia.
Elliott, R. F., G. W. Vander Noot, R. L. Gilbreath & H. Fisher, 1971. Effect of dietary protein level on compositional changes in sow colostrum and milk. J. Anim. Sci. 32, 1128-1137.
Elsley, F.W.H., 1971. Nutrition and lactation in the sow. In: Lactation (ed. I.R. Falconer), pp. 393-411. Butterworths, London, U.K.
Fowler, V.R. & B.P. Gill, 1989. Voluntary food intake in the young pig. In: The Voluntary Food Intake of Pigs (eds. J.M. Forbes, M.A. Varley & T.J. Lawrence), pp. 51-60. Occasional Publication No. 13, British Society of Animal Production, Edinburgh, U.K.
Fraser, D., 1984. The role of behavior in swine production: A review of research. Appl. Anim. Ethol. 11, 317-339.
Fraser, D. & R. Morley Jones, 1975. The 'teat order' of suckling pigs. 1. Relation to birth weight and subsequent growth. J. Agric. Sci. 84, 387-391.
Harrell, R.J., M.J. Thomas & R.D. Boyd, 1993. Limitations of sow milk yield on baby pig growth. In: Proceedings of the 1993 Cornell Nutrition Conference for Feed Manufacturers, pp. 156-164. Department of Animal Science and Division of Nutritional Sciences of the New York State College of Agriculture and Life Sciences, Cornell University, Ithaca, NY, USA.
Hartman, D.A., T.M. Ludwick & R.F. Wilson, 1962. Certain aspects of lactation performance in sows. J. Anim. Sci. 21, 883-886.
Hartmann, P.E., C.S. Atwood, D.B. Cox & S.E.J. Daly. 1995. Endocrine and
autocrine strategies for the control of lactation in women and sows. In: Intercellular Signaling in the Mammary Gland (eds C.J. Wilde, M. Peaker & C.H. Knight), pp. 203-225. Plenum Press, New York and London.
Hartmann, P.E. & M.A. Holmes, 1989. Sow lactation. In: Manipulating Pig Production II (eds. J.L. Barnett & D.P. Hennessy), pp. 72-97. Australasian Pig Science Association, Werribee, Victoria, Australia.
Head, R.H. & I.H. Williams, 1995. Potential milk production in gilts. In: Manipulating Pig Production V (eds D.P. Hennessy & P.D. Cranwell), p. 134. Australasian Pig Science Association, Werribee, Victoria, Australia.
Hemsworth, P.H., C.G. Winfield & P.D. Mullaney, 1976. Within litter variation in the performance of piglets to three weeks of age. Anim. Prod. 22, 351-357.
Herpin, P. & J. Le Dividich, 1995. Thermoregulation and the environment. In: The Neonatal Pig: Development and Survival (ed M.A. Varley), pp. 57-95. CAB International, Wallingford, Oxon, U.K.
Hodge, R.M.W., 1974. Efficiency of food conversion and body composition of the preruminant lamb and the young pig. Br. J. Nutr. 32, 113-126.

Houle, V.M., E.A. Schroeder, S.C. Laswell & S.M. Donovan, 1996. Small intestinal disaccharidase activities are up-regulated, whereas peptidase activity is decreased by orally administered insulin-like growth factor-1 in the neonatal piglet. FASEB J. 10, A728 (Abstr.).
Houle, V.M., E.A. Schroeder, Y-K. Park, J. Odle & S.M. Donovan, 1995. Orally administered insulin-like growth factor-1 (IGF-I) stimulates neonatal piglet intestinal development. FASEB J. 9, A580 (Abstr.).
Hoy, St. & B. Puppe, 1992. Effects of teat order on performance and health in growing pigs. Pig News Info. 13, 131N-136N.
Kennaugh, L.M. & P.E. Hartmann, 1995. Total creatine in sow's colostrum and milk. In: Manipulating Pig Production V (eds D.P. Hennessy & P.D. Cranwell), p. 130. Australasian Pig Science Association, Werribee, Victoria, Australia.
King, R.H., B.P. Mullan, F.R. Dunshea & H. Dove, 1997. The influence of piglet body weight on milk production of sows. Livest. Prod. Sci. 47, 169-174.
King, R.H., M.S. Toner & H. Dove, 1989. Pattern of milk production in sows. In: Manipulating Pig Production II (ed J.L. Barnett & D.P. Hennessy), p. 98. Australasian Pig Science Association, Werribee, Victoria, Australia.
Koldovsky, O., 1996. Hormones and growth factors in milk. Ann. Nestlé 54, 105-112.
Lecce, J.G., D.O. Morgan & G. Matrone, 1964. Effect of feeding colostral and milk components on the cessation of intestinal absorption of large molecules (closure) in neonatal pigs. J. Nutr. 84, 43-48.
Livingstone, R.M., G.A. Lodge, I.A.M. Lucas, R.M. MacPherson & S.J. MacPherson, 1959; cited in Lucas, I.A.M. & G.A. Lodge, 1961. Nutrition of the Young Pig. Technical Bulletin No. 22. Commonwealth Agricultural Bureaux, Farnham Royal, UK.
Lucas, I.A.M. & G.A. Lodge, 1961. Nutrition of the Young Pig. Technical Bulletin No. 22. Commonwealth Agricultural Bureaux, Farnham Royal, UK.
McCauley, I., A. Billinghurst, P.O. Morgan & S.L. Westbrook, 1995. Manipulation of endogenous hormones to increase growth of pigs. In: Manipulating Pig Production V (eds D.P. Hennessy & P.D. Cranwell), pp. 52-61. Australasian Pig Science Association, Werribee, Victoria, Australia.
Mellor, D.J. & F. Cockburn, 1986. A comparison of energy metabolism in the newborn infant, piglet and lamb. Quart. J. Exp. Physiol. 71, 361-379.
Morgan, C.J., A.G. Cutts, M.C. McFadyen & D. Kelly, 1996. Characterization of IGF-I receptors in the porcine small intestine during post-natal development. J. Nutr. Biochem. 7, 339-347.
Moughan, P.J., M.J. Birtles, P.D. Cranwell, W.C. Smith & M. Pedraza, 1992. The piglet as a model animal for studying aspects of digestion and absorption in milk-fed human infants. World Rev. Nutr. Diet. 67, 40-113.
Mount, L.E., 1968. The Climatic Physiology of the Pig. Edward Arnold, London, U.K.
Newburg, D.S., 1997. Do the binding properties of oligosaccharides in milk protect human infants from gastrointestinal bacteria? J. Nutr. 127, 980S-984S.
Noblet, J. & M. Etienne, 1987. Body composition, metabolic rate and utilisation of milk nutrients in suckling piglets. Reprod. Nutr. Dev. 27, 829-839.
Odle, J., R.T. Zijlstra & S.M. Donovan, 1996. Intestinal effects of milkborne growth factors in neonates of agricultural importance. J. Anim. Sci. 74, 2509-2522.
Okai, D.B., F.X. Aherne & R.T. Hardin, 1977. Effects of sow nutrition in late gestation on the body composition and survival of the neonatal pig. Can. J. Anim. Sci. 57, 439-448.
Pluske, J.R. & I.H. Williams, 1996. Split weaning increases the growth of light piglets during lactation. Aust. J. Agric. Res. 47, 513-523.
Pluske, J.R., I.H. Williams & F.X. Aherne, 1995a. Nutrition of the neonatal pig. In: The Neonatal Pig: Development and Survival (ed M.A. Varley), pp. 187-235. CAB International, Wallingford, Oxon, U.K.

Pluske, J.R., I.H. Williams, A.C. Cegielski & F.X. Aherne, 1995b. Stomach cannulation of pregnant gilts for nutrition studies during lactation. Can. J. Anim. Sci. 75, 497-500.
Pluske, J.R., I.H. Williams, L.J. Zak, E.J. Clowes, A.C. Cegielski & F.X. Aherne, 1998. Feeding primiparous lactating sows to induce three divergent metabolic states. 3. Milk production and piglet growth. J. Anim. Sci. (In press).
Reale, T. A., 1987. Supplemental liquid diets and feed flavours for young pigs. MAgrSc Thesis, University of Melbourne.
Revell, D.K., I.H. Williams, J.L. Ranford, B.P. Mullan & R.J. Smits, 1995. Body fatness reduces voluntary food intake and alters plasma metabolites during lactation. In: Manipulating Pig Production V (eds D.P. Hennessy & P.D. Cranwell), p. 128. Australasian Pig Science Association, Werribee, Victoria, Australia.
Spencer, G.S.G., 1986. Immuno-neutralization of somatostatin and its effects on animal production. Domest. Anim. Endocrinol. 3, 55-68.
Sun, Y.X., G.L. Drane, S.D. Currey, N.D. Lehner, J.M. Gooden, R.M. Hoskinson, P.C. Wynn & G.H. McDowell, 1990a. Immunization against somatotropin release inhibiting factor improves digestibility of food, growth and wool production in crossbred lambs. Aust. J. Agric. Res. 41, 401-411.
Sun, Y.X., S.E. Sinclair, P.C. Wynn & G.H. McDowell, 1990b. Immunization against somatotropin release inhibiting factor increases milk yield in lambs. Aust. J. Agric. Res. 41, 393-400.
Toner, M.S., R.H. King, F.R. Dunshea, H. Dove & C.S. Atwood, 1995. The effect of exogenous somatotropin on lactation performance of first-litter sows. J. Anim. Sci. 73, 167-172.
Tritton, S.M., R.H. King, R.G. Campbell & A.C. Edwards, 1993. The effects of dietary protein on lactation performance of first-litter sows. In: Manipulating Pig Production IV (ed E.S. Batterham), p. 265. Australasian Pig Science Association, Werribee, Victoria, Australia.
van der Steen, H.A.M. & P.N. de Groot, 1992. Direct and maternal breed effects on growth and milk intake of piglets: Meishan versus Dutch breeds. Livest. Prod. Sci. 30, 361-373.
Westbrook, S.L., A.M. Ali & G.H. McDowell, 1994. Passively-acquired antibodies to somatotropin release inhibiting factor (SRIF) increase appetite and growth of milk-fed lambs. Aust. J. Agric. Res. 45, 293-302.
Westbrook, S.L., K.D. Chandler & G.H. McDowell, 1993. Immunization of pregnant ewes against somatotropin release inhibiting factor increases growth of twin lambs. Aust. J. Agric. Res. 44, 229-238.
Widdowson, E.M., V.E. Colombo & C.A. Artavanis, 1976. Changes in the organs of pigs in response to feeding for the first 24 h after birth. II. The digestive tract. Biol. Neonate 28, 272-281.
Widdowson, E.M. & D.E. Crabb, 1976. Changes in the organs of pigs in response to feeding for the first 24 h after birth. I. The internal organs and muscles. Biol. Neonate 28, 261-271.
Wilde, C.J., C.V.P. Addey, L.M. Boddy-Finch & M. Peaker, 1995. Autocrine control of milk secretion: from concept to application. In: Intercellular
Signaling in the Mammary Gland (eds C.J. Wilde, M. Peaker & C.H. Knight), pp. 227-237. Plenum Press, New York and London.
Williams, I.H., 1976. Nutrition of the young pig in relation to body composition. PhD Thesis, University of Melbourne.
Williams, I.H., 1995. Sow's milk as a major nutrient source before weaning. In: Manipulating Pig Production V (eds D.P. Hennessy & P.D. Cranwell), pp. 107-113. Australasian Pig Science Association, Werribee, Victoria, Australia.
Xu, R-J., 1996. Development of the newborn GI tract and its relation to colostrum/milk intake: a review. Reprod. Fert. Dev. 8, 35-48.

Xu. R-J., D.J. Mellor, M.J. Birtles, B.H. Breier & P.D. Gluckman, 1994. Effects of oral IGF-I or IGF-II on digestive organ growth in newborn piglets. Biol. Neonate 66, 280-287.

Xu, R-J. & T. Wang, 1996. Gastrointestinal absorption of insulin-like growth factor-1 in neonatal pigs. J. Pediatr. Gastroenterol. Nutr. 23, 430-437.

4 Metabolic precursors for milk synthesis

R. Dean Boyd and Ronald S. Kensinger

4.1 Introduction

Mammary glands are the primary users of absorbed nutrients in lactating sows and virtually dictate dietary needs (Bauman and Currie, 1980; Boyd and Touchette, 1997). At least 70% of the total energy requirement is needed to support lactation (Aherne and Williams, 1992). More than 90% of absorbed amino acids are needed for milk synthesis and mammary growth during lactation. Indeed, the requirement of mammary tissue for milk substrates (or precursors) is so dominant that the sow is seemingly an appendage to the udder. Inadequate diets or feeding management can result in extensive use of body reserves (adipose, body protein, bone) which will compromise subsequent pig output in younger females (Boyd and Touchette, 1997).

This chapter is devoted to a review of the metabolic precursors that are used to synthesize milk nutrients in sows. The classical techniques that were developed by James Linzell to study precursor uptake and metabolism by the mammary gland have been extensively applied to the ruminant. Application to the lactating sow is very limited so the nature of this review is by no means comparable to the classic review in ruminants (Annison, 1983). These methods are discussed, and the precursor - milk nutrient relationships applied to the elite sow, to illustrate how dramatic the precursor need is when compared with the sow of the early 1970's (6.25-7.50 kg milk/d). Milk output will become increasingly important because optimized preweaning growth decreases nursery mortality under commercial conditions and can shift the growth curve to market by up to 15 d (Mahan and Lepine, 1991; Harrell et al., 1993).

4.2 Milk constituents and blood precursors

Milk is a complex biological fluid. It contains a wide array of molecules that provide for the nutritive, immunological and developmental needs of the neonate (Hartmann and Holmes, 1989). The most abundant constituent is water and much of the rest is carbohydrate, protein and lipid. An impressive array of pathogen protective and polypeptide growth factors are present. The latter appear to mediate growth and development of the newborn (Burrin et al., 1992). Milk enzymes may also benefit neonatal digestion and assimilation of milk components. Some may protect the mammary gland against infection during lactation.

Milk contains approximately 4.9% lactose, 5.6% protein and 6.8% fat respectively (Pluske et al., 1995; see Chapter 3). Lactose provides about 50% of the glucose requirement of the nursing pig (Boyd, unpublished calculations) which is essential to survival, especially during the initial 2-3 days of age. Fat contributes the greatest amount to gross energy (65%) and provides essential fatty acids for cellular development. The relatively low protein and high fat content of milk results in a low protein:energy ratio (3.70 g lysine/Mcal gross energy) which encourages deposition of body fat for insulation and energy reserves. However, we believe that this constrains protein deposition and thus growth rate in the neonatal pig (Williams, 1976).

Lactose is the predominant carbohydrate in milk. Carbohydrates that are present in small amounts include the components of lactose (glucose, galactose) and oligosaccharides. Lactose is the major osmotic constituent and, in combination with salts and proteins, causes milk to be iso-osmotic with blood plasma (Jenness, 1985). It appears that lactose formation is a determinant of milk yield through osmotic pull of water into the gland. Blood glucose is the primary precursor for lactose synthesis (accounts for ≥ 70%), with the residual derived from glycerol, lactate and extra-mammary conversion of dispensable amino acids to glucose.

Protein components of colostrum and milk are diverse (see Hartmann and Holmes, 1989). Approximately 96-97% of total milk nitrogen is in the form of protein bound amino acids (Klobasa et al., 1987) with 2-3% of the non-protein nitrogen as urea and free amino acids (Wu and Knabe, 1995). Ninety-five percent of sow milk proteins are synthesized in the mammary gland from amino acid precursors that are extracted from the blood. This suggests that free and protein bound amino acids (and possibly di- and tri-peptides) cross the mammary epithelial membrane intact.

Milk lipid is composed mainly of triglycerides with small proportions of di- and mono-glycerides, phospholipids, cholesterol, fat-soluble vitamins and free fatty acids (Jenness, 1985). Fatty acids in milk are derived from blood triglycerides and de novo synthesis in the mammary gland (Linzell et al., 1969). Mammary tissue of the sow is capable of synthesizing saturated fatty acids with 14 to 18 carbons and of desaturating palmitic and stearic fatty acids to the corresponding monounsaturated fatty acids (Spincer and Rook, 1968). Five fatty acids account for approximately 95% of milk fatty acids: palimitic, palmitoleic, stearic, oleic and linoleic acids (Seerley and Poole, 1974; Jenness, 1974). Linoleic acid cannot be synthesized and must be provided preformed in the diet. A proper mix of saturated to unsaturated fatty acids is essential for high fat digestibility. Micelle development is important for digestion by intestinal lipase but an improper balance of fatty acids types will decrease micelle formation.

4.3 Methods used to identify milk precursors

The study of mammary uptake and metabolism of blood precursors for milk synthesis is in its infancy in sows. Techniques that have proven invaluable to the identification of precursors for milk synthesis involve the A-V procedure and use of a radioactive precursor. The former involves determining the amount of precursor transported into the mammary gland by subtracting the venous concentration from the arterial concentration (arterial-venous difference, A-V). Radioactivity can then be used to trace the transfer of a labeled precursor to milk nutrients. For example, we could determine the amount of leucine taken up daily (g/d) by the mammary gland but we could not say how much was used for protein synthesis as compared to energy generation (oxidation to ATP) or for fatty acid synthesis without the use of 'labels'. Concepts and methodologies for these techniques have been presented in seminal reviews (Linzell, 1974; Linzell and Annison, 1975; Annison, 1983).

The A-V technique provides a quantitative measure of precursor uptake from the blood as it passes through the mammary gland. It requires (1) simultaneous measure of the difference in precursor concentration of arterial and venous blood and (2) measurement of blood flow (BF) rate to the mammary gland. Uptake (U) is then computed by the equation $U = (A - V) BF$. If this estimate is coupled with isotopic techniques, the amount of specific milk nutrients formed from transported precursors can be estimated. Extraction ratio (E) by mammary tissue is a qualitative measure of transfer that is possible without blood flow information. It is calculated as follows:

$$E = (A - V) / A$$

The A-V technique requires accurate sampling of blood that is entering and leaving the glands. A valid arterial sample can be taken from any artery because systemic blood is well mixed so that composition is identical at the various arterial sites. However, great care is required in placement of venous cannula to ensure that blood is exclusively sampled from mammary glands since the composition of venous blood varies with the tissue being drained. For example, the carotid artery and right anterior mammary vein were used in recent studies on amino acid uptake in sows (Trottier et al., 1997).

Blood flow must be determined in conscious animals and under stable conditions because movement can introduce considerable variation in the rate. Estimates have been made using a variety of techniques such as the dilution of an infused non-metabolizable substance, use of electromagnetic probes and by application of the Fick principle. The latter has been applied in ruminants (Davis and Bickerstaffe, 1978) and may be beneficial in studies with sows where anatomical differences pose a greater challenge to accurate BF estimates. This method is based on direct transfer of a precursor from blood to milk without metabolism to other products. Calcium and certain amino acids are examples (Annison, 1983). Mammary blood flow may be calculated as follows using the Fick principle:

BF, ml/h = milk nutrient output, mg/h / nutrient A-V, mg/ml

The vascular system of the ruminant mammary gland is straightforward compared to the more diffuse system of the sow (Linzell, 1974). Ruminant glands are located in the inguinal region with the main arterial supply and venous drainage accounted for by two vessels (pudic artery, caudal epigastric vein). The mammary system of sows extends over the entire abdominal wall. Blood leaving the glands of sows use two different pathways. Anterior glands are drained by two large veins (abdominal veins) that run parallel to each row of glands. Blood exits the posterior glands by way of the same veins but in a caudal direction. Cannulation of the anterior venous end seems preferable since glands are more apt to remain functional and productive. A thorough description of the mammary circulatory system for sows was published recently by Trottier and co-workers (1995).

4.4 Blood precursors used for milk synthesis

Our knowledge of the importance of various blood precursors for milk synthesis in pigs is largely the result of the pioneering work of Linzell and Spincer (Linzell et al., 1969; Spincer et al., 1969; Spincer and Rook, 1971) who used the A-V technique. This type of research has been undertaken almost exclusively in ruminants because of the more obvious importance of milk production. There are some important differences that limit application to the pig (e.g., rumen production of VFA and limited glucose absorption). Boyd and co-workers (1995) provided convincing evidence that enhancement of lactation is important to the pig industry. They used the pioneering work to illustrate how an understanding of precursor - milk product relationships allows us to predict nutrient need with increases in milk output. Fortunately, the study of nutrient uptake and metabolism by mammary tissue of lactating sows has been revived by recent studies (Trottier et al., 1997; Nielsen et al., 1997; Hurley et al., 1996).

Glucose, triglyceride fatty acids and amino acids represent approximately 95% of the total carbon mass taken up by sow mammary tissue (Table 4.1). Spincer and co-workers (1969) reported that glucose accounted for 61%, amino acids 24%, triglyceride fatty acids 12% and acetate 1% of total uptake. These are in good agreement with results computed from a report by Linzell et al., (1967 - see Spincer et al., 1969). Percent extraction of non-esterified fatty acids (-6%), lactate (2%) and other metabolites (eg., βHBA, citrate) suggest an insignificant role in milk nutrient synthesis. The contribution of NEFA as a precursor is conceivably more important in early lactation and with large litters when negative energy balance and body fat

Table 4.1. Relative uptake of plasma constituents by the mammary gland of lactating sows[1]

Constituent	A-V[2] difference (mg/dl)	Percent extraction	Relative uptake[3] (% total)	Uptake for Milk synthesis[4] (g/dl milk)
Glucose	37.5	31	61	14.1
Acetate	0.6	46	1	0.2
Triacylfatty acids	7.2	16-23	12	2.7
Amino acids	15.1	23-41	24	6.2
β-hydroxybutyrate	0.2	11	-	-
Lactate	1.4	12	2	0.5
Citrate	0	0	-	-

[1] Summarized from Spincer et al., 1969.
[2] Arterial Venous difference in concentration of plasma constituents.
[3] Percent of the total mass (mg) of constituents extracted.
[4] Assumes 375 ml plasma flow through the udder per 1 ml of milk secreted.

mobilisation occur. The net contribution of acetate is small even though extraction rate is high (46%) because of a typically low blood concentration.

Incorporation of plasma-derived triglyceride fatty acids (TGFA) into milk fat seems to be quantitatively less important for the sow than for the goat when comparing mammary uptake to milk content. This suggests that de novo synthesis of milk fat is greater for pigs, and from glucose as opposed to acetate and βHBA as observed for ruminants (Spincer et al., 1969). In lactating dairy cows, there is a positive relationship between arterial TGFA concentration and A-V difference. This suggests that raising blood TGFA levels by dietary means would lead to increased uptake by the mammary gland (Baldwin and Smith, 1983). We expect this relationship to hold for lactating sows since increased dietary fat intake results in greater milk fat concentration and milk output (Boyd et al., 1981).

A simplified overview of the absorbed metabolites from dietary energy and protein is shown in Figure 4.1. Metabolism of the primary precursors for milk synthesis is shown as a frame of reference for sections 4.4 and 4.6. Metabolism is integrated among tissues to support milk synthesis. Adaptations occur late in pregnancy so that the mammary is given priority for glucose. Adipose and muscle use less glucose, while lives synthesis of glucose and reincorporation of NEFA (from adipose) into triglycerides becomes even more important (see legend).

Spincer and co-workers (1969) computed the precursor requirement for milk synthesis using the multiple of A-V (mg/dL) and an estimate of blood flow (375 mL

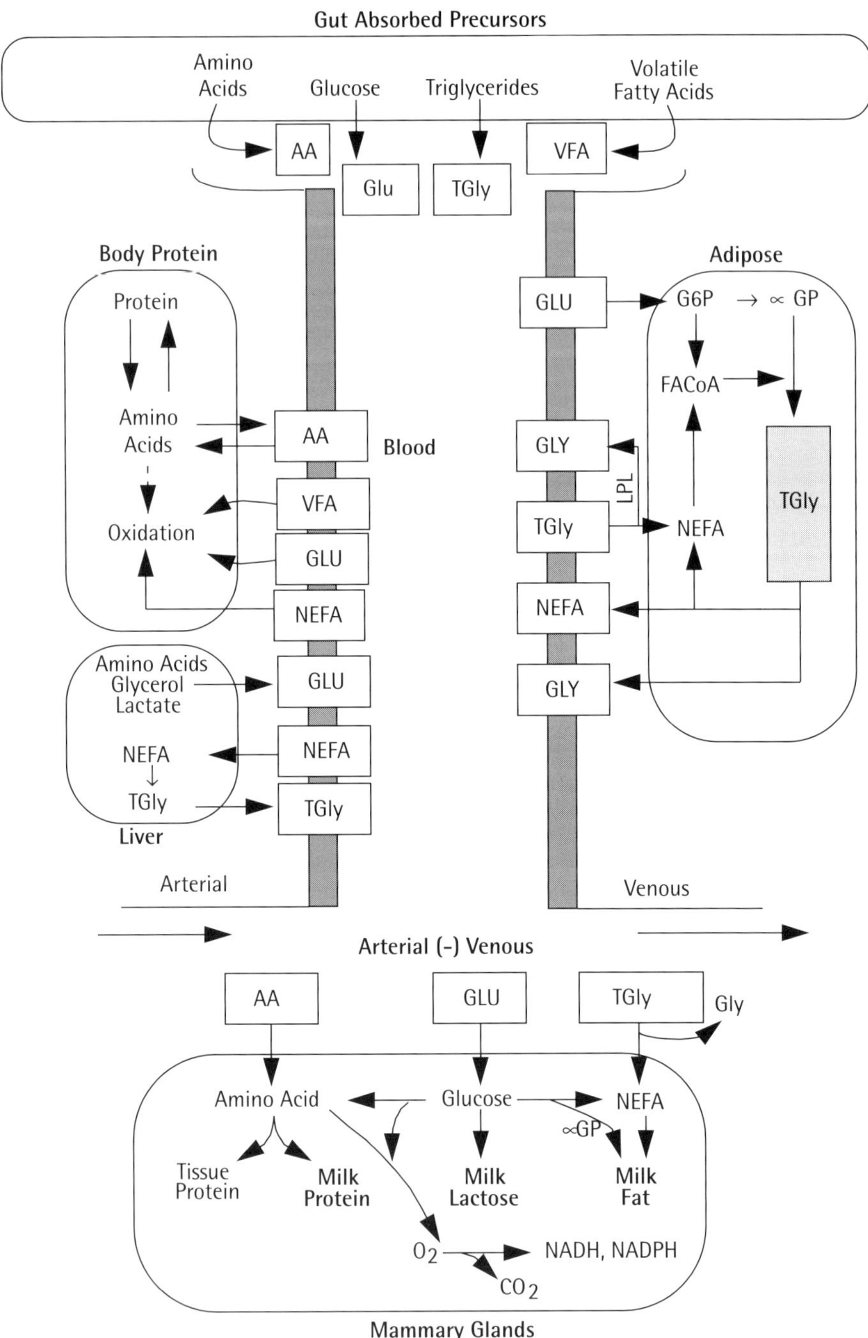
Gut Absorbed Precursors
Amino Acids
Glucose
Triglycerides
Volatile Fatty Acids
AA
Glu
TGly
VFA
Body Protein
Protein
Amino Acids
Oxidation
AA
Blood
VFA
GLU
NEFA
Amino Acids
Glycerol
Lactate
NEFA
TGly
Liver
GLU
NEFA
TGly
Arterial
Adipose
GLU
G6P
∝ GP
FACoA
GLY
LPL
TGly
NEFA
TGly
NEFA
GLY
Venous
Arterial (-) Venous
AA
GLU
TGly
Gly
Amino Acid
Glucose
NEFA
∝GP
Tissue Protein
Milk Protein
Milk Lactose
Milk Fat
O2
NADH, NADPH
CO2
Mammary Glands

Figure 4.1. Simplified overview of the partition of absorbed metabolites of energy and protein among body tissues of the lactating sow. (drawn by S. Shoulders) Glucose (GLU), amino acids (AA) and Triglycerides (TGly) represent 95% of gut absorbed metabolites that are taken up by mammary tissue. Volatile fatty acids (VFA) are not absorbed from the gut in significant amounts under most circumstances. Mammary uptake of each precursor is determined by the difference in precursor concentration of arterial and venous blood if multiplied by the rate of blood flow through the mammary system. Adipose, liver, muscle and perhaps bone respond in a highly coordinated manner to support rather than compete with the mammary for GLU and other nutrients (Newsholme and Leech, 1983). For example, adipose tissue is less responsive to insulin stimulation for GLU uptake so that more is available to the mammary. Adipose TGly is mobilized as nonesterified fatty acids (NEFA) and glycerol (GLY) and reincorporated by liver to TGly for use by mammary tissue. NEFA mobilisation from adipose can be used by the large muscle mass to conserve GLU for mammary use. Liver generates GLU from various precursors that are absorbed from the gut (glucogenic AA) or arise from tissue metabolism (GLY, lactate). Other abbreviations: G6P, glucose 6 phosphate; ∝GP, alpha glycerol phosphate; FACoA, fatty acyl CoA; LPL, lipoprotein lipase.

plasma flow through glands per mL of milk secretion). They estimated that 14.1 g glucose was needed per 100 mL of milk. This compares to 6.2 g of amino acids and 2.7 g triglycerides (Table 4.1). This type of information can be used to make dynamic estimates of precursor need for different milk production levels. The relevance of this is illustrated in section 4.9.

4.5 Energetic efficiency of milk synthesis from precursors

The energetic efficiency of milk synthesis from plasma precursors is high. Estimates for lactating rats and cows are 87% and 86% respectively (Baldwin and Yang, 1974; Pucinski, 1976 as calculated by Baldwin and Miller, 1991). Experimental estimates have not been made using blood precursors relative to milk products for the lactating sow but the theoretical efficiency is similar. We calculated this to be 89% (Table 4.2) using information from Table 4.1 and by assuming an average milk composition of 4.8% lactose, 5.5% protein and 6.8% fat. The theoretical efficiency would be slightly higher if minor constituents of milk were considered (1-2%). Efficiency will also vary with fat output, which is the most variable component among milk nutrients. Residual energy is accounted for by the partition of protein for mammary growth and energy for tissue maintenance. This means that the maintenance energy requirement of the mammary gland is less than 10% of the total.

Table 4.2. Estimation of the energetic efficiency of milk synthesis in the sow mammary gland[1,2]

	Uptake/dl Milk			Output/dl Milk	
Precursor	Mmol	Kcal	Product	Mmol	Kcal
Glucose	78.2	52.5	Lactose	13.3	18.0
Triacylglycerol	2.9	20.9	Fat	7.25	47.4
Amino acids	42.8	24.2	Protein	37.9	21.7
Total	-	97.6		-	87.1

[1] Precursors account for 97% of total uptake as computed from Spincer et al., 1969. Composition of milk assumed to be: Lactose, 4.8%; fat, 6.8%; protein, 5.5%.
[2] Efficiency = (kcal output/kcal uptake) x 100.

4.6 Mammary uptake and metabolism of precursors

4.6.1 Glucose

Glucose is known to be a major substrate for milk synthesis in farm animals (Rook and Thomas, 1983). It is pre-eminent among precursors for lactating sows (Table 4.1). We estimated that 69% of the glucose used by sows is needed to support a milk yield of 9.0 kg/d and that the proportion increases with increases in milk yield (Boyd et al., 1995). Linzell and co-workers (1969) reported that 26% of arterial glucose was removed with each pass through mammary tissue. This compares with an estimate of 31% by Spincer et al., (1969). Absorbed glucose is used to meet maintenance energy needs of the mammary gland; it is a precursor for lactose and glycerol synthesis and is a substrate for fatty acid synthesis. Glucose oxidation must also provide at least 65% of the energy needed to fuel fatty acid synthesis (NADPH) and other processes through ATP.

Linzell and co-workers (1969) used labelled glucose carbon ([U-^{14}C]-glucose) to trace its' metabolic partition within the mammary. They observed that 53% was used for lactose synthesis ($\geq$ 70% is synthesized from glucose) and 34% was oxidized to CO_2. The remainder (13%) was used for the synthesis of glycerol (40% from glucose), fatty acids and amino acids. De novo synthesis of milk fatty acids from glucose is extensive but the net contribution of glucose to amino acid carbon appears to be minor. The proportion of blood derived fatty acids vs gland synthesized fatty acids in milk triglycerides is not yet clear. Glucose accounted for 54% of mammary CO_2. Extensive use of glucose for NADPH generation is anticipated but has not to our knowledge been estimated (Bauman et al., 1970).

4.6.2 Lipids

There is little information on the mammary uptake and metabolism of blood lipids for species other than the cow and goat. In sows, fatty acid uptake occurs largely from the triglyceride fraction since non-esterified fatty acid (NEFA) extraction appears to be negligible (-6%, Spincer et al., 1969). Approximately 16-23% of arterial triglyceride fatty acids (TGFA) were removed by mammary tissue which represents 12% of the total mass (Table 4.1) or about 22% of total energy (Table 4.2). Fatty acids are liberated from circulating triglycerides by lipoprotein lipase activity in mammary capillaries (Barry et al., 1963). The principal fatty acids of blood triglycerides, under normal conditions, are palmitic, stearic, oleic and linoleic acids. The A-V difference for glycerol is small relative to TGFA uptake. Glycerol from glucose and hydrolyzed triglycerides is acted upon by glycerol kinase to form α-glycerol phosphate, which is the backbone of milk triglycerides.

We expect that about 50% of the fatty acids in sow's milk are taken up from blood with the remaining 50% being synthesized de novo in mammary cells. The fatty acid profile of milk triglycerides will reflect predominant fatty acids of body fat when sows are in negative energy balance (mobilizing large amounts of fatty acids) or diet fatty acids if fats are added (Pond and Houpt, 1978). Sow milk does not contain 4-10 carbon fatty acids as observed for ruminants (Jenness, 1974). The shortest chain length fatty acid of quantitative significance is myristic acid (14:0). This is unfortunate since 8 to 10 carbon fatty acids would benefit the metabolically vulnerable newborn pig (Lepine et al., 1989).

4.6.3 Amino Acids

Mammary uptake of amino acids is extraordinary and accounts for more than 90% of whole-body utilisation. The majority are used for milk protein synthesis, however, uptake exceeds the amount secreted in milk. This is especially true for the branched-chain amino acids (leucine, isoleucine, valine) and arginine and suggests that amino acids are being used for other purposes. Mammary absorbed amino acids (AAabs) may serve the following roles:

AAabs=Milk protein+Mammary protein (growth+maintenance)+Milk lipid+Energy

Trottier and co-workers (1997) estimated that 25% of absorbed essential amino acids (49 g) was retained daily. A similar estimate was reported for lactating cows (Guinard et al., 1994). Positive A-V nitrogen and carbon balance suggests that mammary growth (hypertrophic) is occurring during lactation. Positive balance of individual amino acids could also suggest use for other metabolic purposes. They may be used for the synthesis of nutritionally dispensable amino acids (Mepham, 1980; Peeters and Roets, 1987; Clark et al., 1978), functional proteins, energy to fuel lactose synthesis and to provide energy and carbon for fatty acid synthesis (Annison, 1983). Glucogenic amino acids are probably not used for glucose synthesis in mammary tissue since this process appears to be confined to the liver and to some extent the kidney (Scott et al., 1975).

Protein partition to support mammary growth during lactation should not be ignored. Mammary growth during lactation occurs to a variable extent among species. Nursing intensity is a major stimulant in litter bearing species (Tucker, 1987).

Amino acid supply to mammary tissue is a function of arterial concentration, blood flow rate and extraction efficiency (extraction %). Plasma free amino acids constitute the major form available to the mammary gland, however, extraction from erythrocytes has been reported for some amino acids. For this reason, blood is preferable to plasma which can be misleading for some amino acids (Hanigan et al., 1991). Peptide bound amino acids also appear to make contributions to the mammary pool based on information from the goat (Backwell et al., 1996),

Table 4.3. Percent arterial extraction and uptake (A-V) of plasma amino acids and glucose by the mammary glands of lactating sows

	Extraction %[1]		A-V, umol/L[1]	
Amino acid[2]	Linzell[3]	Trottier[3]	Linzell	Trottier
Leucine	30.0	37.0	69.4	64.9
Valine	18.0	23.4	66.6	42.6
Lysine	28.0	53.0	54.0	37.3
Arginine	26.0	34.5	47.1	42.0
Isoleucine	30.0	39.9	43.5	32.8
Threonine	22.0	20.9	31.9	31.4
Phenylalanine	25.0	24.6	26.6	22.0
Histidine	26.0	15.7	26.4	11.5
Methionine	36.0	31.2	12.7	10.2
Tryptophan	-	13.5	-	9.9
Glutamate	37.0	33.4	126.4	75.5
Glucose	26.0	21.0	13.5	19.3

[1] % extraction = [(arterial - venous concentrations) / arterial concentration] 100; A-V is the difference in metabolite concentration in plasma which is interpreted as mammary uptake (see text).

[2] Nutritionally indispensable amino acids except for glutamate.

[3] A - V differences for amino acids and glucose obtained from Linzell et al., (1969). Trottier et al., (1997) used for amino acids and Trottier et al. (1994) used for glucose.

but measurement of peptide uptake is not feasible because reliable and reproducible methodology is lacking (Bequette and Backwell, 1997).

Substantial A-V differences have been observed for all nutritionally indispensable amino acids in the lactating sow (Table 4.3). The extraction rate varied from 18 to 39% in the pioneering studies by Linzell et al., (1969) and Spincer et al., (1969). It ranged from 14 to 53% in a recent report by Trottier and co-workers (1997). The highest extraction percentage and absolute uptake was observed for the nutritionally dispensable amino acid glutamate. This is consistent with the relative abundance of glutamate in the milk (2.62 x lysine).

Figure 4.2 shows that mammary uptake for each nutritionally essential amino acid meets or exceeds the amount secreted in milk. This is not true for every dispensable amino acid as some appear to be secreted in milk to a greater extent than absorbed. This observation is consistent with dairy cattle (Clark et al., 1978) and and early work with pigs (Linzell et al., 1969, calculated by Boyd et al., 1995) and suggests that their synthesis may occur in the gland. Lysine, methionine and

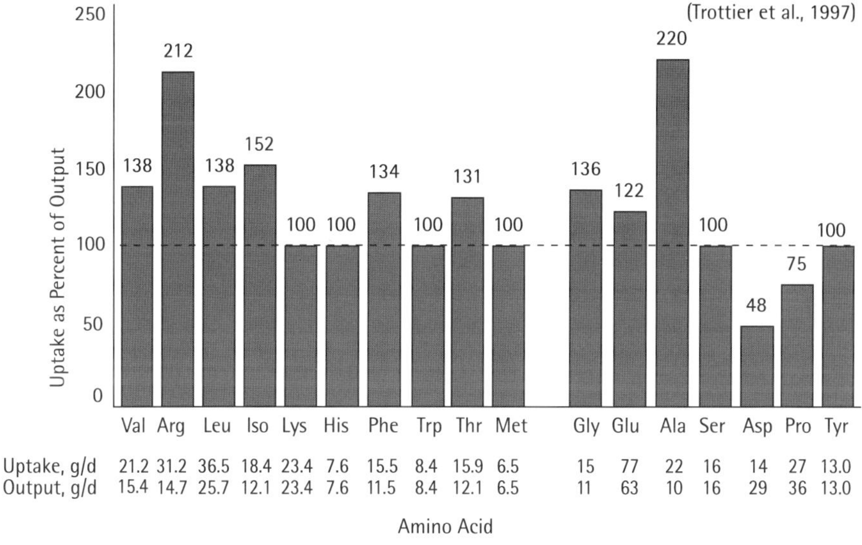

Figure 4.2. Relative uptake of amino acids by sow mammary glands.
Uptake of nutritionally essential and non-essential amino acids were determined using plasma samples (Trottier et al. (1997). Milk output of the amino acids was estimated indirectly by using the reported values for mammary retention which was determined by the authors using daily amino acid uptake minus daily milk amino acid output. The average plasma flow through the mammary during lactation was determined to be 4,275 (± 386) L/d and was based on application of the Fick principle. Perfect balance between uptake and output equals 100%.

histidine appear to be directly transferred into milk. Almost twice as much arginine is absorbed as secreted. Leucine, isoleucine and valine are transported in excess of that needed as milk protein. Arginine and branch-chain amino acids have been shown to contribute energy for metabolism, carbon for milk fat synthesis and carbon and nitrogen for dispensable amino acids in ruminants (Wohlt et al., 1977; Clark et al., 1978; Mepham, 1982). For example, in cow mammary tissue arginine is the precursor for proline. The large retention of glutamate and alanine and large release of aspartate (Trottier et al., 1997) also suggest transamination and conversion to other amino acids.

We used data from Table 4.3 to compute the ratio of amino acid uptake relative to lysine (Table 4.4). This ratio allows us to rank each amino acid for presumed importance to the mammary gland and provides the basis for identifying potentially limiting amino acids in diets (shown later). The amino acid to lysine ratio was also computed for milk protein. The pattern appears to be relatively similar when comparing mammary uptake and milk protein composition but the relative uptakes of leucine, valine, isoleucine and arginine by the mammary are higher than expected from milk amino acid composition. This suggests that the involvement of branched-chain amino acids and arginine in mammary metabolism is

Table 4.4. Comparison of the amino acid pattern using mammary uptake and sow's milk

Amino acid[1]	A-V, g/d[2]	Amino acid to lysine Ratio	
		A-V[3]	Sow Milk[3]
Leucine	36.5	156	114
Valine	21.2	90	78
Lysine	23.4	100	100
Arginine	31.2	133	66
Isoleucine	18.4	79	59
Threonine	15.9	68	59
Phenylalanine	15.5	66	56
Histidine	7.6	32	40
Methionine	6.5	28	28
Tryptophan	8.4	36	19
Glutamate	54.2	232	262

[1] Nutritionally indispensable amino acids except for glutamate.

[2] A - V differences in g/d taken from Trottier et al. (1997).

[3] Ratio of amino acids to lysine with lysine set = 100. Amino acid pattern in sow's milk taken from King et al., (1993).

greater than suggested by the milk pattern. Arginine is of particular interest since the A-V ratio is about twice that observed for milk protein (1.33 vs 0.66). This illustrates the shortcoming of using the milk amino acid pattern as the basis for the ideal pattern for lactation. Tissue growth and metabolic requirements for individual amino acids are not even considered by such an approach.

Hurley and co-workers (1996) used slices of mammary tissue to study the metabolism of leucine, valine and lysine in more detail. Incorporation into protein accounted for 80% of radioactivity for leucine and 82% for valine. Valine appears to be extensively oxidized to carbon dioxide (17%), while leucine contributes to fat synthesis (9%). They did not account for the conversion to other amino acids in the protein fraction. The use of lysine for protein was high (90%) but not exclusive. This emphasizes that the dietary requirement for amino acids involves more than protein synthesis (milk, mammary tissue). Their contribution to the energy requirement and to fat synthesis could be significant when considered collectively. However, it is also not clear whether this aspect of the requirement is obligatory.

A review of the metabolic pathways for milk substrate metabolism and sites of milk synthesis is beyond the scope of this chapter. This information is available in the excellent review by Rook and Thomas (1983).

4.7 Transport mechanisms for mammary uptake of precursors

The mammary gland of a high producing sow must be one of the most active tissues in the body with respect to transport. For example, mammary tissue of a sow that produces 10 kg of milk per day will take up approximately 1410 g glucose/d and 620 g protein/d. This represents about 70% of the glucose utilized by the sow daily (Boyd et al., 1995). Obviously, an efficient system for transport is needed. Our understanding of the mechanisms of glucose, amino acid and triglyceride transport is in its infancy, even in the ruminant where the motive for studying mammary metabolism is more obvious.

4.7.1 Glucose

Six glucose transporters have been identified for facilitative transport across mammalian cell membranes. They are characterized by differences in tissue distribution and hormone sensitivity (Bell et al., 1990). It appears that mammary glands of non-ruminants and ruminants rely mostly on the high capacity GLUT 1 transporter for access to blood glucose (Bell and Bauman, 1997). GLUT 1 transporters are the predominant glucose carriers in rat mammary tissue (Madon et al., 1990; Camps et al., 1994). They increase during development, decrease with bromocryptine-induced decline in prolactin and milk secretion (Fawcett et al., 1992), and decrease upon weaning (Camps et al., 1994). This suggests that the GLUT 1 transporter is under endocrine control. GLUT 4 is present in mammary tissue of virgin rats and is known to be an insulin stimulated transport system in adipose tissue (Camps et al., 1994). However, there is a relative lack of GLUT 4 expression in lactating rat mammary tissue (Flint, 1995).

Our knowledge about glucose transporters and uptake regulation in porcine mammary tissue is modest indeed. Reynolds and Rook (1977) and Holmes et al., (1988) observed that insulin infusion did not enhance glucose use by lactating sow mammary glands. Chronic glucose administration to lactating sows resulted in an increase in milk yield in one report (Reynolds and Rook, 1977), but more acute glucose infusion did not cause a difference in glucose uptake as observed by Holmes et al., (1988). While more research is needed in this area, the weight of evidence suggests that glucose uptake is regulated primarily by intramammary demand which is similar to the ruminant (Bell and Bauman, 1997). Miller (1996) observed an increase in the level of GLUT 1 transcripts in sow mammary tissue from 5 d pre-partum to 2 d post-partum with a further increase by d 14 of lactation (Table 4.5). This corresponded with an increase in milk production and suggests that GLUT 1 gene expression, and perhaps transport activity, in the mammary gland is regulated.

Kensinger and co-workers (1996) did not observe an increase in GLUT 1 gene expression in sow mammary tissue cultured with prolactin, insulin and cortisol, whereas, expression of the milk protein gene β-casein was increased dramatically. While these hormones may not affect GLUT 1 gene expression, they may affect glucose uptake in some manner. Their impact on glucose utilisation is more clear. A 2 to 3 fold increase in glucose use for fat synthesis and oxidation was observed in mammary tissue cultures containing insulin, cortisol and prolactin (Jerry et al., 1989).

Table 4.5. Relationship between levels of GLUT1 transcript (2.8 kb) in porcine mammary tissue and level of milk production[1]

Item	Day of Lactation		
	-5	2	14
GLUT1 mRNA	6.79	13.01	33.85
Milk Yield, kg/day	–	5.5	10.3

[1] Adapted from Miller, 1996.

4.7.2 Amino Acids

Baumrucker (1985) wrote a comprehensive review of the seven amino acid transport systems and those known to occur in mammary tissue. Mammalian amino acid transport systems and the amino acids that they were named for include: ASC (ala, ser, cys), A (ala), L (leu), N (gln, his, asn), Y+ (lys, arg), Anionic (asp, glu) and GLY (gly). There is evidence that all but the Anionic and N system exist in mammary tissue. It is also clear that mammary tissue can derive cysteine through mechanisms involving δ-glutamyl transpeptidase, glutathione and red blood cells (Baumrucker, 1985). We have begun to appreciate the ability of mammary glands to take up blood peptides as a source of amino acids (Bequette and Backwell, 1997), however, the transport mechanism is less clear. Future A-V difference work needs to consider less traditional means by which mammary tissue can obtain amino acids (peptide bound and blood cell as carrier) in order to refine our understanding of amino acid uptake versus output.

4.7.3 Fatty Acids

Fatty acid uptake occurs largely from the triglyceride fraction since percent NEFA extraction appears to be very low (Spincer et al., 1969). Fatty acids are liberated from circulating triglycerides by lipoprotein lipase (LPL) in mammary capillaries (Barry et al., 1963) and then transported as NEFA. There is no question that LPL activity is important since it is increased more than 100 fold in rodent mammary tissue at the time of parturition (McBride and Korn, 1963). The magnitude of LPL change in porcine mammary tissue is not yet known. The rate of mammary synthesis of fatty acids from glucose increases dramatically from 3 d pre-farrow to 4 d post-farrow. Kensinger and co-workers (1982) reported a 93-fold increase in synthesis which coincides with a coordinated increase in the GLUT 1 transporter (Miller, 1996).

4.8 Coordination or competition for milk precursors?

We pose two questions to set the stage for a discussion of how the body allocates nutrients to support the extraordinary demands of lactation. Does the mammary gland compete with other organs and tissues for precursors? What drives milk synthesis; nutrient availability to the mammary gland or mammary metabolic activity (i.e., push - pull mechanism)?

Bauman and Currie (1980) argued that nutrient use is a coordinated process that minimizes the need for competition among tissues. They taught that the partitioning of nutrients involves two types of regulation, homeostasis and homeorhesis. The latter was defined as the 'coordinated changes in metabolism of body tissues necessary to support a physiological state.' This concept helps to explain how nutrient use by tissues is altered to support the changing priorities of pregnancy and lactation.

Perhaps the most obvious example of homeorhesis in domestic animals is the transition from pregnancy to lactation, where extensive changes in the metabolism of maternal organs and tissues occur in late pregnancy. This insures that the mammary gland will be supplied with the nutrients necessary for milk synthesis (Bauman and Currie, 1980). The net effect is to shift nutrient use from adipose storage and fetal growth (anabolic) to a predominantly catabolic disposition. This change was beautifully illustrated by the declining response of adipose tissue to insulin and increasing response to epinephrine in late pregnant and lactating females (Vernon, 1989). These changes cause a shift from energy storage, which is characteristic of pregnancy, to a state in which adipose tissue is more responsive to the energy needs of lactation. The result is less adipose use of glucose and greater availability of NEFA (Figure 4.1). Both are supportive rather than competitive with the mammary gland. While it is clear that body protein is mobilized to support lactation, similar mechanisms have not been illustrated for body protein pools such as skeletal muscle.

The most impressive feature of homeorhetic control is the simultaneous influence on many tissues and organs and its mediation through altered tissue responses to homeostatic signals such as insulin. Hormones such as somatotropin, prolactin and placental lactogen may play predominant roles in mediating changes in tissue response but a simultaneous decline in the level of progesterone may be equally important (Bauman and Currie, 1980). The vast array of changes that may occur are best illustrated by studies with somatotropin and are summarized by Bell and Bauman (1997). The changes in adipose, muscle, liver, pancreas and mammary are shown in Table 4.6.

We believe that milk secretion is driven largely by the metabolic capacity of mammary tissue (i.e., pull mechanism). It is doubtful that increased blood nutrient level drives milk nutrient output (i.e., push mechanism), however a low nutrient concentration limits output if arterial extraction efficiency is unable to fully compensate (Baldwin and Smith, 1983). Peel and co-workers (1982) tested the 'push mechanism' by increasing blood glucose and amino acids through post-ruminal infusion in lactating cows fed adequately balanced diets. They were unable to increase milk or lactose output. Lewis and Speer (1973) illustrated that a single amino acid deficiency could limit milk yield and milk protein output in lactating sows. Bequette and Backwell (1997) reported on the effects of a single amino acid limitation in lactating goats. The deficiency was induced by intra-abomasal infusion of a complete amino acid mixture ± histidine. Deletion of histidine resulted in a decrease in arterial plasma histidine and milk protein output. Interestingly, mammary extraction rate increased at least 4-fold (from about 20 to 95%) and blood flow increased in an effort to maintain histidine uptake when histidine was deleted.

Table 4.6. Effects of Bovine Somatotropin on Glucose Metabolism and Related Processes in Specific Tissues in Lactating Ruminants[1]

Tissue		Process
Mammary	↑	milk synthesis
	↑	lactose synthesis
	↑	glucose uptake
	NC	GLUT 1 mRNA
	↑	blood flow consistent with increase in milk yield
Liver	↑	hepatic gluconeogenesis
	↓	ability of insulin to inhibit gluconeogenesis
Adipose	↓	Lipogenesis
	↓	ability of insulin to stimulate lipogenesis
	↓	glucose uptake
	↓	GLUT4 mRNA
Muscle	↓	glucose uptake
	↑	lactate output
	↓	glucose oxidation (inferred)
	↓	insulin receptor abundance and tyrosine kinase activity[b]
	↓	GLUT4 mRNA
Pancreas	NC	basal or glucose-stimulated secretion of insulin
	NC	basal or insulin/glucose-stimulated secretion of glucagon

[1] Adapted from (Bell and Bauman, 1997). ↑ = increased, ↓ = decreased, NC= no change.
[2] Demonstrated in nonlactating animals and consistent with observations on lactating animals.

Mammary blood flow is probably part of the coordinated response to support the metabolic demand for milk secretion. Bequette and Backwell (1997) cited data that support the concept that blood flow is driven, at least in part, by the mammary requirement for substrates. They observed that frequent milking of unilateral glands (8 times daily for 5 d) resulted in increases in milk yield and that these were associated with similar increases in blood flow to that side of the mammary gland. Blood flow to the contralateral gland (milked once daily) corresponded to the lower milk yield. This suggests that blood flow was regulated locally and in response to metabolic activity of the gland. The mechanism is presently unclear but local regulation appears to be very important (Hartmann et al., 1997).

In summary, the capacity for milk secretion is ultimately determined by the metabolic activity of mammary cells. The number of secretory cells and the amount and activity of cell enymes determine the metabolic ability of mammary tissue. However, maximum rates of milk synthesis depend on a continuous provision of precursors. Substrate concentrations within the secretory cell depend on the level in arterial blood which will ultimately limit enzymatic reactions for milk synthesis when blood flow rate (precursor delivery rate) and extraction efficiency by the gland can no longer compensate for deficiencies. Proper coordination of extra-mammary tissues (eg., adipose, muscle, liver) and food intake occur to provide adequate substrate supply. This summary is consistent with concepts presented in seminal reviews (Rook and Thomas, 1983; Bauman and Currie, 1980; Bauman and Elliot, 1983).

4.9 Dynamics of precursor needs in relation to milk output

This chapter concludes with theoretical estimates of glucose and amino acid (amount and pattern) needs for an elite modern sow. A sow producing 7.5 kg milk/d was also used as a standard for comparison (NRC, 1988). The purpose is to illustrate how improvements in milk secretion alters the requirement for the most critical nutrients. The precursor - milk product relationships in Tables 4.1 and 4.4 were used to derive estimates.

Milk output varies in direct proportion to the number of pigs nursed (Auldist and King, 1995). Sows also differ in the degree to which they express their capacity for milk production. This was illustrated in a recent study with 100 sows (Boyd and Touchette, 1998). Milk production was estimated using the relationship of 4 g milk output / 1 g pig gain. Average yield was predicted to be 10.8 kg/d for the 20 d lactation. However, the top 10 sows produced an average of 13.6 kg milk/d, while the bottom one-third averaged 9.6 kg/d (Figure 4.3). This is a 42% difference in milk secretion. The mammary requirement for nutrients is very different for the two groups.

We estimate that elite sows (13.6 kg milk/d) use 83% of their net energy requirement to support milk production. Mammary uptake of glucose is expected to be 1.96 kg glucose/d which is 76% of the whole body requirement (Table 4.7). The reference sow (7.5 kg milk/d) used 72% and 63% of energy and glucose, respectively to support milk synthesis. Glucose availability is critical to milk synthesis and is a direct function of feed intake (Annison, 1983). Sows that produce more milk require more feed so feeding management is very important. The quantitative requirement for amino acids is also substantial. Almost 95% of the daily lysine requirement would be needed for milk synthesis. This shows that the mammary gland dominates the amount and pattern of amino acids. Milk fat output, for the elite sow, is

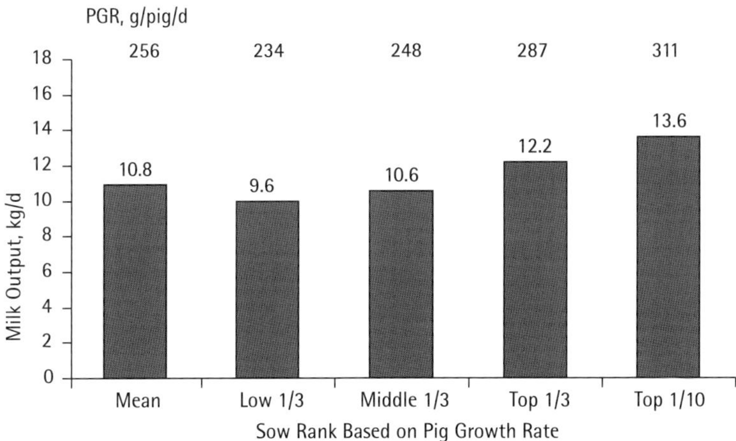

Figure 4.3. Milk production estimates for prolific sows using pig growth rate (PGR) (Boyd and Touchette, 1998).
Milk production was determined indirectly in 100 sows (litters 1-3) by measuring litter weight gain at 5 d intervals. Litters were standardized to 11 pigs each and weaned an average of 10.2 pigs per litter. Milk output was estimated using the relationship of 4 g milk per 1 g pig gain. Average yield was predicted at 10.8 kg/d for the 20 d lactation. The difference among sows in expressed capacity for milk production is illustrated (number on each baris estimate in kg/d).

extraordinary (952 g/d) and may pose an unnecessarily high energetic cost (requiring greater mobilisation from adipose and greater mammary use of glucose). Sow milk appears to be deficient in amino acids relative to energy and this may limit the rate of piglet growth. The lysine: energy ratio is below the requirement for optimum growth of artificially reared neonatal pigs (F. Dunshea, personal communication) and weaned pigs (NRC, 1998). Constraint of mammary fat synthesis after days 3-5 (very young pig benefits from high fat-insulation) may benefit the sow and enhance neonatal growth through increased protein deposition.

The net lysine requirement for sows producing 13.6 kg milk/d is 58 g/d. Adequate levels of other amino acids must be provided and can be estimated by comparing the ratio of mammary uptake for each amino acid to lysine (ideal pattern). The most important contribution of A-V difference data for amino acids is that it becomes the ideal for assessing potential dietary limitations to milk synthesis (Table 4.4). This concept is illustrated by comparing amino acid patterns of two diets to the pattern of mammary uptake (Table 4.8). A percent dietary lysine of 0.95% is typical for the modern lactating sow. Formulating to 0.95% lysine changes the dietary margin for valine, isoleucine and arginine when compared to a 0.60% lysine diet (previously typical). However, apparent deficiencies need to be

Table 4.7. Estimated needs for first limiting nutrients and milk nutrient output for the Elite Modern Sow (13.6 kg milk/d). Compared to a previous standard

Item	Milk Yield kg/d		Milk nutrient output kg/d[5]	
	7.5	13.6[1]		13.6
Net Energy, Mcal/d[2]			Energy, Mcal GE/d	15.5
Maintenance(NEm)	4.5	4.5	Lactose, g/d	612
Milk (NEp)	11.8	21.9	Protein, g/d	762
Glucose, g/d[3]			Fat, g/d	952
Maintenance	620	620	Lysine : Mcal GE	3.68
Mammary Uptake	1058	1960		
Protein, g/d				
Mammary Uptake	465	843		
Net Lysine, g/d[4]				
Maintenance	2.5	2.5		
Milk	32.1	55.5		

[1] Supports 3.48 kg/d litter growth (Boyd and Touchette, 1998).

[2] NEm = 86.6 Mcal/d/$BW^{0.75}$. Assume NE = 0.82 ME and that average body weight (bw) is 195 kg. NEp = 1.92 Mcal ME/kg milk x 0.82.

[3] Glucose use for maintenance = 2.21 mg glucose/minute/kg bw (Linzell et al., 1969). Glucose uptake = 14.1 g/dL milk (see Table 1).

[4] Maintenance lysine = 49 mg/kg $bw^{.75}$; Assumes milk is 5.7% protein, milk protein is 7.5% lysine and that 100% of mammary uptake is secreted in milk.

[5] Composition of milk assumed: Lactose, 4.5%; fat, 7.0%; protein 5.6% and assumed protein is 7.5% lysine. Energy density of milk, 1.14 Mcal gross energy/kg milk per Noblet and Etienne, 1987.

verified through experiments. An apparent arginine deficiency could be misleading because the sow can synthesize it to some extent (NRC, 1998). It is also unclear whether the relative amounts of isoleucine, leucine and valine uptake is obligatory, and whether an apparent deficiency of one might be compensated for by increased extraction or increased use of another branch-chain amino acid.

In summary, comparison of the elite modern sow (13.6 kg milk/d) to a standard of the past (7.5 kg/d) illustrates how an increasing proportion of energy, glucose and amino acids is needed for milk synthesis. The pattern of mammary amino acid uptake is not expected to be very different, but the pattern provided by diets formulated to meet increasing lysine needs undergoes marked changes. For this reason the order of limiting amino acids for diets is expected to change with improvements in milk production.

Table 4.8. Using the mammary pattern of amino acid uptake to identify possible dietary limitations

Amino Acid	Mammary A-V Pattern[1]	Dietary Lysine, %[2,3]	
		0.60	0.95
Lysine	100	100	100
Leucine	156	221	171
Valine	90	97	85
Arginine	133	123	123
Isoleucine	79	79	74
Threonine	68	75	67
Phenylalanine	66	84	73
Histidine	32	59	49
Methionine	28	39	31
Tryptophan	36	21	22

[1] Lysine set = 100. Each amino acid taken up per day set as a ratio to lysine from Table 4.4.
[2] Diets formulated to total lysine level using corn, soybean meal (48% protein) and lysine HCl (0.075% of diet). Ratio of each amino acid to lysine used net digestible values for amino acids (NRC 1998).
[3] 0.60% lysine provides 32 g total lysine/d at 5.30 kg feed/d and supports 1300 g litter growth/d. 0.95% lysine provides 53 g total lysine/d at 5.6 kg feed/d and supports 2500 g litter growth/d.

4.10 References

Aherne, F.X. & I.H. Williams, 1992. Nutrition for optimizing breeding herd performance. Vet. Clinics North America: Food Animal Practice 8:589.

Annison, E.F., 1983. Metabolite utilization by the ruminant mammary gland. In: T.B. Mepham (Ed.), Biochemistry of Lactation, Chap. 13. Elsevier Science Publishers.

Backwell, F.R.C., B.J. Bequette, D. Wilson, J.A. Metcalf, M.F. Franklin, D.E. Beever, G.E. Lobley & J.C. MacRae, 1996. Evidence for the utilization of peptides for milk protein synthesis in the lactating dairy goat in vivo. Am. J. Physiol. 271:R955.

Baldwin, R.L., & N.E. Smith, 1983. Adaptations of metabolism to various conditions: Milk production. In: P.M. Riis (Ed.), Dynamic Biochemistry of Animal Production, Chap. 14. Elsevier Press, New York, NY.

Baldwin, R.L., & P.S. Miller, 1991. Mammary gland development and lactation. In: P.T. Cupps (Ed.), Reproduction in Domestic Animals, Chap 11. Academic Press Inc., New York, NY.

Baldwin, R.L. & Y.T. Yang, 1974. Enzymatic and metabolic changes in the development of lactation. In: B.L. Larson and V.R. Smith (Ed.), Lactation: A Comprehensive Treatise. Vol. II. p. 349. Academic Press, New York.

Barry, J.M., W. Bartley, J.L. Linzell & D.S. Robinson, 1963. The uptake from the blood of triglyceride fatty acids of chylomicra and low-density lipoproteins by the mammary gland of the goat. Biochem. J. 89:6.
Bauman, D.E., R.E. Brown & C.L.Davis, 1970. Pathways of fatty acid synthesis and reducing equivalent generation in mammary gland of rat, sow and cow. Arch. Biochem. Biophys. 140:237.
Bauman, D.E. & W.B. Currie, 1980. Partitioning of nutrients during pregnancy and lactation: A review of mechanisms involving homeostasis and homeorhesis. J. Dairy Sci. 63:1514.
Bauman, D.E. & J.M. Elliot, 1983. Control of nutrient partitioning in lactating ruminants. In: T.B. Mepham (Ed.), Biochemistry of lactation, Elsevier Science Publishers.
Baumrucker, C.R., 1985. Amino acid transport systems in bovine mammary tissue. J. Dairy Sci. 68:2436.
Bell, A.W. & D.E. Bauman, 1997. Adaptations of glucose metabolism during pregnancy and lactation. J. Mammary Biol. and Neoplasia. 2:265.
Bell, G.I., T. Kayano, J.B. Buse, C.F. Burant, J.Takeda, D. Lin, D. Fukumoto & S. Seino, 1990. Molecular biology of mammalian glucose transporters. Diabetes Care 13:198.
Bequette, B.J. & F.R.C. Backwell, 1997. Amino acid supply and metabolism by the ruminant mammary gland. Proc. Nutr. Soc. 56:593.
Boyd, R.D. & K.J. Touchette, 1997. Current concepts in feeding prolific sows. Proc. 13th annual North Carolina swine nutrition conference, pp. 55.
Boyd, R.D. & K.J. Touchette, 1998. Milk production curves for Camborough 22 sows estimated using piglet growth rate. PIC USA Technical Memo 171.
Boyd, R.D., R.S. Kensinger, R.J. Harrell & D.E. Bauman, 1995. Nutrient uptake and endocrine regulation of milk synthesis by mammary tissue of lactating sows. In: H.A. Tucker, J.E. Pettigrew and D. Petitclerc (Ed.), Supply of Precursors and Synthesis of Milk Components in Normal, Extreme and Disease States. Proc. Second Int. Workshop on the Biology of Lactation in Farm Animals.
Boyd, R.D., B.D. Moser, E.R. Peo, Jr. & A.J. Lewis, 1981. Effect of tallow and choline chloride addition to the diet of sows on milk composition, milk yield and preweaning pig performance. J. Anim. Sci. 54:1
Burrin, D.G., R.J. Shulman, R.J. Reeds, T.A. Davis & K.R. Gravitt, 1992. Porcine colostrum and milk stimulate visceral organ and skeletal muscle protein synthesis in neonatal pigs. J. Nutr. 122:1205.
Camps, M., S. Vilaro, X. Testar, M. Palaci & A. Zorzano, 1994. High and polarized expression of GLUT 1 glucose transporters in epithelial cells from mammary gland: Acute down-regulation of GLUT 1 carrier by weaning. Endocrinol. 134:924.
Clark, J.H., H.R. Spires & C.L. Davis, 1978. Uptake and metabolism of nitrogenous components by the lactating mammary gland. Fed. Proc. 37:1233.
Davis, S.R. & R. Bickerstaffe, 1978. Mammary glucose uptake in the lactating ewe and the use of methionine arteriovenous difference for the calculation of mammary blood flow. Aust. J. Bio. Sci. 31:133.
Fawcett, H.A.C., S.A. Baldwin & D.J. Flint, 1992. Hormonal regulation of the glucose transporter: Glut1 in the lactating rat mammary gland. Biochem. Soc. Trans. 20:17S.
Flint, D.J., 1995. Hormonal regulation of uptake and metabolism of milk precursors in normal lactating mammary gland. In: H.A. Tucker, J.E. Pettigrew and D. Petitclerc (Ed.), Supply of Precursors and Synthesis of Milk Components in Normal, Extreme and Disease States. Proc. Second Int. Workshop on the Biology of Lactation in Farm Animals.
Guinard, J., H. Rulquin & V. Verite, 1994. Effect of graded levels of duodenal infusions of casein on mammary uptake in lactating cows. I. Major nutrients. J. Dairy Sci. 77:2221.

Hanigan, M.D., C.C. Calvert, E.J. DePeters, B.L. Reiss & R.L. Baldwin, 1991. Whole blood and plasma amino acid uptakes by lactating bovine mammary glands. J. Dairy Sci. 74:2484.

Harrell, R.J., M.J. Thomas & R.D. Boyd. 1993. Limitations of sow milk yield on baby pig growth. Proc. Cornell Nutr. Conf., p. 156.

Hartmann, P.E. & M.A. Holmes, 1989. Sow lactation. In: J.L. Barnett and D.P. Hennessy (Ed.), Manipulating Pig Production II. Proc. Australasian Pig Sci. Assoc., Vol. 2, p. 72.

Hartmann, P.E., N.A. Smith, M.J. Thompson, C.M. Wakeford, P.G. Arthur, 1997. The lactation cycle in the sow: physiological and management contradictions. Livestock Prod. Sci. 50:75.

Head, R.H., N.W. Bruce & I.H. Williams, 1991. More cells might lead to more milk. In: E.S. Batterham (Ed.), Manipulating Pig Production III. Proc. Australasian Pig Sci. Assoc., Vol. 3, p. 76. (Abstr.).

Holmes, M.A., C. Maughan, A. Paterson, G. Bryant-Greenwood, G. Rice & P.E. Hartmann, 1988. The uptake of glucose by the mammary glands of lactating sows. Proc. Nutr. Soc. Aust. 13:113.

Hurley, W.L., R.A. Easter & J.M. Bryson, 1996. Amino acid utilization by porcine mammary tissue: Branched-chain amino acids. National Pork Producers Research Investment Report, USA, p.477.

Jenness, R., 1974. The composition of milk. In: B.L. Larson and V.R. Smith (Ed.), Lactation: A Comprehensive Treatise. Vol. III, p. 3. Academic Press, New York, New York.

Jenness, R., 1985. Biochemical and nutritional aspects of milk and colostrum. In: B.L. Larson (Ed.), Lactation. p.164, Iowa State Univ. Press, Ames Iowa.

Jerry, D.J., R.K. Stover & R.S. Kensinger. 1989. Quantitation of prolactin-dependent responses in porcine mammary explants. J. Anim. Sci. 67:1013.

Kensinger, R.S., R.J. Collier, F.W. Bazer, C.A. Ducsay & H.N. Becker, 1982. Nucleic acid, metabolic and histological changes in gilt mammary tissue during pregnancy and lactogenesis. J. Anim. Sci. 54:1297.

Kensinger, R.S., J. Rittenhouse Pruss & L.C. Griel Jr., 1996. Prolactin increases β-casein but not GLUT 1 gene expression in porcine mammary tissue. FASEB J. 10:A728 (Abstr.)

King, R.H., C.J. Rayner & M. Kerr, 1993. A note on the amino acid composition of sow's milk. Anim. Prod. 37:500.

Klobasa, F., E. Werhahn & J.E. Butler, 1987. Composition of sow milk during lactation. J. Anim. Sci. 64:1458.

Lepine, A.J., R.D. Boyd, J.A. Welch & K.R. Roneker, 1989. Effect of colostrum intake or medium-chain triglyceride supplementation on plasma glucose, non-esterified fatty acids and survival of neonatal pigs. J. Anim. Sci. 67:983.

Lewis, A.J. & V.C. Speer, 1973. Lysine requirement of the lactating sow. J. Anim. Sci. 37:104.

Linzell, J.L., 1974. Mammary blood flow and methods of identifying and measuring precursors of milk. In: B.L. Larson and V.R. Smith (Eds.), Lactation. Academic Press, New York, NY, Vol I p. 143.

Linzell, J.L. & E.F. Annison, 1975. Methods of measuring the utilization of metabolites absorbed from the alimentary tract. In: I.W. McDonald and ACI Warner (Eds.), Digestion. and Metababolism in the Ruminant. Univ. of New England Pub. Unit, Armidale, Australia, p. 306.

Linzell, J.L., T.B. Mepham, E.F. Annison & C.E. West, 1967. Mammary metabolism in the lactating sow. Biochem. J. 103:42DP (Abstr).

Linzell, J.L., T.B. Mepham, E.F.Annison & C.E.West, 1969. Mammary metabolism in lactating sows: arteriovenous differences of milk precursors and the mammary metabolism of [^{14}C]glucose and [^{14}C]acetate. Br. J. Nutr. 23:319.

Madon, R.J., S. Martin, A. Davies, H.A.C. Fawcett, D.J. Flint & S.A. Baldwin, 1990. Identification and characterization of glucose transport proteins in plasma membrane and Golgi vesicle enriched fractions prepared from lactating rat mammary gland. Biochem. J. 272:99.
Mahan, D.C. & A.J. Lepine, 1991. Effect of pig weaning weight and associated feeding programs on subsequent performance to 105 kilograms body weight. J. Anim. Sci. 69:13.
McBride, O.W. & E.D. Korn, 1963. The lipoprotein lipase of mammary gland and the correlation of its activity to lactation. J. Lipid Res. 4:17.
Mepham, T.B., 1980. Amino acid utilization by the lactating mammary gland. J. Dairy Sci. 65:287.
Miller, H.M., 1996. Aspects of nutrition and metabolism in the periparturient sow. Ph D Dissertation, Univ. Alberta, Alberta Canada.
Newsholme, E.A., & A.R. Leech. 1983. Biochemistry for the medical sciences. John Wiley & Sons Ltd., New York, New York.
Nielson, T.T., N.L. Trottier, C. Bellaver, H.H. Stein & R.A. Easter, 1997. Effect of litter size on mammary gland amino acid uptake in lactating sows. Livest. Prod. Sci. 50:167 (Abstr).
Noblet, J. & M. Etienne, 1987. Metabolic utilization of energy and maintenance requirements in lactating sows. J. Anim. Sci. 67:774.
Noblet, J., & M. Etienne, 1989. Estimation of sow milk nutrient output. J. Anim. Sci. 67:3352.
NRC., 1998. Nutrient Requirements of Swine (10th Revised Edition). National Academy Press, Washington, DC. USA, In Press.
Pan, Y., P.K . Bender, R.M. Akers & K.E. Webb, 1996. Methionine containing peptides can be used as methionine sources for protein accretion in cultured C_2C_{12} and MAC-T cells. J. Nutr. 126:232.
Peel, C.J., T.J. Fronk, D.E. Bauman & R.C. Gorewit, 1982. Lactational response to exogenous growth hormone and abomasal infusion of a glucose-sodium caseinate mixture in high yielding dairy cows. J. Nutr. 112:1770.
Peeters, G. & E. Roets, 1987. Amino acids as precursors of milk proteins. Ann. Med. Vet. 131:169.
Pluske, J.R., I.H. Williams & F.X. Aherne, 1995. Nutrition of the neonatal pig. In: M.A. Varley (Ed.), The Neonatal Pig: Development and Survival, p. 187. CAB International, Wallingford, Oxon UK.
Pond, W.G. & K.A. Houpt, 1978. Lactation and the mammary gland. In Biology of the Pig, p. 181-191. Comstock Publishing Assoc., Ithaca NY.
Pucinski, T., 1976. A dynamic simulation model of rat metabolism. Ph D. thesis. Univ. California, Davis.
Reynolds, L. & J.A.F. Rook, 1977. Intravenous infusion of glucose and insulin in relation to milk secretion in the sow. Brit. J. Nutr. 37:45.
Rook, J.A.F. & P.C. Thomas, 1983. Milk secretion and its nutritional regulation. In: J.A.F. Rook and P.C. Thomas (Ed.), Nutritional Physiology of Farm Animals, p. 314. Longman Inc., New York, New York.
Scott, R.A., D.E. Bauman & J.H. Clark, 1975. Cellular gluconeogenesis by the lactating bovine mammary gland. J. Dairy Sci. 59:50.
Seerley, R.W., & D.R. Poole, 1974. Effect of prolonged fasting on carcass composition and blood fatty acids and glucose of neonatal swine. J. Nutr. 104:210.
Spincer, J., & J.A.F. Rook, 1971. The metabolism of [U-^{14}C]glucose, [1-^{14}C]palmitic acid and [1-^{14}C]stearic acid by the lactating mammary gland of the sow. J. Dairy Res. 38:315.
Spincer, J., J.A.F. Rook & K.G. Towers, 1969. The uptake of plasma constituents by the mammary gland of the sow. Biochem. J. 111:727.

Trottier, N.L., C.F. Shipley & R.A. Easter, 1997. Plasma amino acid uptake by the mammary gland of the lactating sow. J. Anim. Sci. 75:1266.
Trottier, N.L., C.F. Shipley & R.A. Easter, 1994. Arteriovenous differences for amino acids, urea nitrogen, ammonia and glucose across the mammary gland of the lactating sow. J. Anim. Sci. 72 (Suppl. 1):332 (Abstr.).
Trottier, N.L., C.F. Shipley & R.A. Easter, 1995. A technique for venous cannulation of the mammary gland system in the lactating sow. J. Anim. Sci. 73:1390.
Tucker, H.A. 1987. Quantitative estimates of mammary growth during various physiological states: A review. J. Dairy Sci. 70:1958.
van Kempen, G.J.M., C. Geerse, M.W.A. Verstegen & J. Mesu, 1985. Effect of feeding level on milk production of sows during four weeks of lactation. Netherlands J. Agric. Sci. 33:23.
Vernon, R.G., 1989. Endocrine control of metabolic adaptation during lactation. Proc. Nutr. Soc. 48:23.
Vernon, R.G. & C.M. Pond, 1997. Adaptations of maternal adipose tissue to lactation. J. Mammary Biol. and Neoplasia 2:231.
Wang, S., K.E. Webb & R.M. Akers, 1996. Peptide bound methionine can be a source of methionine for the synthesis of secreted proteins by mammary tissue explants from lactating mice. J. Nutr. 128:1662.
Webb, K.E. Jr., D.B. Dirienzo & J.C. Mathews, 1993. Recent developments in gastrointestinal absorption and tissue utilization of peptides. J. Dairy Sci. 76:351.
Williams, I.H., 1976. Nutrition of the young pig in relation to body composition. Ph D thesis, University of Melbourne, Melbourne Australia.
Wohlt, J.E., J.H. Clark, R.G. Derrig & C.L. Davis, 1977. Valine, leucine and isoleucine metabolism by lactating bovine mammary tissue. J. Dairy Sci. 60:1875.
Wu, G. & D.A. Knabe, 1995. Free and protein-bound amino acids in sow's colostrum and milk. J. Nutr. 124:415.

5 Genetic influences on milk quantity

D.D.S. Mackenzie and D.K. Revell

5.1 Introduction

Common lore suggests that certain breeds of pig produce more milk than others and this is assumed to be based on a genetic superiority for milk production. There is, however, very little quantitative information on the genetic basis for variation in milk yield in the sow. This is far from unusual in that it is only in a limited number of species used for dairying, predominantly ruminants, that there are sufficient data on production to allow sound inferences to be made about their genetic merit for milk yield. The lack of data in the sow is, in part, because physiological and logistical factors make it difficult to obtain direct estimates of milk production.

Consideration of the well established variation in lactational capacity between different breeds of cattle allows one to envisage genetically-based variation in both milk yield and composition in the sow. Of even greater importance, the development of dairy breeds of cattle illustrates quite dramatically the plasticity of the mammal to respond to environmental challenges. It is probable that the lactational ability of the progenitor of modern dairy cattle was no more than that required to nourish a single calf. Artificial selection for high milk production represented a change in the environment that favoured the survival of certain genotypes so that now the milk production of individual cows is far in excess of the requirements of the young. More importantly, the response to selection in the cow is such that it encourages belief in a similar potential in swine. This is a belief of practical relevance since it is apparent that milk production by the sow limits the growth of the piglet so that the weight of a piglet at weaning may be only 50 - 60% of its potential (Hodge, 1974; Harrell *et al.*, 1993).

An important difference exists between farmed dairy animals and those that suckle their offspring throughout their lactation. In the case of dairy animals, milk removal from the mammary gland is normally more complete, through the use of either machine or hand-milking methods, than with suckled mothers. Incomplete milk removal is probably common with newborn offspring during early lactation in that the capacity of the offspring to remove milk would be expected to be below the mother's potential to produce it. Retained milk triggers feedback mechanisms that operate to reduce milk yield, an effect that can be seen over the entire lactation (cf. Peaker, 1995). Hence, with suckling animals, this down-regulation in early lactation nullifies the expression of the full genetic potential for total lactation milk production. This may be particularly important in the sow where individual piglets usually feed from the same teat (Hartmann *et al.* 1995). This aspect will be considered in more detail later, as it is likely to have profound effects on our ability to select sows that possess a higher genetic potential for milk output.

This chapter reviews the genetics of milk production in the sow but, because of a lack of specific data, the major emphasis is placed on discussing how putative genetic variation in milk production might be identified and exploited to increase the productivity of the pig industry.

5.2 Genotype and milk production in the sow

There is a wealth of data on milk yield, or estimates of milk yield based on piglet (litter) growth rates but differences in experimental design, nutrition, litter size and other environmental factors frequently confound genetic effects and very few studies have attempted to separate the genetic from the environmental effects. In the absence of specific estimates, comparisons of production measured under uniform conditions provide the best means of comparing the genetic merit of breeds or groups of individuals. On this understanding Figure 5.1 was compiled from estimates of milk production reported in the literature. Excluded from Figure 5.1 are data obtained under conditions where milk output was clearly below potential such as those from sows fed low-quality diets or suckling small litters. Diet composition was not always available for the earlier work quoted in Figure 5.1, but the more recent data presented were obtained from sows fed a lactation diet containing at least 16.0% crude protein. Litter sizes of the suckling sows presented in Figure 5.1 were at least 8 pigs per litter. Estimates of milk yield based on piglet growth rates were not used in Figure 5.1, given the potential variation between genotypes in the efficiency of converting milk to piglet weight gain. All the data chosen were from experiments where measurements of milk yield were obtained by machine milking or by isotope dilution.

From an inspection of Figure 5.1, it is apparent that the rate of gain in milk yield over the past 2-3 decades is remarkable. The modern sows clearly outperform any of the earlier sows to such an extent that primiparous sows now produce more milk than mature sows from two decades ago. Comparison of the data presented by Elsley in 1971 with those reported in the 1990s, and depicted by the shaded portion of Figure 5.1, indicates that daily milk yield has increased by approximately 3 kg. This represents an annual increase in the daily milk production of approximately 100 g or 1-2% per year.

The different breeds depicted in Figure 5.1 are not represented evenly across time from two or more decades ago until the present, which means that some of the increases in milk production shown may be attributed to a predominance of higher producing breeds in the later years. The 'white breeds' (e.g., Large White and Landrace), however, are, represented across all periods, and do show a marked increase in milk yield over the past two decades.

It is instructive to compare this estimate of genetic improvement in sow milk yield with increases attained in the dairy cow. Rates of gain of up to 2.0% per annum have been predicted for artificially bred cows sired by proven bulls (Robertson and Rendel, 1950) while increases in yield of 1.5 - 1.7% per annum have been reported from controlled experiments (Hickman, 1971; Legates and Myers, 1988) and somewhat smaller gains have been achieved in commercial practice (Van Tassell and Van Vleck, 1991). Despite the lack of a direct selection procedure for milk production in sows, and despite sows suckling for the duration of lactation rather than being machine- or hand-milked, the apparent rate of gain in milk output appears comparable to that obtained with dairy cows where breeding schemes have been developed specifically to enhance milk production. Two explanations may be advanced for this rather surprising result. Possibly, given that our calculations are based on phenotypic data, we have overestimated the rate of genetic gain because the environmental conditions (such as nutrition, housing and disease status) in the more recent experiments were better than those under which the experiments were conducted two or more decades ago. Alternatively, as a result of the various selection programmes used in pig breeding over the past decades, indirect selection for milk output, as outlined in Section 5.5, has been more effective than anticipated. Data currently available do not permit a ready resolution of the issue.

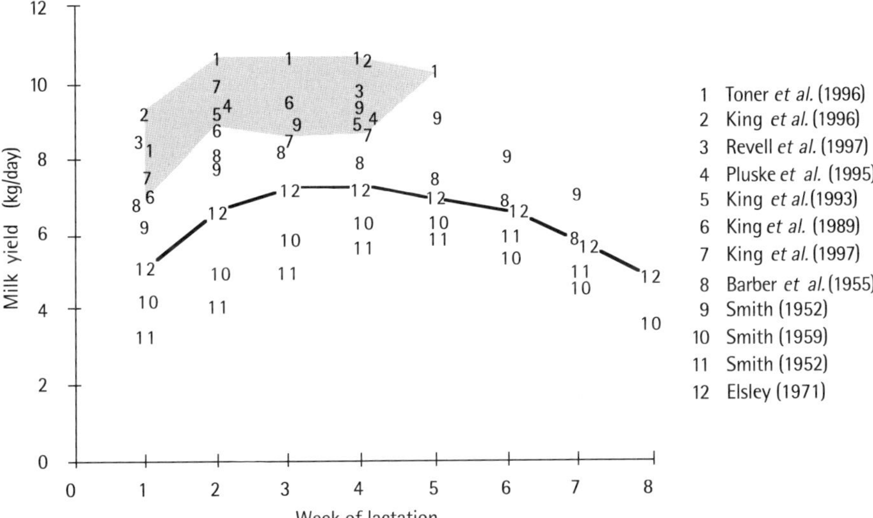

Figure 5.1. A comparison of milk yield recorded in the literature from 1952 to 1997. The shaded region represents milk yield obtained from gilts or sows during the 1990s. The line joining the points from reference number 12 is that compiled by Elsley (1971) and is probably the best set of data to reflect milk yield of the 1960s.

The estimated 1-2% annual gain for the sow is for the improvement in milk yield only, as no account has been made for possible changes in milk composition. However, there is no evidence that the composition of sow's milk has changed much over the past two to three decades. For example, milk protein content, and the responses of milk protein to increasing dietary crude protein, are almost identical in the 1990s (King *et al.*, 1993) as they were in the 1960s (Holden *et al.*, 1968). Over the wide range in dietary crude protein covered in these studies (from 6 to 24%) the concentration of milk protein did not vary outside the narrow range of 5.0 to 5.9%.

5.3 The biological basis for genetic variation in milk production

It is of interest to reflect on the biological processes that might change in response to a selection programme that alters milk production. Metabolic adaptations of the lactating sow have been discussed by Boyd *et al.* (1995) so comments will be confined to the potential for changing milk yield and composition, the amount and activity of the secretory tissue and the control of secretion.

5.3.1 Milk synthesis and secretion

A comparison of the composition and yield of milk across species is evocative. It is clear that there is tremendous variation in milk composition across species as exemplified by the differences between milk from human beings, pigs, cows, seals and rabbits. Over a range of mammals the concentration of fat varies 25 fold, protein by 15 fold and lactose is barely detectable or absent in some milks (Jenness, 1974; Oftedal, 1984). There is also variation within species and although it is best demonstrated in the bovine there are sufficient data to suggest that genetically based variation in composition is present in other species as well. Given the appropriate selection pressure it should be possible to change the composition of sow's milk.

The nature of the response will be determined by the relationship between milk yield and yield of the solids components. Milk yield is determined primarily by the volume of water that accompanies the solutes, i.e., ions and other solids components (cf. Peaker, 1977, 1978). The glandular epithelium acts as a semipermeable membrane restricting the movement of most solutes but allowing the passive movement of water to maintain similar osmotic pressures on both sides of the epithelium. Thus the osmotic pressure of the milk is similar to that of blood and other body fluids and as a consequence varies within very narrow limits. The major ions in the milk, such as sodium, potassium and chloride, are also maintained at constant concentrations by specific, albeit poorly understood, mechanisms. The osmotic pressure exerted by the other solutes is equal to that of the milk less that exerted by the ions. In those species that secrete it, lactose, a solute of relatively small molecular weight, is produced in substantial amounts and represents the major osmole in milk. The concentration of lactose varies little because the total osmotic pressure of the milk is constant and the concentration of the ionic solutes is held constant. Within a species the concentration of lactose is the least variable of the three major solids components, lactose, protein and fat. Coefficients of variation for lactose concentration in bovine milk from healthy udders at peak lactation usually do not exceed 5%. There is little variation between individuals and even between breeds of cow. Extrapolating to the sow, it is expected that the lactose concentration will remain unchanged in response to selection for increased milk or solids yield.

As a consequence of the relationship between the water, ions and lactose, the amount of lactose produced determines the volume of milk produced. Thus a 10% increase in lactose yield will induce a 10% increase in milk yield. Selection for milk yield means selection for an increase in lactose yield. Therefore, the concentrations of protein and fat are dependent on what happens to the yields of these components. If their yields are unchanged while that of lactose increases, then their concentrations will fall. In other words, changes in fat and protein concentrations reflect changes in their yield relative to that of lactose. Furthermore, there are positive genetic correlations between milk yield and yields of both protein and fat in dairy cattle (Touchberry, 1974) which suggest that the synthesis and secretion of lactose and protein, and lactose and fat are co-ordinated. Nevertheless there is some independence especially for the synthesis of fat in that the correlations are less than unity. Thus estimates of the correlations between protein and milk yield vary, between 0.82 and 0.93, and those for fat and milk yield, between 0.66 and 0.87. This is also reflected by the relative size of the coefficients of variation for the concentration of protein and fat in bovine milk from cows in mid lactation which are often greater than 10% and 15%, respectively. Similar relationships might be expected in the sow so that it should be possible to increase the yields of lactose, protein and fat independently but the greatest progress would probably be made by increasing all three together.

It is well established that in dairy cows there is a negative genetic correlation between milk yield and concentration of milk protein or milk fat while there is a positive relationship between the yield of fat or protein and their concentrations in the milk (Touchberry, 1974). Consequently, on the one hand, selection for milk yield alone results in concomitant increases in protein and fat yield but the increases are less than that of milk yield and the concentration of fat and protein decreases. These changes reflect an increase in synthesis of all three of the solids components but a relatively greater increase in the synthesis of lactose compared to that of fat and protein. On the other hand, selection for fat yield increases both fat concentration and milk yield but the increase in milk yield is more modest than that achieved by selecting for milk yield alone. Protein concentration and protein yield are also increased. In this case increases in fat and protein yield have been greater than that of lactose yield reflecting a relative diversion of gluconeogenic precursors away from lactose synthesis.

It has been suggested that the protein concentration in sow's milk is too low relative to the fat concentration to support maximum growth of the piglet. Perhaps this reflects more spartan living conditions of ancient pigs so that a supply of energy to maintain body temperature of the piglet was more important than maximising lean body growth. Changing the proportion of fat to protein may be possible but may occur only gradually if the positive genetic correlation between the yields of fat and protein observed in the cow also occurs in the sow.

5.3.2 Amount and activity of mammary tissue

Reliable estimates of the volumes of milk produced by a range of species are difficult to obtain but milk yield and mammary weight scale approximately to body weight raised to the power of 0.75, such that milk volume per unit of mammary gland tissue is remarkably constant across species (Hanwell and Peaker, 1977). On this basis there would appear to be more scope for changing milk composition than genetically increasing milk volume if body weight and hence mammary weight are held constant. Furthermore, there are several-fold differences in the energy content of milk across species (Oftedal, 1984). Nonetheless selection for milk production in the dairy cow has produced an udder that is larger than expected on a cross species basis. Indeed an increase in udder size may account for all the increase in milk production of the cow since it is not clear whether there has been any increase in activity per unit of mammary gland tissue (Hanwell and Peaker, 1977). Thus it is uncertain whether selection for an increased yield of milk energy will be achieved by increasing the amount or activity of the mammary gland of the sow.

5.3.3 Genetic variation in the control of milk secretion

Rather than select sows directly on the basis of milk yield it might be possible in future to select animals on how they control the rate of milk secretion. If it is accepted that milk secretion per unit weight of tissue is relatively constant it follows that the amount of mammary gland tissue present will largely determine the amount of milk produced. In most species, including the pig, a large proportion of the secretory tissue is developed during pregnancy so that at parturition the dam probably has the potential to produce more milk than is required by the young. Milk production and nutrient requirements will be brought into balance probably by the operation of an autocrine mechanism controlling production at the glandular level (Wilde *et al.* 1995; Hartmann *et al.* 1995). This is a very parsimonious system in that the young are fed adequately and the dam wastes no energy in producing excess milk. It is easy to envisage that such a mechanism will be of particular importance in the pig where each piglet tends to suck the same gland at each feed and local regulation of milk supply would have significant advantages. The downside, however, is that although production increases as the young grow, the full potential of the dam may not always be realised. By the time the demand of the piglet has reached the initial potential of the gland, production by the gland may have been irreversibly down-regulated.

Identification of sows which are better able to regain the functionality of the tissue down-regulated during early lactation might lead to improved litter growth rates. Although a much greater understanding of the mechanisms of autocrine control is required before this can be used, it nevertheless does hold considerable promise for the future. For example selection of sows might be based on the concentration of the feedback inhibitor of lactation or some related parameter.

5.4 Identification of animals of superior genetic merit for milk production

The traditional approach to assessing the genetic merit of an animal for a particular trait is to measure the phenotypic expression of the trait itself. This has the major advantage that the contribution of all the genes has been integrated during the development of the animal. For many traits, however, the phenotypic expression is often strongly influenced by environmental factors and the actual genotype of the animal remains obscure. In animal improvement programmes this imprecision in assessing the genetic merit of the individual is circumvented by using statistical techniques to plan the breeding of relatively large populations of animals.

A further disadvantage of using measures of the phenotype for breeding is that the expression of some traits is restricted to certain members of the population. Thus milk production is expressed only by females after a pregnancy. In dairy cattle breeding this has led to the progeny test for bulls so that, ironically, the genetic merit of the bull for milk production is generally much more accurately known than that for the cow. A progeny test does, however, take time and consequently bulls are generally 5 - 6 years of age while the cow is generally 2.5 - 3 years of age before the animals of superior genetic merit are identified. Thus mating for producing the next generation of parents is delayed for a significant time after the minimal breeding age for both sexes. This means generation intervals in dairy cattle breeding programmes are longer than biologically necessary.

These disadvantages will also be present, if not in the same magnitude, in any scheme to improve milk production in sows by selecting on the basis of milk production data. Although the generation time for pigs is lower than that for cattle, the need for gilts to be maintained in the breeding herd for at least one cycle, and fed appropriately during pregnancy and lactation, makes phenotypic assessment of milk yield a costly exercise.

5.4.1 Measurement of milk yield

There are considerable practical difficulties in obtaining the requisite data on milk yield and composition in the sow. Perhaps the most significant difficulties are encountered in obtaining reliable estimates of milk output and of the true potential milk yield. Estimating milk output from piglet (litter) growth rate relies on an accurate figure for the conversion of milk to piglet weight gain. This method may be suitable within a single experiment, but it is fraught with potential errors (Lewis *et al.*, 1978), and can vary significantly between sows and between stages of lactation within an experiment (D.K. Revell and J.R. Pluske, unpublished data). An alternative method is the isotope dilution method (Pettigrew *et al.*, 1987), but adopting this technique on a large scale in breeding programmes would be cost-prohibitive.

The practical difficulty in determining a sow's potential milk yield arises because the demand of the piglets during early lactation has not reached its peak (see Boyd *et al.*, 1995). If milk is not completely removed from the gland, the autocrine mechanism probably inhibits milk synthesis. An experimental method to minimise the extent of down-regulation of milk synthesis due to incomplete milk removal early in lactation is to replace newborn piglets with older piglets that remove more milk during each drinking bout (e.g. Head and Williams, 1995; King *et al.*, 1997). The resultant milk yield should be closer to the genetic potential of the sow, but the practical problems of cross-fostering older piglets onto newly farrowed sows in a large scale breeding programme limit the usefulness of this technique.

The disadvantages of traditional breeding programmes such as those used with dairy cattle, and the practical problems associated with measuring milk yield of sows, means that alternative systems should be explored for their possible application in pig breeding.

5.4.2 Gene mapping

It is well accepted that a production variable such as milk yield is controlled by a number of genes. Animal breeders base much of their work on the so-called infinitesimal model in which a very large number of genes are postulated, each having a small effect. The success of the animal breeders in the application of this concept in breeding programmes testifies to its soundness. Nevertheless it is generally accepted that variation is due to a finite number of genes with variable effects; those with the largest effect are referred to as quantitative trait loci (QTL). There is controversy over the number of these major genes that would be necessary to account for continuous characteristics that behave as expected for the infinitesimal model (Mackay, 1995). Furthermore, how the expression of any individual gene contributes to milk production remains largely unknown. In a sense, most if not all of the genetic constitution of a lactating animal contributes to her ability to produce a certain volume of milk of a unique composition.

Considerable effort is being exerted to identify major genes by using gene mapping techniques in dairy cattle. Once identified, classical animal breeding techniques will be applied to bring together as many of the most desirable genes as possible in individual animals. This, in itself, is not a trivial task as parents will have a combination of desirable and less desirable genes. Moreover it may even be that the weighting of individual genes will vary depending upon the combination of other genes present in the animal (Haley, 1995).

Theoretically, validated QTL would be extremely useful in the pig industry. They would allow the selection for breeding of both sows and boars of high genetic merit for milk production before puberty without having to measure milk yield. It is extremely unlikely, however, that suitable indicators will be available in the medium term. Moreover, to identify and verify suitable parameters would require independent data on milk production from a large number of sows, which is not conceivable at this time.

5.4.3 Phenotypic indicator traits

Another approach is to identify markers or phenotypic indicator traits (PITs) that are expressed in animals of both sexes before puberty and that are highly correlated with genetic merit for milk production (Meuwissen and Van Arendonk, 1992). In principle these could be anything from sequences of DNA in the genome through a myriad of parameters reflecting the expression of the genes, including the concentration of hormones, metabolites, activities of enzymes etc. Early examples of the use of PITs were the efforts of breeders to select animals on the basis of 'type'. Thus the conformation, colouring and temperament of dairy stock have all been given credence over the years. With time these have generally proved to be poor predictors of genetic merit either because they are too influenced by environmental factors or because their connections with milk production are too remote or even non-existent.

More recently, searches for indicator traits have been rationalised following the development of the concept that suitable traits would most likely be found on the pathway between the DNA of the major gene(s) and actual milk production. Furthermore since a number of major genes might be contributing along quite different pathways the best place to look for PITs would be in processes that immediately precede milk production. Thus it has been argued that the function and control of metabolic processes that are essential for the production of milk might provide suitable indicator traits. Further, since many metabolic processes are under tight homeostatic control and may not exhibit much variation under resting conditions it is considered that the ability of animals to respond to perturbations of their normal metabolism might be particularly revealing (cf. Woolliams and

Lovendahl, 1991). Searches have been carried out by several groups by comparing the response of animals in lines of dairy cattle differing in genetic merit for milk production or using bulls that were entering progeny test programmes. Several of these studies have shown significant correlations between genetic merit for milk production and basal glucose concentration or the release of insulin in response to an intravenous glucose tolerance test (Woolliams and Lovendahl, 1991; Xing *et al.* 1991). To date these responses have not been used in a breeding trial partly because the genetic correlations with milk yield and the PITs have not been high enough to predict a significant improvement in the rate of genetic improvement relative to that achievable by conventional methods.

The difficulty of using this approach in the selection of sows is similar to that for the QTL. That is, verification requires access to reliable estimates of milk production in sows. Furthermore although the data for the cattle trials are promising they are far too equivocal to justify a detailed search in the pig.

5.5 Relationships between milk output and other selection criteria

Given the difficulties in measuring milk output directly, improvements in the milk production of sows that can be attributed to improved genetics have occurred largely through the use of selection criteria that are indirectly related to milk production. Very few selection programmes have involved direct selection for milk yield of sows and, since the indirect effect of any particular selection criterion on milk output is probably quite small, a number of factors must collectively account for most of the estimated genetic gain of 1-2% per annum. It is of interest then, to consider the possible relationships between milk yield and other traits, although it is not always possible to quantify the genetic correlations.

5.5.1 Selection for increased growth rate

Food intake

The highly successful application of animal breeding techniques that has resulted in an increase in growth rate and a reduction in backfat of pigs (e.g., see Vangen and Kolstad, 1986) may also have altered milk production in either direction, depending on the actual selection criterion or criteria. Selection programmes that have focused on reducing backfat may have reduced voluntary food intake and, in such cases, we would expect both voluntary food intake and milk production of lactating sows to also be reduced or the efficiency of milk production increased. There is support for both responses. Piglet growth rate was reduced by 30 g/day following seven generations of selection of gilts for low food intake relative to a control group that was not subjected to any selection pressure (Kerr and Cameron, 1996). In contrast, piglets sucking gilts selected for high food intake did not grow any faster than piglets on control sows, suggesting that low food intake of sows can inhibit milk yield below that for unselected animals, rather than high food intake enhancing milk yield. Alternatively, Revell and Williams (1993), comparing milk production and food intake of sows in the 1970s with that of the 1990s, concluded that the modern genotypes with *ad libitum* feeding produce about 35% more milk, but do not eat much more than sows on restricted feeding regimens 20 years earlier. Hence it would appear that the efficiency of milk production in the modern sow has been improved, as she is able to produce more milk despite little increase in food intake.

Gilts selected for improved growth rate or improved lean tissue growth rate, rather than for reduced backfat, are likely to exhibit an increase in milk production. This concept is supported by the positive and significant genetic correlation of 0.52 found between average daily gain during performance tests from 30 to 85 kg live weight and the weaning weight of a litter produced by the performance-tested gilts (Kerr and Cameron, 1996). The weaning weight of a litter will reflect a range of factors, including both the capacity of the sow to produce milk and the capacity of the litter to remove milk. Nevertheless, an improved weaning weight is consistent with an increase in milk production in gilts or sows of fast-growing genotypes, especially as the intake of creep feed by piglets is often low and variable (Pluske *et al.*, 1995).

Weaning weight

Higher milk yields from fast-growing genotypes may reflect the close relationship between post-weaning growth rate and weaning weight (e.g., Harrell *et al.*, 1993). It is probable that, on average, pigs which grow faster during the grower or finisher phases are weaned at a heavier weight than slower-growing counterparts. Successful breeding programmes based on the criterion of pig growth rate, as discussed above, are likely to have indirectly led to selection for a heavier weaning weight which, in turn, will have been related to an increased milk consumption during the suckling phase.

Prepubertal growth rates

It is possible that the rate of growth of the gilt around the time of puberty may influence her subsequent milk production. In dairy cattle (Little and Kay, 1979; Sejrsen et al, 1982) and goats (Bowden et al., 1995) rapid rates of growth in the prepubertal period are associated with substantial reductions in milk production in all subsequent lactations. The aetiology of this phenomenon is still unclear but recent reports suggest that heifers fed a diet with an adequate protein:energy balance are unaffected and that the deleterious effect is associated with an excessive deposition of fat during the prepubertal period. Therefore it is tempting to speculate that gilts may be similarly affected and that part of the reason for the improved milk production of the modern sow is a better balance of protein:energy in the diet during this critical period of growth.

5.5.2 Selection for increased litter size

Milk output is influenced by the stimuli from the sucking piglets (Auldist and King, 1995), and hence we might expect that increasing litter size would enhance milk output. Much interest was generated in the possible improvements in sow productivity to be attained by crossing European breeds (such as the Large White) with the highly prolific Chinese breeds of the Taihu group, i.e. Meishan and Jiaxing. Although the Chinese breeds produce about 5 extra piglets at birth and about 3 extra pigs at weaning, it appears from litter weight gains that they may produce only 5% (Sellier & Legault, 1986) to 14% (Sinclair *et al.*, 1996) more milk than the European breeds. Although increasing sow prolificacy may enhance overall productivity of a production enterprise, it does not necessarily reflect significantly more milk per sow. Furthermore, it is unlikely that the gains in milk yield that have occurred over the past few decades can be attributed to an increase in litter size. A comparison of the response in milk yield to litter size obtained about three decades ago with that obtained more recently reveals that, for any given litter size, modern sows produce about 2 kg/day more milk (Auldist and King, 1995).
If litter size cannot fully explain the improvement in milk yield over recent decades, then perhaps the nursing demand of litters has increased. Barber *et al.* (1955) recorded the average interval between sucklings with litters aged between 6 and 31 days as 51-54 minutes. More recently, Auldist *et al.* (1995) observed suckling intervals of between 44 and 52 minutes, depending on litter size and stage of lactation. Hence, suckling intervals during the first two weeks of lactation appear to have been reduced by about 7 minutes, but during later lactation (weeks 3 and 4), there is no evidence for more frequent suckling. A reduction of 7 minutes during early lactation would permit 4.5 extra suckling bouts during a 24 hour period and, assuming the amount of milk consumed during each suckling bout remained constant, it would represent an increase of 16% in daily milk output during early lactation. As milk yield during early lactation has increased by perhaps 60% over the past few decades (Figure 5.1), more frequent suckling could perhaps explain 20-30% of this increase.

5.5.3 Selection of pigs with an increased mature body size

An alternative hypothesis to explain the increase in milk yield over the past few decades is that modern genotypes have a larger body size and more mammary tissue. It has been suggested that changes in growth rate, protein deposition and maintenance requirements of pigs over the past 20 years can be explained solely by changes in body size (Williams, 1995). However, an increase in mature body size, which has undoubtedly occurred over the past few decades, does not fully explain the higher milk yields of modern sows compared to their predecessors. The modern gilt, which is still growing during her first reproductive cycle, now produces at least 20% more milk than the mature sow a few decades ago (see Figure 5.1) even though she is smaller than mature sows from 20 years ago and is physiologically younger, suggesting that more mammary tissue alone is unlikely to explain the increase in milk yield. Nevertheless data which would allow the comparison of mammary gland weight, corrected for body weight, across time are not available.

5.6 Biochemical and nutritional consequences of increased milk production

The topic has been well covered by Boyd *et al.* (1995) in their full and stimulating review on nutrient uptake and regulation of milk synthesis in the sow. Selection of sows that produce greater yields of lactose, protein and fat but proportionally greater amounts of protein will lead to particular demands on those aspects of their metabolism supplying amino acids to the glands. Revell *et al.* (1998) found that primiparous sows of a 'modern-genotype' were not able to completely buffer a shortfall in dietary protein by mobilising more body protein. Similarly, under the conditions of high milk demand associated with large litters in late lactation, the capacity to mobilise body stores, which is influenced by genotype, will affect milk output (Sauber *et al.*, 1994).

Genetic differences in milk output may also be associated with differences in the partitioning of energy and/or protein between maternal tissue and milk during lactation, and hence the extent to which genetic differences are exhibited will depend on the dietary conditions employed and the age of the sows (i.e. degree of maturity). For example, in situations where maternal requirements for protein are less, such as in mature sows compared with growing (immature) gilts or sows, or in Meishan sows compared with European White breeds (Sinclair *et al.*, 1996), milk yield per unit of dietary protein is likely to be higher. Such considerations need to be borne in mind when making comparisons between parities and genotypes in assessing the capacity for milk production.

5.7 Conclusion

For the present time it would appear that the only practicable step for increasing milk production in sows is to select indirectly on the basis of the weight gain of their litters. Similarly boars can be progeny tested by measuring the weaning weight of the litters of their daughters. The biology is difficult to interpret since such data reflect milk solids production by the sow, efficiency of food conversion by the piglet, its appetite and growth potential. Nevertheless selection on this basis would be expected to result in the most advantageous balance of increased yields in each of the major solids components. As our understanding of the genetic control of milk production improves, and advancements in technologies such as gene mapping, embryo transfer and transgenics become more accessible to animal breeders, more direct methods of improving milk output will become more feasible.

5.8 References

Auldist, D.E. & R.H. King, 1995. Piglets' role in determining milk production in the sow. In: Manipulating Pig Production V. Hennessy, D.P. & P.D. Cranwell (eds). Australasian Pig Science Association, Werribee, Victoria. 114-118.

Auldist, D.E., D. Carlson, L. Morrish, C. Wakeford & R.H. King, 1995. Effect of increased suckling frequency on mammary development & milk yield of sows. In: Manipulating Pig Production V. Hennessy, D.P. & P.D. Cranwell (eds). Australasian Pig Science Association, Werribee, Victoria. 137.

Barber, R.S., R. Braude & K.G. Mitchell, 1955. Studies on milk production of Large White pigs. J. Agr. Sci. 46, 97-118.

Bowden, C.E., K. Plaut & R.L. Maple, 1995. Effect of plane of nutrition on mammary gland development in prepubertal goats. In: Intercellular Signalling in the Mammary Gland. Wilde, C.J., M. Peaker & C.H. Knight (eds). Plenum Press, New York & London. 71-72.

Boyd, R.D., R.S. Kensinger, R.J. Harrell & D.E. Bauman, 1995.Nutrient uptake & endocrine regulation of milk synthesis by mammary tissue of lactating sows. J. Anim. Sci. 73 Suppl. 2, 36-56.

Elsley, F.W.H., 1971. Nutrition & lactation in the sow. In: Lactation. Falconer, I.R. (ed.). Butterworths, London. 393-411.

Haley, C.S., 1995. Livestock QTLs - bringing home the bacon? Trends Gen. 11, 488-492.

Hanwell, A. & M. Peaker, 1977. Physiological effects of lactation on the mother. Symp. Zool. Soc. Lond. 41, 297-312.

Harrell, R.J., M.J. Thomas & R.D. Boyd, 1993. Limitations of sow milk yield on baby pig growth. Proceedings of the 1993 Cornell Nutrition Conference for Feed Manufacturers, Cornell University, Ithaca, NY. 156-164.

Hartmann, P.E., C.S. Atwood, D.B. Cox & S.E.J. Daly, 1995. Endocrine & autocrine strategies for the control of lactation in women & sows. In: Intercellular Signalling in the Mammary Gland. Wilde, C.J., M. Peaker & C.H. Knight (eds). Plenum Press, New York & London. 203-225.

Head, R.H. & I.H. Williams, 1995. Potential milk production in gilts. In: Manipulating Pig Production V. Hennessy, D.P. & P.D. Cranwell (eds). Australasian Pig Science Association, Werribee, Victoria. 134.

Hickman, C.G., 1971. Response of selection of breeding stock for milk solids production. J. Dairy Sci. 54, 191-198.

Hodge, R.M.W., 1974. Efficiency of food conversion & body composition of the preruminant lamb & the young pig. Br. J. Nutr. 32, 113-126.

Holden, P.J., E.W. Lucas, V.C. Speer & V.W. Hays, 1968.Effects of protein level during pregnancy & lactation on reproductive performance in swine. J. Anim. Sci. 27, 1587-1590.

Jenness, R., 1974. The composition of milk. In: Lactation . A comprehensive treatise. Vol. III. Larson, B.L. & V.R.Smith (eds). Academic Press, New York, London. 3-107.

Kerr, J.C. & N.D. Cameron, 1996. Responses in gilt post-farrowing traits & pre-weaning piglet growth to divergent selection for components of efficient lean growth rate. Anim. Sci. 63, 523-531.

King R.H., B.P. Mullan, F.R. Dunshea & H. Dove 1997. The influence of piglet body weight on milk production of sows. Livest. Prod. Sci. 47, 169-174.

King, R.H., J.E. Pettigrew, J.P. McNamara, J.P. McMurtry, T.L. Henderson, M.R. Hathaway & A.F. Sower, 1996. The effect of exogenous prolactin on lactation performance of first-litter sows given protein-deficient diets during the first pregnancy. Anim. Repr. Sci. 41, 37-50.

King, R.H., C.J. Rayner & M. Kerr, 1993. A note on the composition of sow's milk. Anim. Prod. 57, 500-502.

King, R.H., M.S. Toner & H. Dove, 1989. Pattern of milk production in sows. In: Manipulating Pig Production II. Barnett, J.L. & D.P. Hennessy (eds.). Australasian Pig Science Association, Werribee, Victoria. 98.

King, R.H., M.S. Toner, H. Dove, C.S. Atwood & W.G. Brown, 1993. The response of first-litter sows to dietary protein level during lactation. J. Anim. Sci. 71, 2457-2463.

Legates, J.E. & R.M, Myers, 1988. Measuring genetic change in a dairy herd using a control population. J. Dairy Sci. 71, 1025-1033.

Lewis, A.J., V.C. Speer & D.G. Haught, 1978. Relationship between yield & composition of sows' milk & weight gains of nursing pigs. J. Anim. Sci. 47, 634-638.

Little, W. & R.M. Kay 1979. The effects of rapid rearing & early calving on the subsequent performance of dairy heifers. Anim. Prod. 29, 131-142.

Mackay, T.F.C., 1995. The genetic basis of quantitative variation: numbers of sensory bristles of *Drosophila melanogaster* as a model system. Trends Gen. 11, 464-470.

Meuwissen, T.H.E. & J.A.M. Van Arendonk, 1992. Potential improvement in rate of genetic gain from marker-assisted selection in dairy cattle breeding schemes. J. Dairy Sci. 75, 1651-1659.

Oftedal, O.T., 1984. Milk composition, milk yield & energy output at peak lactation: a comparative review. Symp. Zool. Soc. Lond. 51, 33-85.

Peaker, M., 1977. The aqueous phase of milk: ion & water transport. Symp. Zool. Soc. Lond. 41, 113-134.

Peaker, M., 1978. Ion & water transport in the mammary gland. In: Lactation. A comprehensive treatise. Vol. IV. Larson, B.L. (ed.). Academic Press, New York, London. 437-462.

Peaker, M., 1995. Autocrine control of milk secretion: development of the concept. In: Intercellular Signalling in the Mammary Gland. Wilde, C.J., M. Peaker & C.H. Knight (eds.)., Plenum Press, New York & London.193-202.

Pettigrew, J.E., S.G. Cornelius, R.L. Moser, & A.F. Sower, 1987. A refinement & evaluation of the isotope dilution method for estimating milk intake by piglets. Livest. Prod. Sci. 16, 163-174.

Pluske, J.R., I.H. Williams, E.C. Clowes, L.J. Zak, A.C. Cegielski & F.X. Aherne, 1995. Super-alimentation of gilts during lactation. In: Manipulating Pig Production V. Hennessy, D.P. & P.D. Cranwell (eds.). Australasian Pig Science Association, Werribee, Victoria. 129.

Revell, D.K. & I.H. Williams, 1993. A review - Physiological control & manipulation of voluntary food intake. In: Manipulating Pig Production IV. Batterhamn, E.S. (ed.). Australasian Pig Science Association, Attwood, Victoria. 55-80.

Revell, D.K., I.H. Williams, B.P. Mullan, J.L. Ranford & R.J. Smits, 1998. Body composition at farrowing & nutrition during lactation affects the performance of primiparous sows. II. Milk composition, milk yield & piglet growth. J. Anim. Sci. (in press).

Robertson, A. & J.M. Rendel, 1950. The use of progeny testing with artificial insemination in dairy cattle. J. Gen. 50, 21-31.

Sauber, T.S., R.C. Ewan & N.H. Williams, 1994. Maximum lactational capacity of sows with a high & low genetic capacity for lean tissue growth. J. Anim. Sci. 72 Suppl. 1, 364.

Sellier, P. & C. Legault, 1986. The Chinese prolific breeds of pigs: examples of extreme genetic stocks. In: Exploiting New Technologies in Animal Breeding. Genetic Developments. Smith, C., J.W.B. King & J.C. McKay (eds.). Oxford University Press, Oxford. 153-162.

Sejrsen, K., J.T. Huber, H.A. Tucker & R.M. Akers, 1982. Influence of nutrition on mammary development in pre- & postpubertal heifers. J. Dairy Sci. 65, 793-800.

Sinclair, A.G., S.A. Edwards, S. Hoste, A. McCartney & V.R. Fowler, 1996. Partitioning of dietary protein during lactation in the Meishan synthetic & European White breeds of pig. Anim. Sci. 62, 355-362.

Smith, D.M., 1952. Yield & composition of milk of New Zealand Berkshire sows. N. Z. J. Sci. Tech. 34, 65-75.

Smith, D.M., 1959. The yield & composition of milk from sows fed on three ration levels. N. Z. J. Agric. Res. 2, 1071-1083.

Toner, M.S., R.H. King, F.R. Dunshea, H. Dove & C.S. Atwood, 1996. The effect of exogenous somatotropin on lactation performance of first-litter sows. J. Anim. Sci. 74, 167-172.

Touchberry, R.W., 1974. Environmental & genetic factors in the development & maintenance of lactation. In: Lactation . A comprehensive treatise. Vol. III. Larson, B.L. & V.R. Smith (eds.). Academic Press, New York, London. 349-382.

Vangen, O. & N. Kolstad, 1986. Genetic control of growth, composition, appetite & feed utilisation in pigs & poultry. In: 3rd World Congress on Genetics Applied to Livestock Production. Dickerson, G.E. & R.K. Johnson (eds.). University of Nebraska Board of Regents, Lincoln, Nebraska. 367-380.

Van Tassell, C.P. & L.D. Van Vleck, 1991. Estimates of genetic selection differentials & generation intervals for four paths of selection. J. Dairy Sci. 74, 1078-1086.

Wilde, C.J., C.V.P. Addey, L.M. Boddy-Finch & M. Peaker, 1995. Autocrine control of milk secretion: from concept to application. In: Intercellular Signalling in the Mammary Gland. Wilde, C.J., M. Peaker & C.H. Knight (eds.). Plenum Press, New York & London. 227-237.

Williams, I.H., 1995. Sows' milk as a major nutrient source before weaning. In: Manipulating Pig Production V. Hennessy, D.P. & P.D. Cranwell (eds.). pp. 107-113 Australasian Pig Science Association, Werribee, Victoria.

Woolliams, J.A. & P. Lovendahl, 1991. Physiological attributes of male & juvenile cattle differing in genetic merit for milk yield: a review.Livest. Prod. Sci. 29, 1-16.

Xing, G.Q., D.D.S. Mackenzie & S.N. McCutcheon, 1991. Diurnal variation in plasma metabolite & hormone concentrations & response to metabolic challenges in high breeding index and low breeding index Freisian heifers fed at two allowances. N. Z. J. Agric. Res. 34, 295-304.

6 Energetic efficiency of milk production

J. Noblet, M. Etienne, J.-Y. Dourmad

6.1 Introduction

The productivity of sows has increased considerably over the last 30 years related to a reduction in the duration of lactation and genetic selection for a higher prolificacy. In addition, piglet weight gain over the suckling period has increased even though the consumption of creep feed is negligible over the three to four week lactation period. This means that daily litter weight gain and related sow milk production have become much higher (see Chapter 16) with a subsequent higher demand for energy and nutrients. Furthermore, the mature weight of sows has increased with an associated higher demand for energy at maintenance. The appetite of lactating sows, however, has not increased in proportion with their higher energy requirements. Mobilisation of body reserves becomes more acute then, with possible detrimental effects on reproductive traits. In this review, we will consider approaches used to quantify the energy requirements of lactating sows, the effects of energy supply on their performance and some factors of variation of appetite and energy intake in lactating sows.

6.2 Energy requirements of lactating sows

Establishment of the energy requirements of lactating sows requires the determination of their energy expenditures (maintenance and milk production) and the efficiencies of utilisation of energy from the diet and from body reserves. One first difficulty for estimating these values is the necessity of keeping the piglets with the sow in order to maintain milk production. In this case, it is necessary to divide the total heat production, as measured for instance in a respiration chamber, between the sow and its litter. Methods have been proposed by Verstegen *et al.* (1985), Beyer (1986), Noblet and Etienne (1987a) and Everts (1994). A more sophisticated method based on the direct and continuous measurement of net oxygen uptake by the lungs of the lactating sow, according to blood flow and arterio-venous differences in oxygen concentration (Giles *et al.*, 1991) is quite attractive as a way of overcoming this difficulty (Lorschy *et al.*, 1993). The second difficulty in studying energy metabolism in lactating sows is related to the impossibility of a physiological and direct measurement of milk production (see Chapter 16).

6.2.1 Maintenance energy requirements

According to Beyer (1986) and Noblet and Etienne (1987a), metabolizable energy requirements for maintenance (MEm) average 460 kJ per kg $BW^{0.75}$ per day in lactating sows. A slightly higher value (490 kJ/kg $BW^{0.75}$ per day) was suggested by Verstegen *et al.* (1985) in second parity sows. In addition, there are indications from the results of Beyer (1986) that MEm would increase with parity number; but this change has not been clearly explained. In comparison with pregnant sows, lactating sows are given high feeding levels with a subsequent lower critical temperature (LCT) (see Chapter 15). Therefore, in most housing systems, lactating sows are above their LCT with no additional requirements for cold thermoregulation. Similarly, their level of physical activity is usually low or, at least, varies little resulting in no additional energy cost for physical activity (Noblet *et al.*, 1993). Consequently, literature MEm values for lactating sows obtained under favourable environmental conditions can be considered applicable to most practical conditions.

6.2.2 Requirements for milk production

Methods such as the weigh-suckle-weigh technique or the isotope dilution techniques have been used under strictly controlled experimental conditions to estimate milk production of sows (see Chapter 16). However, they are not applicable under practical or routine conditions and alternative methods such as the relationships between growth of the litter and milk production have been proposed. The accuracy of the prediction is improved when variation in composition of the gain occurs as a result of nutritional treatments that will affect milk composition or genetic characteristics of the piglets (Table 6.1).

Composition of sow's milk is affected by many factors such as the stage of lactation, the composition of feed, the intensity of mobilisation of body reserves and genetics (see Chapter 1). Its energy content is, therefore, variable. However, an average value of 4.8 kJ/g, as suggested by Noblet and Etienne (1986), can be

Table 6.1. Prediction of energy output in milk (Emilk, kJ/d/piglet) from body weight (BW, kg), daily growth of the piglet (ADG, g/d) and energy content in piglet weight gain (Eg, kJ/g)

Equation no.	Equation[2]	R^2	Reference[1]
1	Emilk = 548 + 10.50 x ADG + 301 x BW	.80	1
2	Emilk = 640 + 10.63 x ADG + 329 x BW	.88	2
3	Emilk = 20.6 x ADG - 376	.87	2
4	Emilk = 17.1 x ADG + 230 x Eg - 2030	.97	2

[1] References 1 and 2 correspond to Beyer (1986) and Noblet and Etienne (1989), respectively.
[2] Equations 1 and 2 are applicable to short (3 to 5 d) periods during lactation while equations 3 and 4 can be used for predicting Emilk over total lactation (20 to 25 days).

used as a conversion factor. Furthermore, as illustrated in Table 6.2, it can be estimated that each kg of piglet gain requires about 3.8 kg of milk, 0.7 kg of milk dry matter or 18.4 MJ of milk energy. These different ratios can be used to readily obtain estimates of milk output. The mean energy content of piglet gain is about 10 MJ per kg (Noblet and Etienne, 1987b). Finally, it should be stressed that, in comparison with most other growing mammals, the gross efficiency of utilisation of sow's milk for gain is quite high since about 50 to 55% of milk energy and 85 to 90% of milk nitrogen are converted into piglet gain, respectively (Noblet and Etienne, 1986).

Very few estimates of efficiency of utilisation of ME for energy production in sow's milk are available. The highest value (79%) was obtained by Beyer (1986) and the lowest (68%) by Verstegen *et al.* (1985). Intermediate values were given by Burlacu *et al.* (1993) and Noblet and Etienne (1987a) (72%) and Hoffmann *et al.* (1990) (75%). A 72% mean value can then be proposed. In addition to dietary energy, energy from body reserves is frequently used for meeting total energy requirements for lactation (Table 6.2). The efficiency of utilisation of body energy for milk energy is quite high (88 to 90% according to Beyer, 1986 and Noblet and Etienne, 1987a). This value is in agreement with the preferential mobilisation of body fat (Etienne *et al.*, 1985, Beyer, 1986; Everts, 1994) and the probable direct incorporation of fatty acids in milk fat (Salmon-Legagneur, 1964).

Table 6.2. Mean components of energy balance in sows over lactation[1]

Parity	1	3
Mean lactation body weight, kg	168	207
Litter size, n	9.5	10.6
Litter weight gain, g/d	1880	2810
Milk production, kg/d	7.1	NA
Litter energy gain, MJ/d	18.7	28.5
Energy balance, MJ/d		
ME intake	59.6	69.7
Heat production	34.1	NA
Milk energy	34.1	NA
Maternal balance	-8.5	-19.6

[1] Adapted from Noblet and Etienne (1986 and 1987a; d1 to d21)) and Everts (1994; d4 to d25) for data of columns 1 and 2, respectively; NA: not available.

6.2.3 Total lactation energy requirements

Total metabolizable energy requirements of lactating sows (MEl) correspond to the addition of maintenance energy requirements and requirements for milk production. According to the values cited above, MEl (MJ/day) is then equal to: 0.460 x BWs $^{0.75}$ + Emilk/0.72; BWs corresponds to the sow body weight after farrowing. Emilk over total lactation can be estimated from Equation 3 in Table 6.1, so that MEl = 0.460 x BWs $^{0.75}$ +28.6 x Litter gain (kg/d) - 0.52 x Litter size. Illustrations of the approach are given in Table 6.3 for a conventional sow (10 piglets and average milk potential) and an improved sow (higher prolificacy and high milk potential). This table indicates that lactation energy requirements are 3 to 4 times higher than pregnancy requirements. In addition, under most practical conditions, MEl is above spontaneous feed energy intake, so that part of this requirement is met by mobilisation of body energy reserves (see following paragraphs).

Table 6.3. Effect of sow body weight and litter performance on daily ME requirements of lactating sows over total lactation (MJ/d)

Litter weight gain, kg/d	2.0[1]		3.0[1]	
Sow BW, kg	200	250	200	250
ME for maintenance	24.5	28.9	24.5	28.9
ME for production	52.0	52.0	79.6	79.6
Total requirements				
MJ ME	76.5	80.9	104.1	108.5
kg of feed[2]	5.9	6.2	8.0	8.3

[1] 10 and 12 piglets for 2 and 3 kg/d, respectively.
[2] 13.0 MJ ME per kg of feed.

6.3 Effects of energy supply on performance of lactating sows

6.3.1 Effects of energy supply on milk production and litter growth

The effect of lactation energy supply on milk nutrient output has been determined in a small number of recent experiments. Most measurements have been taken at one or two stages of the lactation period and therefore only quite rarely at regular intervals over total lactation (van Kempen *et al.*, 1985; Noblet and Etienne, 1986). However, under usual rearing conditions for suckled piglets (i.e.

at or above their thermoneutral zone and with reduced physical activity), litter growth rate can be considered a reliable indicator of milk nutrient output. Therefore, to assess most literature studies on this topic, litter growth will be used as a criterion to estimate the effects of energy supply on milk production of the sow. From a methodological point of view, it should also be noticed that variations of energy intake are often induced by changes in feeding level without any adaptation in the composition of feeds. In other words, variations of energy supply are often confounded with proportional variations of protein supplies. Results of Tokach *et al.* (1992) suggest that the minimum lysine to energy ratio for maximum milk yield would be slightly increased at low energy supplies. Therefore, attention should also be paid to daily supplies of protein and amino acids relative to milk yield when different energy supplies are compared. Finally, there might be confusion between the effects of energy intake and changes in the nature of nutrients supplied to the sow. One illustration is provided by studies in which different inclusion levels of fat induced variations of total energy intake but also amounts of fat and starch (Schoenherr *et al.*, 1989; Coffey *et al.*, 1994).

From a review of the literature, Henry and Etienne (1978) concluded that live weight of each piglet in the litter when weaned at 42 days of age was increased by about 25g for each additional daily MJ of DE. More recent studies conducted over shorter lactations (20 to 30 days) confirm this overall tendency for heavier piglets with higher energy intakes (Reese *et al.*, 1982; Nelssen *et al.*, 1985; van Kempen *et al.*, 1985; Brendemuhl *et al.*, 1987; Mullan and Williams, 1989). Williams (1995) in a compilation of recent literature studies suggested an increase of daily piglet growth of about 1g for each additional daily MJ of DE to the sow (i.e. 25 to 30 g higher weight gain at weaning per additional daily MJ of DE), which is comparable to the value obtained by Henry and Etienne (1978) over a longer lactation. But the magnitude of the response is quite variable with absolutely no significant response of litter weight gain to variation of energy intake in some studies (King and Williams, 1984a and 1984b; Reese *et al.*, 1982; Noblet and Etienne, 1986). Similarly, the response of lactating sows to overfeeding (by stomach cannula) is quite variable: Pluske *et al.* (1995) (cited by Williams, 1995) observed no additional weight gain of the litter when ME intake was increased from 75 to 104 MJ/d while Matzat *et al.* (1990) (cited by Williams, 1995) obtained a linear relationship between piglet growth and energy intake.

In fact, the effect of energy supply on milk production and litter weight gain must be considered in connection with the amount of 'available' body reserves of the sow. Indeed, energy restriction has usually only negligible effects on litter growth in early lactation, the sow being able to compensate by a higher mobilisation of its body reserves in order to maintain milk nutrient output. In such a situation, a higher body weight loss and a reduction of backfat thickness are observed. Similarly, overfeeding does little to improve milk production if body condition of the sow is satisfactory. However, with advancement of lactation at low energy intakes and progressive depletion of body reserves, the effects of energy level on growth of the litter become significant (Table 6.4). Similarly, van Kempen *et al.* (1985) and Noblet and Etienne (1986) observed that the effect of energy restriction on milk nutrient output and more especially on fat production became significant or more pronounced during the third week of lactation. An excellent illustration of the close relationship between the effect of energy restriction on milk production and the level of sow body reserves is given by O'Grady *et al.* (1973, 1975). These authors applied variable energy intakes (52 to 84 MJ DE /day) during the lactation period over three successive parities, feeding level being similar for all sows during pregnancy. At first parity, neither litter weight at 21 days of age nor production of milk constituents at 24 days of lactation were significantly affected by lactation energy intake. At second parity and to a larger extent at third parity, the energy restricted sows had significantly lighter piglets and lower milk outputs than those fed at more liberal feeding levels. These sows were also lighter with less lean and highly reduced body fat after their third lactation. This indicates that lactating sows are able to maintain their milk production and compensate an energy deficit by an increased body energy mobilisation as long as their body reserves, and especially body fat reserves, are not depleted to a large extent.

More generally, sows have become leaner with progressive selection and have, therefore, lower amounts of fat reserves. This means that their ability to compensate for lactation energy deficit has become lesser or, in other words, they may be more rapidly affected by nutritional deficits and exhibit more frequent reproduction problems associated with excessive mobilisation of their body reserves.

Table 6.4. Effect of lactation energy supply and stage of lactation on litter growth

Reference	King and Dunkin, 1986b			Mullan and Williams, 1989	
Energy intake, MJ DE/d	27	45	63	27	60
Growth of piglet, g/d					
Weeks 1 to 3	177	185	193	196	224
Week 4	156	193	193	159	210

Milk composition is dependent on several factors (see Chapter 1). With regard to the effect of dietary energy supply during lactation, changes in milk composition are directly related to the nature and the importance of mobilisation of body reserves. As illustrated in Table 6.5 and by the results of O'Grady *et al.* (1973) and van Kempen *et al.* (1985), milk solids content and more especially fat content are increased when mobilisation of body reserves is accentuated. The consequence is that more fat is exported in milk, even on a daily basis, with a sub-

Table 6.5. Effect of energy restriction on milk yield and composition and litter weight gain in lactating sows over a 21-d lactation (adapted from Noblet and Etienne, 1986)

Energy intake, MJ DE/d	60	44
Milk composition		
Dry matter, %	17.8	19.1
Fat, %	6.9	8.0
Nitrogen, %	0.74	0.78
Energy, kJ/g	4.78	5.32
Milk yield		
kg/d	7.1	6.6
Fat, g/d	490	532
Energy, MJ/d	34.1	35.2
Litter weight gain, g/d	1879	1843
Composition of litter weight gain		
Protein, %	16.1	15.9
Fat, %	14.3	15.9

sequent higher adiposity of the piglets at weaning. However, this fat enrichment of milk has little or negligible consequences on piglet growth since it is generally accepted that the main limiting factor for piglet growth is the supply of protein and amino acids (Williams, 1995).

As a whole, these results indicate that milk production and litter growth are positively related to lactation energy supply. The dependency, however, is attenuated as long as the sow body condition is satisfactory.

6.3.2 Effects of energy supply on sow body tissues

The most common and most accessible indicators of body composition changes in lactating sows are body weight and backfat thickness changes. However, the most important criteria to be considered are the changes in weight of tissues. Even the weights of udder, uterus and digestive tract are significantly changed over lactation, most weight change concerns lean and adipose tissues. Whittemore and Yang (1989) have suggested the following relationship between backfat thickness and weight of adipose tissues: each 1 mm backfat thickness change is associated with a change of about 1.8 kg of weight of adipose tissues. The corresponding change in body lipid content would be 1.3 to 1.5 kg according to Whittemore and Yang (1989) and Dourmad *et al.* (1997). These values can be used to estimate the partition of total BW loss between lean tissue and adipose tissue losses, the mass of lean tissue being estimated as the difference between total weight change and adipose tissue weight change.

Most recent studies indicate that a moderate degree of dietary protein restriction does not affect milk yield. A subsequent increased mobilisation of lean tissue will be directly dependent on the balance between protein supplies and protein needs for milk production (Dourmad et al., 1997). In the case of a significant protein shortage and subsequent high mobilisation of lean tissue, milk production will be depressed (Ranford *et al.*, 1994; Chapter 7). It is also clear from the literature that, with adequate protein supplies, variation in mobilisation of body tissues induced by energy restriction during lactation mainly affects adipose tissues (Nelssen *et al.*, 1985; King and Dunkin, 1986a and 1986b; Brendemuhl *et al.*, 1987 and 1989; Table 6.6). Finally, in a situation of energy and protein deficit, observed for instance with sows having high milk productions and relatively low energy intakes, both lean and fat tissues will be mobilised. This simplified presentation illustrates that lean tissue mobilisation depends primarily on the adequacy of protein supplies for protein requirements, while fat tissue loss is directly related to the difference between energy intake and energy requirements. The extent of the mobilisation will be dependent on the importance of the nutritional deficit and also on the response of the sow in terms of milk production. In other words, sows are either able to mobilise large amounts of body reserves, thereby maintaining their milk production, or reduce their milk production following a nutrient restriction resulting in a moderate mobilisation of body reserves.

There is general agreement that lactating sows do not maintain their milk production when the loss of lean or fat tissue becomes too great. However, there is no indication about the minimum levels of lean and/or adipose tissues and the mechanisms which induce a reduction of milk production and a subsequent preservation of sow body tissues. It can also be suggested that these levels are probably dependent on the milk production potential of the sow or, more generally, on its genetic characteristics. In conclusion, milk production in sows has a higher priority than maintaining the sow body tissues, with a limit to the intensity of mobilisation which is dependent on sow characteristics. This priority is more

Table 6.6. Effect of energy restriction on composition of body weight loss in lactating sows over a 21-d lactation (adapted from Etienne et al., 1985)[1]

Energy intake, MJ DE/d	60	44
Tissue weight loss (kg/21 days):		
Lean	9.5	11.2
Adipose	1.6	6.8

[1] Daily protein supplies were similar in both groups.

accentuated at the beginning of lactation which usually coincides with higher levels of body reserves and hormonal levels more favourable to driving the nutrients towards milk production.

6.4 Factors of variation of energy intake in lactating sows

An approach for estimating the energy requirements of lactating sows was proposed in Part 6.2; its application illustrates that energy requirements during lactation are mainly dependent on milk production level. In Part 6.3, it was clearly demonstrated that energy intake affects milk yield and, to a much larger extent, changes in body composition of lactating sows. There is clear evidence that body reserves can partly compensate for the nutrient and energy deficits and contribute to maintaining the level of milk production. Under most practical conditions, lactating sows lose body weight during the lactation period, even under *ad libitum* feeding conditions. This indicates that supplies of nutrients do not usually meet the requirements of the sow. In addition, nutritional requirements have increased over the last two decades related to an increase of litter size and higher weaning weight of piglets. This change emphasises the risk of an accentuated difference between requirements and spontaneous intake of the lactating sow allowed by its ingestion capacity and the environment. It becomes important to quantify the respective effects of most factors which affect voluntary feed intake (VFI) of lactating sows to maximise nutrient intake and minimise depletion of body reserves and subsequent reproductive difficulties. More details about the specific effects of some factors (climatic conditions in Chapter 15; genetics in Chapter 5) are given elsewhere in this text and review papers on the regulation of VFI in lactating sows are available (O'Grady *et al.*, 1985; Dourmad, 1988).

6.4.1 Stage of lactation

It is usually recommended that the amount of feed over the first days of lactation be restricted, especially in order to help adaptation to new lactation feeds and reduce the occurrence of post-partum agalactia (Neil, 1996). Energy intakes are then, relatively low over the first week of lactation. Under *ad libitum* feeding initiated just after farrowing, most authors observe a steady increase of feed intake with a plateau after the third week of lactation (Table 6.7). From a limited number of studies, NRC (1988) proposed the following relationship between DE intake (MJ/d) and stage of lactation (Stage, days): $DE = 56.0 + 2.5 \times Stage - 0.072 \times Stage^2$. It must be stressed that the level of production (litter size, milk production, ...) in these studies was lower than in most present situations. Recent results of Neil *et al.* (1996) would even suggest that the plateau is attained at the second week of lactation with a tendency for lower VFI during the fourth and fifth weeks of lactation, especially in third or fourth parity sows.

The experiment of Stahly *et al.* (1979) indicates that VFI after the first week of lactation is not affected by feeding regimen (*ad libitum vs* restricted) during the first week of lactation. However, results of Neil (1996) suggest that, between day 3 and day 30 of lactation, sows fed restrictedly for 3 days after farrowing and *ad libitum* thereafter consume significantly less feed (8.1 kg/d) than sows fed *ad libitum* immediately after farrowing (8.3 kg/d). From both studies, it is clear that sows fed *ad libitum* throughout lactation consume more feed than those whose feed is restricted over the first days of lactation. Finally, this linear increase of feed intake over lactation is not observed in all situations. Typical feed intake patterns have been described by Koketsu *et al.* (1996). These authors, and more recently, Zak *et al.* (1997) also suggested relationships between feed intake pattern and levels of hormones or metabolites and reproductive traits during the subsequent pregnancy.

Milk yield increases over lactation (Chapter 16). Is the change of VFI as described above related to this variable nutritional demand? In fact, most papers report mean values over total lactation and from the literature there is limited information available for comparing the kinetics of change of VFI over lactation and the corresponding change of milk yield or energy requirements. A theoretical approach of Revell and Williams (1993) would suggest that energy balance is negative throughout lactation, the deficit being accentuated during the third or the fourth week of lactation. These authors also suggest that over longer lactations, the nutritional deficit would become smaller and the balance could even be positive.

Table 6.7. Effect of stage of lactation and sow body condition at farrowing on voluntary feed intake during lactation

	Experiment 1[1]		Experiment 2[2]	
Body condition at farrowing	Lean	Fat	Lean	fat
Body weight after farrowing, kg	186.0	212.8	150.4	161.0
Backfat thickness after farrowing, mm	23.6	29.2	17.0	24.8
Voluntary feed intake, kg/d				
Week 1	4.69	3.67	4.1	2.8
Week 2	4.55	4.03	5.9	3.8
Week 3	5.02	4.76	6.1	4.7
Week 4	5.09	4.87	6.4	5.4

[1] Adapted from Dourmad (1991 and 1993); lean and fat sows were fed 1.8 and 2.7 kg per day over pregnancy, respectively.
[2] Adapted from Revell *et al.* (1994); lean and fat sows received daily 1.7 kg of a 14.5% crude protein diet and 2.3 kg of a 5.8% crude protein diet, respectively.

6.4.2 Litter size

As indicated by O'Grady *et al.* (1985), litter size has a positive effect on VFI, in connection with a positive effect of litter size on milk yield. The statistical relationship they established from measurements conducted on a large number of sows (VFI, g/d = A + 224 x N - 8 x N^2 where A corresponds to the intercept and the effects of other factors and N is the number of piglets) suggests that the increase per additional piglet is more important for smaller litters (145 and 65 g/d for 5 and 10 piglets, respectively) and becomes negligible above 12 piglets. Over the maximum practical range for litter size (6 to 14 piglets), the total increase of VFI would be about 500 g/day according to these authors. Similarly, VFI is positively correlated to milk yield *per se* (at a similar litter size). According to Dourmad (1991), the daily VFI increase would be 45g per additional daily MJ of milk.

From the results of Auldist and King (1995), it can be calculated that each additional piglet results in an increased daily milk production of about 0.6 kg. This value is comparable to that suggested by Elsley (1971). If we assume that the mean energy content of milk is 5 MJ/kg and that the efficiency of utilisation of ME for milk energy is 72%, this increased production is equivalent to an additional requirement of about 4.2 MJ of ME or 350 g/d of feed for each additional piglet. For between 6 and 14 piglets, the daily feed requirement would be increased by about 2.8 kg. The comparison of corresponding additional VFI (+0.5 kg: see above) and additional requirements due to increased litter size indicates that the effect of litter size on VFI is quite negligible, in comparison with the increased nutrients demand. Furthermore, from a practical point of view, results of Neil *et al.* (1996) on 60 sows followed over four parities, indicate that VFI is largely independent of litter size and milk yield.

6.4.3 Parity

From a compilation of literature results, Dourmad (1988) showed an important increase of VFI between the first and the second lactation (+0.6 kg) and no important change afterwards. Recent results of Neil *et al.* (1996) obtained over four successive parities and 5 weeks of lactation and those of Coffey *et al.* (1994), measured for a large number of sows kept for three parities confirm this conclusion (Table 6.8). From observations on a large number of sows, O'Grady *et al.* (1985) proposed an equation for estimating the effect of parity number (P) on VFI: VFI = A + 297 x P - 22 x P^2. This equation indicates that, under their experimental conditions, VFI increased in a curvilinear fashion with parity number, with no further increase after the 6th parity. The total increase between parity 1 and parity 6 would be 715g/d. This amount is close to what Dourmad (1988) and Neil *et al.* (1996) suggested as the increase between parity 1 and parity 2. Increase in parity number is also associated with heavier females (Table 6.8), larger litters and subsequently higher energy requirements. Results of Neil *et al.*

(1996) and Neil and Ogle (1996) indicate that the additional feed intake over successive parities, is higher than additional requirements (Table 6.8). This approach also illustrates that the nutritional deficit and body weight loss are the most pronounced in first-parity sows with a subsequent higher occurrence of reproductive problems after the first lactation.

Table 6.8. Effect of parity number on body weight, feed intake and performance of lactating sows (adapted from Neil et al., 1996, Neil and Ogle, 1996 and Neil, personal communication)[1]

Parity	1	2	3	4
Sow body weight, kg[2]	171	190	210	219
Feed intake, kg/d	6.2	6.8	7.3	7.7
Body weight loss, kg	16	8	9	3
Backfat thickness change, mm	-1.2	-0.3	-0.1	+0.6
Litter size	9.9	7.6	9.4	9.5
Litter weight gain, g/d	1950	1700	2010	2010
Additional feed requirements, kg/d[3]	-	-0.4	+0.4	+0.5

[1] Mean of two groups of sows fed diets with either 14.7 or 10.8% crude protein during pregnancy; lactation lasted 5 weeks.
[2] At day 7 of lactation.
[3] g/day of feed containing 12 MJ of ME/kg; calculated as additional ME requirements due to increased body weight (460 kJ/kg $BW^{0.75}$) and increased litter weight gain (25 MJ per kg of gain); Parity 1 is used as the initial value for ME requirements.

6.4.4 Sow body condition

Using a multiple regression approach, O'Grady *et al.* (1985) confirmed that lactation feed intake was inversely related to the importance of pregnancy net weight gain (Salmon-Legagneur, 1965). Similar conclusions were reported more recently by Coffey *et al.* (1994) and Dourmad (1993) (see Tables 6.7 and 6.9). From measurements conducted on primiparous sows, Dourmad proposed that VFI during lactation is reduced by about 50 g for each additional daily MJ of DE during pregnancy. Revell *et al.* (1994) fed sows rather extreme diets during pregnancy in order to achieve comparable net weight gains but with quite different body composition at farrowing (Table 6.7). Their results indicate that the effect of higher feed allowances during pregnancy would be mainly due to the higher amount of body fat at farrowing. Similar conclusions were obtained by Hulten *et al.* (1996), with sows exhibiting a more intense catabolic state of their fat reserves when their backfat thickness at farrowing was high. These last authors also indicate that the catabolic state was the highest during the first week after farrowing. This observation is quite consistent with a higher depressive effect of high backfat thickness at farrowing on VFI during the first days or the first week after farrowing (Table 6.7). All these observations point to a major role for body fat in the regulation of VFI in lactating sows; some mechanisms have been proposed (Revell and Williams, 1993). Recent investigations on leptin could also help to explain the role of body fat mass on VFI.

A recent feeding technique for pregnant sows consists of supplying bulky diets at high feeding levels in order to reduce stereotypic behaviour and improve the welfare of sows (Robert *et al.*, 1993; Brouns *et al.*, 1994; Ramonet *et al.*, 1997). Results of Farmer *et al.* (1996) also show that at similar pregnancy energy intakes, VFI during lactation was higher in sows receiving higher feeding levels during pregnancy from low energy diets.

Even though higher feed intakes during pregnancy are associated with a higher weight loss and a lower VFI during lactation, feed intake and, to a smaller extent, body weight gain over the total reproductive cycle (pregnancy + lactation) are significantly higher than under restricted pregnancy feed intakes (Table 6.9). However, low VFI during lactation induces a shortage of energy but also of protein and other essential nutrients. The energy deficit can be compensated by a higher mobilisation of fat reserves (Experiment 2 in Table 6.9). However, the ability of lactating sows to compensate for a shortage of protein by mobilisation of their protein mass is limited, with subsequent reduced milk yield and a higher occurrence of reproduction problems. Overfeeding during pregnancy is also not recommended because of the increased frequency of farrowing problems in fat sows (Dourmad *et al.*, 1994). Therefore, the best strategy during lactation appears to be to feed the sow as closely as possible to its nutritional requirements in order to limit body weight loss during lactation and not to overfeed during pregnancy.

6.4.5 Characteristics of feed

Since insufficient feed intake during lactation is a major problem in the nutrition of sows, addition of fat in lactation diets has been intensively tested in order to stimulate energy intake. This effect would be more pertinent at high ambient temperatures for attenuating the depressive effect of high ambient temperature on VFI (Schoenherr *et al.*, 1989; Chapter 15). In the collaborative study of Coffey *et al.* (1994) conducted on a large number of animals, VFI was maintained when 9% fat was added in lactation diets and, consequently, the energy intake was higher. However, the overall tendency is a reduction of VFI when dietary energy content is increased. In a review of literature data, Dourmad (1988) estimated that VFI was decreased by 150 g when the ME concentration was increased by 1 MJ/kg. This means that, at an average VFI of 5 kg/d, VFI will be reduced by 300 g (-6%) and ME intake increased by 6 MJ/d (+10%) when ME content varies

Table 6.9. Effect of pregnancy feeding level (low, medium and high) on lactation feed intake and body composition changes over lactation in first parity sows

Experiment[1]	1			2		
Gestation feeding level	L	M	H	L	M	H
Pregnancy feed intake, kg/d	1.5	2.0	2.7	1.80	2.25	2.70
Body weight after farrowing, kg	126	144	171	186	198	213
Backfat thickness after farrowing, mm	19.8	23.1	31.6	23.6	26.4	29.2
Lactation feed intake, kg/d	4.90	4.46	3.40	4.89	4.73	4.30
Total feed intake, kg/d	2.22	2.52	2.85	2.41	2.74	3.02
Litter weight gain, kg/d	1.81	1.95	1.86	2.10	2.08	2.18
Backfat thickness change, mm						
Farrowing to weaning	+0.9	-0.9	-4.3	-8.2	-10.2	-11.4
Mating to weaning	+2.6	+2.8	-0.3	-4.1	-2.2	-0.0
Body weight change, kg						
Farrowing to weaning	-3.6	-15.8	-30.7	-12.2	-19.6	-24.6
Mating to weaning	+18.9	+17.9	+16.2	24.9	33.6	39.7

[1] Adapted from Mullan and Williams (1989) (experiment 1; 31 days lactation; 13.5 MJ DE per kg of feed) and Dourmad (1993) (experiment 2; 28 days lactation; 13.2 MJ DE per kg of feed).
[2] Mean feed intake over pregnancy and lactation.

between 12 and 14 MJ ME per kg. However, fat content of milk is increased with fat supplemented diets (Coffey *et al.*, 1982; Lellis and Speer, 1983), so that a non negligible fraction of the additional energy intake is exported in milk as fat. On the other hand , as in growing pigs, addition of fibre in lactating sow diets stimulates VFI; however, overall energy intakes are reduced. In addition, the effect of fibre on the VFI of lactating sows would be dependent on the origin or the nature of fibre (Zoiopoulos *et al.*, 1982).

Other aspects of feed characteristics such as the mode of presentation (O'Grady and Lynch, 1978), the number of meals (Libal and Wahlstrom, 1983; cited by Dourmad, 1988) can affect VFI of lactating sows. The effects of protein and amino acid content of diets on VFI are considered elsewhere (Chapter 6).

6.4.6 Feeding behaviour of lactating sows

In most studies on VFI in lactating sows, only total daily or weekly feed intakes have been measured with no indication about feeding behaviour parameters such as number of meals, meal duration, meal size and ingestion rate. A first study by

Dourmad (1993) indicated that lactating sows have a predominantly diurnal pattern for feed intake (70 to 75% of feeding activity during the day). For the primiparous sows he studied, 8.7 meals per day and an ingestion rate of about 100 g per minute were recorded. Recent results of Quiniou *et al.* (1998), obtained in multiparous sows kept at 25°C, confirm the diurnal pattern (77% of feed intake during the day); but the number of meals was smaller (7.1 per day) than in the study of Dourmad (1993), their average size was 960 g and the total duration of ingestion was about 50 minutes per day; the ingestion rate was 125 g per minute. Further experiments are required to study the effects of ambient temperature (mean daily temperature, daily variations, etc.) or feed characteristics on feeding behaviour of lactating sows.

6.5 Conclusion

The factorial approach applied to the estimation of energy requirements for lactating sows indicates that the mean lactation energy requirements of modern lactating sows range between 80 and 110 MJ ME per day, which corresponds to between about 6 kg and more than 8 kg of conventional feeds. Under practical conditions, such food intakes are hardly achieved, especially when sows are exposed to hot climatic conditions. In Part 6.3 it has been shown that energy deficit can be compensated for by mobilisation of body reserves but with negative consequences on milk yield and further reproductive performance. The situation is the most critical for first parity sows whose productivity has become quite high with the progress of genetic selection, but whose feed intakes have remained relatively low. In addition, the adoption of a feeding strategy over the reproductive cycle is recommended which covers the specific nutritional requirements of each stage of production . Emphasis should then be given to maximisation of voluntary feed intake during the lactation period, either by adaptation of management techniques, genetic selection or changes in the feed characteristics. This aspect is becoming more critical as the productivity of sows, and, as a result, their nutritional requirements continue to increase steadily.

6.6 References

Auldist, D.E. & R.H. King, 1995. Piglet's role in determining milk production in the sow. In: Manipulating Pig production V, D.P. Hennessy and P.D. Cranwell Ed., APSA, Werribee, Australia, 114-118

Beyer, M, 1986. Untersuchungen zum Energie- und Stoffumsatz von graviden und laktierenden Sauen sowie Saugferkeln - ein Beitrag zur Präzisierung des Energie- und Proteinbedarfes. Promotionsarbeit aus dem Forschungszentrum für Tierproduktion Dummerstorf - Rostock.

Brendemuhl, J.H., A.J. Lewis & E.R. Peo, Jr., 1987. Effect of protein and energy intake by primiparous sows during lactation on sow and litter performance and sows serum thyroxine and urea concentration. J. Anim. Sci., 64, 1060-1069.

Brendemuhl, J.H., A.J. Lewis & E.R. Peo, Jr., 1989. Influence of energy and protein intake during lactation on body composition of primiparous sows. J. Anim. Sci., 67, 1478-1488.
Brouns, F., S.A. Edwards & P.R. English, 1994. Effect of dietary fibre and feeding system on activity and oral behaviour of group-housed gilts. Appl. Anim. Behav. Sci., 39, 215-223.
Burlacu, G., M. Iliescu & P. Caramida, 1983. Efficiency of food utilization by pregnant and lactating sows. 1. The influence of diets with different concentrations of energy on pregnancy and lactation. Arch. Tierernähr., 33, 23-45.
Coffey, M.T., R.W. Seerley & J.W. Mabry, 1982. The effect of source of supplemental dietary energy on sow milk yield, milk composition and litter performance. J. Anim. Sci., 55, 1388-1394.
Coffey, M.T., B.G. Diggs, D.L. Handlin, D.A. Knabe, C.V. Maxwell Jr, P.R. Noland, T.J. Prince & G.L. Cromwell, 1994. Effects of dietary energy during gestation and lactation on reproductive performance of sows: a cooperative study. J. Anim. Sci., 72, 4-9.
Dourmad, J.Y., 1988. Ingestion spontanée d'aliment chez la truie en lactation: de nombreux facteurs de variation. INRA Prod. Anim., 1(2), 141-146.
Dourmad, J.Y., 1991. Effect of feeding level in the gilt during pregnancy on voluntary feed intake during lactation and changes in body composition during gestation and lactation. Livest. Prod. Sci., 27, 309-319.
Dourmad, J.Y., 1993. Standing and feeding behaviour of the lactating sow: effect of feeding level during pregnancy. Appl. Anim. Behav. Sci. 37, 311-319.
Dourmad, J.Y., M. Etienne, A. Prunier & J. Noblet, 1994. The effect of energy and protein intake of sows on their longevity. Livest. Prod. Sci., 40, 87-97.
Dourmad, J.Y., M. Etienne, J. Noblet & D. Causeur, 1997. Prédiction de la composition chimique des truies reproductrices à partir du poids vif et de l'épaisseur de lard dorsal. Application à la définition des besoins énergétiques. Journ. Rech. Porcine Fr., 29, 255-262.
Dourmad, J.Y., J. Noblet & M. Etienne, 1998. Effect of protein and lysine supply on performance, nitrogen balance, and body composition changes of sows during lactation. J. Anim. Sci., 76, 542-550.
Elsley, F.W.H., 1971. Nutrition and lactation in the sow. In: Lactation, I.R. Falconer Ed., Butterworths, London, 393-411.
Etienne, M., J. Noblet & B. Desmoulin, 1985. Mobilisation des réserves corporelles chez la truie primipare en lactation. Reprod. Nutr. Dévelop., 25, 341-344.
Everts, H., 1994. Nitrogen and energy metabolism of sows during several reproductive cycles in relation to nitrogen intake. Ph.D. thesis, Wageningen Agricultural University, The Netherlands.
Farmer, C., S. Robert & J.J. Matte, 1996. Lactation performance of sows fed a bulky diet during gestation and receiving growth hormone-releasing factor during lactation. J. Anim. Sci., 74, 1298-1306
Giles, L.R., J.L. Black, J.M. Gooden & E.F. Annison, 1991. Energy expenditure of growing pigs maintained at high ambient temperature. In: Energy Metabolism of Farm Animals, C. Wenk and M. Boessinger Ed., EAAP No. 58, ETH-Zentrum, Zurich, Switzerland, 52-55.
Henry, Y. & M. Etienne, 1978. Alimentation énergétique du porc. Journ. Rech. Porcine Fr., 10, 119-166.
Hoffmann, L., M. Beyer, R. Schiemann & W. Jentsch, 1990. Energiebedarf gravider und laktierender Sauen. Arch. Anim. Nutr., 40, 279-296.
Hulten, F., M. Neil, S. Einarsson & J. Hakansson, 1993. Energy metabolism during late gestation and lactation in multiparous sows in relation to backfat thickness and the interval from weaning to first oestrus. Acta Vet.. Scand., 34, 9-20.

King, R.H. & I.H. Williams, 1984. The effect of nutrition on the reproductive performance of first-litter sows. 1. Feeding level during lactation, and between weaning and mating. Anim. Prod., 38, 241-257.
King, R.H. & I.H. Williams, 1984. The effect of nutrition on the reproductive performance of first-litter sows. 2. Protein and energy intakes during lactation. Anim. Prod., 38, 249-256.
King, R.H. & A.C. Dunkin, 1986a. The effect of nutrition on the reproductive performance of first-litter sows. 3. The relative effects of energy and protein intakes during lactation on the performance of sow and their piglets. Anim. Prod., 43, 319-325.
King, R.H. & A.C. Dunkin, 1986b. The effect of nutrition on the reproductive performance of first-litter sows. 4. The response to graded increases in food intake during lactation. Anim. Prod., 42, 119-125
Koketsu, Y., G.D. Dial, J.E. Pettigrew & V.L. King, 1996. Feed intake pattern during lactation and subsequent reproductive performance of sows. J. Anim. Sci., 74, 2875-2884.
Lellis W.A. & V.C. Speer, 1983. Nutrient balance of lactating sows fed supplemental tallow. J. Anim. Sci., 56, 1334-1339.
Lorschy, M.L., L.R. Giles, C.R. Smith, J.M. Gooden & J.L. Black, 1993. Food intake, heat production and milk yield of lactating sows exposed to high temperature. In: Manipulating Pig production IV, E.S. Batterham Ed., APSA, Attwood, Victoria, Australia, 81
Mullan, B.P. & I.H. Williams, 1989. The effect of body reserves at farrowing on the reproductive performance of first-litter sows. Anim. Prod., 48, 449-457.
Neil, M., 1996. Ad libitum lactation feeding of sows introduced immediately before, at, or after farrowing. Anim. Sci., 63, 497-505.
Neil, M., B. Ogle & K. Anner, 1996. A two diet system and *ad libitum* lactation feeding of the sow. 1. Sow performance. Anim. Sci., 62, 337-347.
Neil, M. & B. Ogle, 1996. A two diet system and *ad libitum* lactation feeding of the sow. 1. Litter size and piglet performance. Anim. Sci., 62, 349-354.
Nelssen, J.L., A.J. Lewis, E.R. Peo, Jr. & J.D. Crenshaw, 1985. Effect of dietary energy intake during lactation on performance of primiparous sows and their litters. J. Anim. Sci., 61, 1164-1171.
Noblet, J. & M. Etienne, 1986. Effect of energy level in lactating sows on yield and composition of milk and nutrient balance of piglets. J. Anim. Sci., 63, 1888-1896.
Noblet, J. & M. Etienne, 1987. Body composition, metabolic rate and utilization of milk nutrients in suckling piglets. Reprod. Nutr. Dévelop., 27, 829-839.
Noblet, J. & M. Etienne, 1987. Metabolic utilization of energy and maintenance requirements in lactating sows. J. Anim. Sci., 64, 774-781.
Noblet, J. & M. Etienne, 1989. Estimation of sow milk nutrient output. J. Anim. Sci., 67, 3352-3359.
Noblet, J., J.Y. Dourmad & M. Etienne, 1990. Energy utilization in pregnant and lactating sows: modelling of energy requirements. J. Anim. Sci., 68, 562-572.
Noblet, J., X.S. Shi & S. Dubois, 1993. Energy cost of standing activity in sows. Livest. Prod. Sci., 34, 127-136.
NRC, 1988. Nutrient requirements of swine (9th revised edition). National Academy Press, Washington, D.C.
O'Grady, J.F., F.W.H. Elsley, R.M. MacPherson & I. MacDonald, 1973. The response of lactating sows and their litters to different dietary energy alowances. 1. Milk yield and composition, reproductive performance of sows and growth rate of litters. Anim. Prod., 17, 65-74.
O'Grady, J.F., F.W.H. Elsley, R.M. MacPherson & I. MacDonald, 1975. The response of lactating sows and their litters to different dietary energy alowances. 2. Weight changes and carcass composition of sows. Anim. Prod., 20, 257-265.

O'Grady, J.F. & P.B. Lynch, 1978. Voluntary feed intake by lactating sows: influence of system of feeding and nutrient density of the diet. Ir. J. agric. Res., 17, 1-5.
O'Grady, J.F., P.B. Lynch & P.A. Kearney, 1985. Voluntary feed intake by lactating sows. Livest. Prod. Sci., 12, 355-365.
Quiniou, N., D. Renaudeau, S. Dubois & J. Noblct, 1998. Influence des températures élevées sur les performances et le comportement alimentaire de la truie en lactation. Journ. Rech. Porcine Fr., 30, 303-311.
Ramonet, Y., M.C. Salaün & J.Y. Dourmad, 1997. Effets d'une incorporation de parois végétales dans la ration alimentaire sur l'activité comportementale des truies gestantes. Journ. Rech. Porcine Fr., 29, 167-174.
Ranford, J.L., D.K Revell, B.P. Mullan, I.H. Williams & J.K. Toussaint, 1994. Milk yield, but not milk composition, may be influenced by body fatness in primiparous sows. J. Anim. Sci., 72 (Suppl 1), 389.
Reese, D.E., B.D. Moserr, E.R. Peo, Jr., A.J. Lewis, D.W. Zimmerman, J.E. Kinder & W.W. Stroup, 1982. Influence of energy intake during lactation on the interval from weaning to first estrus in sows. J. Anim. Sci., 55, 590-598.
Revell, D.K, I.H. Williams, B.P. Mullan & R.J. Smits, 1994. Body fatness influences voluntary feed intake and liweight loss during lactation in primiparous sows. J. Anim. Sci., 72 (Suppl 1), 389.
Revell, D.K. & I.H. Williams, 1993. Physiological control and manipulation of voluntary food intake: a review. In: Manipulating Pig production IV, E.S. Batterham Ed., APSA, Attwood, Australia, 55-80.
Robert, S., J.J. Matte, C.L. Farmer, C.L. Girard & G.P. Martineau, 1993. High-fibre diets for sows: effects on stereotypies and adjunctive drinking. Appl. Anim. Behav. Sci., 37, 297-309.
Salmon-Legagneur, E., 1964. Relations entre les graisses ingérées, les lipides corporels et les acides gras du lait chez la truie. Ann. Biol. Anim. Bioch. Biophys., 4, 141-155.
Salmon-Legagneur, E., 1965. Quelques aspects des relations nutritionnelles entre la gestation et la lactation chez la truie. Ann. Zootech., 14, HS 1, pp 138.
Schoenherr, W.D., T.S. Stahly & G.L Cromwell, 1989. The effects of dietary fat or fiber addition on yield and composition of milk from sows housed in warm or hot environment. J. Anim. Sci., 67, 482-495.
Stahly, T.S., G.L. Cromwell & W.S. Simpson, 1979. Effects of full *vs* restricted feeding of the sow immediately postpartum on lactation performance. J. Anim. Sci. 49, 50-54.
Tokach, M.D., J.E. Pettigrew, B.A. Crooker, G.D. Dial & A.F. Sower, 1992. Quantitative influence of lysine and energy intake on yield of milk components in the primiparous sow. J. Anim. Sci., 70, 1864-1872.
Van Kempen, G.J.M., C. Geerse, M.W.A. Verstegen & J. Mesu, 1985. Effect of feeding level on milk production of sows during four weeks of lactation. Neth. J. Agric. Sci., 33, 23-34.
Verstegen, M.W.A., J. Mesu, G.J.M. van Kempen & C. Geerse, 1985. Energy balances of lactating sows in relation to feeding level and stage of lactation. J. Anim. Sci., 60, 731-740.
Whittemore, C.T. & H. Yang, 1989. Physical and chemical composition of the body of breeding sows with differing body subcutaneous fat depth at parturition, differing nutrition during lactation and differing litter size. Anim. Prod., 48, 203-212.
Williams, I.H., 1995. Sow milk as a major nutrient source before weaning. In: Manipulating Pig production V, D.P. Hennessy and P.D. Cranwell Ed., APSA, Werribee, Australia, 107-113.
Zoiopoulos, P.E., P.R. English & J.H. Topps, 1982. High-fibre diets for *ad libitum* feeding of sows during lactation. Anim. Prod., 35, 25-33.
Zak, L.J., J.R. Cosgrove, F.X. Aherne & G.R. Foxcroft, 1997. Pattern of feed intake and associated metabolic and endocrine changes differentially affect postweaning fertility in primiparous lactating sows. J. Anim. Sci., 75, 208-216.

7 Dietary amino acids and milk production

R. H. King

7.1 Introduction

Amino acids are required to build protein in the body of the pig, mostly in muscle, to replace proteins lost in the course of protein tissue turnover (maintenance), to replace proteins voided in the form of cells, amino acids and other nitrogenous compounds (endogenous losses) and, in the case of the lactating sow, to supply the nutrients required for milk secretion. Some nine amino acids (lysine, methionine, threonine, tryptophan, histidine, isoleucine, leucine, phenylalanine, valine) cannot be synthesised by the pig itself, and are thus regarded as essential amino acids.

The major use of dietary amino acids in the lactating sow is for the synthesis of milk protein. Upon digestion and assimilation into the blood stream, dietary amino acids together with amino acids liberated from muscle protein, can potentially meet a number of metabolic fates. First, they may be taken up by the mammary gland for use in milk synthesis. They may be incorporated into body proteins such as enzymes, muscle or viscera. Alternatively, they may be catabolised to supply carbon for glucose, which may then be used to synthesize milk lactose and fat, or oxidized to supply energy. In addition, after being taken up by the mammary gland, significant proportions of some essential amino acids may be converted to non-essential amino acids which are subsequently incorporated into milk proteins. The interaction between these metabolic functions shown in Figure 7.1 is likely to vary greatly depending upon the sow's nutritional state, body condition and milk yield. Models of sow metabolism have been proposed which integrate this knowledge of amino acid metabolism in the lactating sow (Pettigrew *et al.*, 1992). However, in contrast to numerous studies available in the dairy cow, relatively lit-

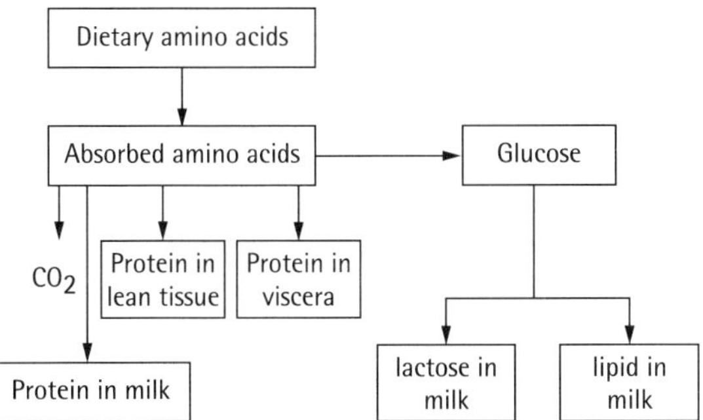

Figure 7.1. Schematic flowchart for a model of amino acid metabolism in lactating sows (from Pettigrew et al. 1993)

tle information is available on the specific amino acid requirements of porcine mammary tissue and mammary uptake and metabolism of amino acids in lactating sows.

Knowledge of the amino acid requirements of lactating sows is presently limited to the results of empirical studies conducted over the past 30 years or so. Anticipated milk yields of 5 to 7 kg/d have often been used to estimate nutrient requirements (ARC, 1981; NRC, 1988). Generally larger, late-maturing genotypes within a species possess greater milk production capacity. Mean daily milk yields of greater than 10 kg are not uncommon for modern sows. In addition to the increased amino acid supply required for milk production, young sows of modern genotypes should still be capable of depositing significant quantities of body protein. Thus, as well as the increased amino acid supply required for milk production, young sows will require additional dietary amino acids to optimise body protein deposition. Consequently, young prolific sows nursing large litters are likely to require amino acid intakes well above those currently recommended.

The extent of body tissue reserves and the ability of the sow to utilise these reserves to support milk production may also complicate assessment of the amino acid requirements of the lactating sow. The requirements for dietary amino acids to maximise milk yield are often lower than those required to maximise N balance during lactation (King *et al.*, 1993b). A reasonable objective during lactation is to optimise N balance rather than maximise milk yield as reproductive performance is likely to be compromised if dietary amino acid intake is not sufficient to meet the needs of maintenance, milk production and tissue deposition, particularly in young sows (Tritton *et al.*, 1996).

7.2 Amino acid requirements of the lactating sow

7.2.1 Lysine

Lysine has often been found to be the first limiting amino acid and, therefore, the protein requirement of lactating sows is often expressed relative to lysine. Estimates of the dietary total lysine requirements of the lactating sow vary considerably. For example, Boomgaardt *et al.* (1972) suggested that the daily lysine requirement of first litter sows was less than 20g whereas the results of Stahly *et al.* (1990) indicated that lactating sows require approximately 47g of lysine/d. Some variation in the reported estimates of protein and lysine requirements of lactating sows may be attributed to parity, dietary energy intake, the ability of the sow to mobilise body reserves and, above all, the different criteria used to estimate amino acids requirements. However, the level of milk production will also have a major influence on the amino acid requirements of lactating sows. Anticipated milk yields of 5 to 7 kg/d have often been used to estimate nutrient requirements (ARC, 1981). The NRC (1988) recommended that lactating sows weighing 165 kg at farrowing required 31.8g lysine/d. This recommendation was based on sows that supported between 0.98 and 1.66 kg of daily litter gain throughout lactation. Pettigrew (1993) collated much of the information published on the lysine requirements of lactating sows and found a close association between the amount of lysine needed to maximise lactational performance and the level of that performance (Figure 7.2). The relationship between lysine requirement (L, g/d) and litter growth rate (LGR, g/d) was described by the equation:

$L = -6.71 + 0.026\ LGR, R^2 = 0.77$ Equation 1

The slope (0.026) indicates that an increase of 100g of litter growth per day requires an additional 2.6g dietary lysine per day. This slope reflects the conversion of dietary lysine into lysine in the body protein of the piglets. Litter growth contains 16% protein or 1.04% lysine (Aumaitre and Duee, 1974; Campbell and Dunkin, 1983) and thus, provided amino acid requirements for maintenance are met, 26 g of the sow's dietary lysine is converted into 10.4 g piglet body lysine reflecting an efficiency of conversion of 0.40. The results of several studies conducted since publication of the review of Pettigrew (1993) have confirmed the higher milk production of modern sows and that levels of dietary lysine in excess of 50-55 g/d are required for these sows to achieve litter growth rates of 2500 g/d (Stahly *et al.*, 1990; Monegue *et al.*, 1993).

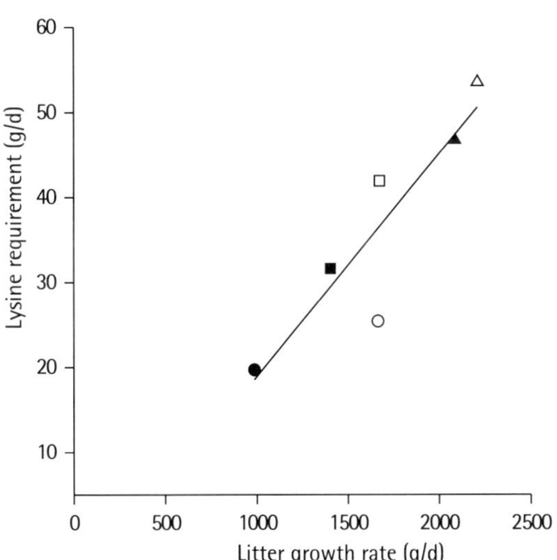

Figure 7.2. Relationship between the dietary lysine requirement of the lactating sow and litter growth rate (from Pettigrew, 1993). ● Boomgaardt et al.,1972, ○ Lewis and Speer, 1973, ■ O'Grady and Hanrahan, 1975, □ Chen et al., 1978, ▲ Stahly et al., 1990, △ Johnston et al., 1991

The negative intercept of Equation 1 reflects the ability of the sow to mobilise her body protein reserves to support milk protein synthesis. Milk protein synthesis appears to have greater priority for amino acids than accretion of body protein, as milk yield is usually maximised at much lower levels of dietary lysine intake than that required for positive N balance (King *et al.*, 1993b). The ability of the sow to mobilise body reserves is likely to depend upon genotype. Not only do modern genotypes have the ability to produce more milk with expected daily litter weight gains in excess of 2 kg in commercial pig production, but the modern sow can also use much more of her protein body stores to support these high levels of milk production. Pettigrew (1993) presented a regression equation similar to Equation 1 based upon the recent data of Tokach *et al.* (1992) and found that the relationship between lysine requirement and litter growth was described by:

$$L = -25.3 + 0.028 \text{ LGR } R^2 = .61 \qquad \text{Equation 2}$$

The similar slope of the relationship is encouraging and indicates that the conversion efficiency of maternal dietary lysine into piglet body lysine remains at about 0.40. But the greater negative intercept in Equation 2 may reflect an increased ability of modern sows to mobilise much more body protein than the older genotypes which contributed to the data set for Equation 1.

In these earlier studies, the dietary lysine requirement for maximum litter growth rate was often similar to the requirement for minimum sow body weight loss or optimum N balance. For example, Lewis and Speer (1973) reported that the estimated dietary lysine required for zero N balance was 29.4 g/d and a similar amount (30.0 g/d) was required to maximise litter weight gain. Similarly, Chen *et al.* (1978) found that piglet weight gain and sow milk yield increased progressively as dietary lysine intake was raised to 29.6 g/d which was also the intake at which N retention reached a maximum.

However, in more recent studies there appear to be greater differences between the lysine required for maximum milk yield and lysine required for maximum N retention (King *et al.*, 1993b; Everts and Dekker; 1994). The experiment of King *et al.* (1993b) was designed primarily to establish lysine requirements of lactating sows based upon N balance, but milk yield and litter growth rate appeared to reach a plateau at much lower dietary lysine levels than those required to maximise N balance; 48.6 g lysine/d was required to maximise N balance whereas the breakpoint in response to litter growth rate and milk yield occurred at about 33 g lysine/d. During lactation, sows were able to utilise body protein reserves relatively easily to support milk production. Up to 20 g N/d was mobilised from body stores to maintain milk production and litter growth rates at acceptable levels (King *et al.*, 1993b).

Genotype may also influence the response of lactating sows to dietary lysine. Sauber *et al.* (1993) observed that litter growth appeared to plateau when daily lysine intake reached 43 g in sows of a high lean genotype. However, sows of a low lean genotype were able to mobilise their own considerable body fat reserves to support milk production and responded to dietary lysine levels up to 55 g/d. Ranford *et al.* (1994) were able to achieve acceptable levels of milk production in fat sows only after supplying relatively high protein diets during lactation to complement the energy supplied by body fat reserves. Thus in situations where dietary energy intake is marginal, fatter sows exhibit a greater ability to mobilise body fat reserves and may respond to higher intakes of dietary lysine by producing more milk and litter gain.

Variation in the amount of milk produced by sows is the most important factor that influences the lysine requirements of lactating sows. Many of the non-dietary factors that influence milk yield are covered in other Chapters. The ability of the sow to mobilise body reserves to support milk production is also likely to be a significant factor that will influence the amount of dietary lysine required to maximise milk production. However, another factor which may affect the response to dietary lysine and interact with the ability of the lactating sow to utilise body reserves, is the dietary energy intake. Tokach *et al.* (1992) found a strong interaction between dietary lysine and ME intake in their effect on milk yield. Sows given higher energy intakes during lactation responded to a much higher level of daily lysine intake than did sows which were restricted in dietary energy intake. Sows receiving 60 MJ ME/day required 45 g lysine/day to maximise milk production whereas more restrictedly fed sows required only 25 g lysine/day to maximise milk yield, albeit at a much lower level (Tokach *et al.*, 1992). Thus the requirement of the lactating sow for dietary lysine will be reduced if milk yield is limited by energy intake and/or mobilisation of body energy reserves.

Obviously, many of the factors discussed earlier will influence the amount of lysine that should be supplied to the lactating sow to enable her to complete a successful lactation and exhibit satisfactory subsequent reproductive performance. Conservative recommendations on dietary amino acid requirements should be based upon the levels required for zero body protein change or N balance during lactation. In empirical studies conducted by Etienne *et al.* (1989) and Dourmad *et al.* (1991), 51 g lysine/d was required to ensure that muscle weight of sows did not change during lactation when they were producing approximately 10 kg milk/d. The factorial approach may also be used to estimate amino acid requirements for zero body N balance. For example, a 145 kg sow producing 10 kg milk/day has a daily digestible lysine requirement of 1.1 g for maintenance (Speer, 1990). Daily output of lysine in milk from this sow would be 38.5 g based upon a milk containing 0.85% N (Whittemore, 1993) and lysine in sow milk being 7.5 g/16 gN (Table 7.1). Assuming that dietary lysine is 85% digestible and that the conversion of digestible N into milk protein N is 70% (Burlacu *et al.*, 1985; Everts, 1994), then

Table 7.1. Estimates of the amino acid composition of sow's milk protein, g/16g N[1]

	Duee and Jung (1973)	Elliott *et al.* (1971)	Dourmad *et al.* (1991)	King *et al.* (1993a)
Lysine	7.75 (1.00)	7.59 (1.00)	7.24 (1.00)	7.09 (1.00)
Arginine	5.00 (.65)	5.12 (.67)	5.36 (.74)	4.62 (.65)
Histidine	2.70 (.35)	3.49 (.46)	3.84 (.53)	2.84 (.40)
Isoleucine	4.25 (.55)	3.83 (.50)	4.20 (.58)	4.22 (.60)
Leucine	8.90 (1.15)	8.76 (1.15)	8.47 (1.17)	8.09 (1.14)
Methionine	2.10 (.27)	1.74 (.23)	1.95 (.27)	1.97 (.28)
Methionine & Cystine	3.90 (.50)	3.00 (.40)	3.62 (.50)	3.29 (.46)
Phenylalanine	4.15 (.54)	4.26 (.56)	3.98 (.55)	3.93 (.55)
Phenylalanine & Tyrosine	8.30 (1.07)	9.09 (1.20)	8.11 (1.12)	7.83 (1.10)
Threonine	4.30 (.55)	4.62 (.61)	4.27 (.59)	4.12 (.58)
Tryptophan	-	1.31 (.17)	1.09 (.15)	1.32 (.19)
Valine	6.20 (.80)	4.80 (.63)	5.00 (.69)	5.46 (.77)
Glycine	3.45 (.45)	3.43 (.45)	3.62 (.49)	3.07 (.43)
Alanine	3.85 (.50)	3.95 (.52)	3.91 (.53)	3.40 (.48)
Serine	5.50 (.71)	5.15 (.68)	5.69 (.77)	4.49 (.63)
Aspartic acid	8.55 (1.10)	7.73 (1.02)	8.57 (1.16)	7.68 (1.08)
Glutamic acid	21.25 (2.74)	20.11 (2.65)	20.41 (2.76)	18.93 (2.67)
Proline	12.20 (1.57)	12.02 (1.58)	12.32 (1.67)	12.21 (1.72)

[1] Figures in parenthesis are amino acid: lysine ratios.

55 g digestible lysine (38.5 ÷ 0.70) or 64.7 g total dietary lysine (55 ÷ 0.85) is required to satisfy the dietary requirements for milk lysine secretion. Thus the lactating sow requires 66 g total lysine (64.7 + (1.1 ÷ .85)) per day to completely satisfy its needs for both milk production and body protein maintenance.

7.2.2 Other amino acids

An ideal amino acid profile has been used in growing pigs to estimate the need for other amino acids, once the requirement for one amino acid, usually lysine, has been established empirically. As the amount of amino acids required for obligatory processes is relatively minor compared to the amount required for milk protein synthesis, the ideal balance of dietary amino acids relative to lysine should be similar to the balance of amino acids in sow's milk. There are several reports of the amino acid composition of sow's milk and although there are some differences in absolute terms, the ratio of the individual essential amino acids expressed relative to lysine are remarkably constant (Table 7.1). The ARC (1981) proposed that the ideal dietary amino acid profile for lactating sows should be based upon the amino acid profile of milk. This proposal assumes that amino acids are used extensively for milk protein synthesis and ignores the possibility that particular amino acids may be used by the mammary gland for other metabolic purposes.

Comparison of the balance of amino acids in sow's milk to that derived from empirical studies (NRC, 1988) shows reasonable agreement for most of the essential amino acids except for leucine and valine (Table 7.2). However, the only empirical experiment upon which the NRC (1988) estimate for leucine is based was that reported by Rousselow *et al.* (1979) who used sows which produced only 4-5 kg milk/day. It is reasonable to assume that higher amounts of dietary leucine would be required for higher and thus more acceptable milk yields. On the other hand, the stated NRC (1988) valine requirement is higher than that based on the ratio in sow milk, which suggests that valine is used for purposes other than the synthesis of milk protein. Furthermore, the results of recent empirical studies have suggested that the dietary valine requirements during lactation are substantially higher than that based on the balance of amino acids in sow's milk. This may be so particularly during periods of high nursing demand. Tokach *et al.* (1993) increased the dietary valine: lysine ratio from 0.67 to 1.00 and found that litter growth rate improved, particularly when sows were suckling large litters. Richert *et al.* (1995) found that high levels of both lysine (1.2%) and valine (120% dietary lysine) were necessary to maximise litter growth and, again, the positive response to valine was restricted to sows with a high level of milk production (Table 7.3).

Evidence for a possibly greater requirement for some amino acids relative to their balance in sow's milk is provided by arterio-venous (A-V) differences observed

Table 7.2. The balance of amino acids (expressed relative to lysine) required by lactating sows

	Sow's Milk	NRC (1988)
Lysine	1.00	1.00
Arginine	0.66	0.67
Histidine	0.40	0.42
Isoleucine	0.55	0.65
Leucine	1.15	0.80
Methionine	0.26	0.26
Methionine & cystine	0.45	0.60
Phenylalanine	0.55	-
Phenylalanine & tyrosine	1.12	1.17
Threonine	0.58	0.72
Tryptophan	0.18	0.20
Valine	0.73	1.00

Table 7.3. Effect of lysine and valine concentrations in sow diets on average litter growth (kg/d) between day 2 and 24 of lactation (Richert et al., 1995)

Dietary lysine (%)	0.8			1.2			
Valine: lysine ratio	0.8	1.0	1.2	0.8	1.0	1.2	SEM
Litter size ≥ 10 pigs	2.18	2.12	2.28	2.36	2.29	2.55	0.06
Litter size < 10 pigs	1.90	1.94	1.89	1.88	2.09	1.81	0.06

in mammary tissue. Boyd *et al.* (1995) reviewed the small amount of data available on A-V differences in sows and suggested that the relative uptake of the branch chain amino acids (valine, isoleucine, arginine and possibly leucine) is greater than their secretion in milk proteins. If so, this suggests that the role of branch-chain amino acids and arginine in mammary metabolism may be quantitatively more significant than that suggested by the milk amino acid pattern.

The early classical work of Linzell *et al.* (1969) and Spincer *et al.* (1969) which was reviewed by Boyd *et al.* (1995) has been questioned by Trottier (1994) who has developed much better techniques for determining the mammary uptake of amino acids. Comparison of the uptake:output ratios for individual amino acids estimated by Trottier (1994) indicates that there was a reasonable balance between uptake and output for most of the amino acids, suggesting their use is exclusively for milk protein synthesis (Table 7.4). Linzell *et al.* (1969) reported that over twice as much valine was absorbed as was secreted in milk protein. However, Trottier (1994) found that the uptake:output ratio for valine was no different from that for the majority of the essential amino acids. These results question the validity of proposing a dietary requirement for valine in excess of that suggested by the amino acid profile in sow's milk. Further fundamental studies are required to determine whether or not valine is used disproportionately by the mammary gland for metabolic or increased maintenance needs.

7.3 Conclusion

The daily dietary lysine requirement for maximum lactational performance in modern sows nursing more than the 9-10 pigs is greater than the ARC (1981) and NRC (1988) recommendations. Moreover, the lactating sow requires a greater daily dietary lysine intake to achieve a positive N balance than it does to maximise lactational performance (King *et al.*, 1993b). Because lysine from mobilised muscle protein contributes to the total needs for milk production (Etienne *et al.* 1985), lactational performance can be maximised even if the intake of dietary

Table 7.4. Estimates of the amino acid uptake from plasma and output in milk

	Linzell *et al.* (1969)[1]			Trottier (1994)		
	Uptake ($g\ d^{-1}$)	Output ($g\ d^{-1}$)	Uptake/ Output (%)	Uptake ($g\ d^{-1}$)	Output[3] ($g\ d^{-1}$)	Uptake/ Output (%)
Lysine	1.56	2.14	73	23.3	22.3	104
Methionine	-	-	-	6.5	5.4	120
Threonine	.96	1.27	75	16.0	12.4	129
Tryptophan	-	-	-	8.6	-	-
Leucine	2.52	2.52	100	36.5	25.5	143
Isoleucine	1.32	1.49	89	18.4	12.0	153
Arginine	1.90	1.42	134	31.3	14.5	215
Histidine	.77	.77	100	7.6	7.9	96
Valine	3.48	1.46	238	21.3	15.6	137
Phenylalanine	1.15	1.18	97	15.5	11.3	137

[1] Uptake and output are on an individual gland basis.
[2] Uptake of nutrients by the whole mammary gland was calculated assuming plasma flow was 4275 ld^{-1} (Trottier, 1994).
[3] (N.L. Trottier, University of Illinois, 1996, personal communication).

lysine is less than that required for milk production. However, restricted amino acid intake and excessive body protein mobilisation during lactation have been associated with the occurrence of post-weaning anoestrus in sows (King and Dunkin, 1986; Brendemuhl *et al.*, 1987).

Calculations using Equation 2 for a sow which produces 10 litres of milk/day and has a litter growth rate of 2.2 kg/day, indicate a requirement of only 36.3 g lysine/day for maximum litter growth rate and milk yield. However, using the factorial approach, a daily intake of 66 g lysine is required to completely satisfy the needs for both milk yield and maintenance. The dilemma for the commercial pig industry is to determine an appropriate feeding strategy for lactating sows commensurate with the greatest profitability. The appropriate and economic feeding strategy for the supply of amino acids to sows during lactation is likely to be intermediate between that required for body N balance and the level at which reproductive and/or lactational performance will be compromised by the depletion of body protein reserves during lactation.

7.4 References

Agricultural Research Council, 1981. The Nutrient Requirements of Pigs. Commonwealth Agricultural Bureaux, Slough, U.K.
Aumaitre, A. & P.H. Duee, 1974. Composition en acides amines des proteines corporelles du porcelet entre la naissance e l'age a huit semanies Ann. de Zootech. 23:231-236
Boomgaardt, J., D.H. Baker, A.H. Jensen & B.G. Harmon, 1972. Effect of dietary lysine levels on 21- day lactation performance of first-litter sows. J. Anim. Sci. 34:408-410.
Boyd, D.R., R.S. Kensinger, R. Harrell & D.E. Bauman, 1995. Nutrient uptake and endocrine regulation of milk synthesis by mammary tissue of lactating sows. J. Anim. Sci. 73 (Suppl 2) 36-56.
Brendemuhl, J.H., A.J. Lewis & E. R. Peo, Jr., 1987. Effect of protein and energy intake by primiparous sows during lactation on sow and litter performance and sow serum thyroxine and urea concentrations. J. Anim. Sci. 64:1060-1069.
Burlacu G., M. Iliescu & P. Caramida, 1985. Efficiency of food utilization by pregnant and lactating sow. Proceedings 10th International Symposium on Energy Metabolism, Sept 15-21, Airlie, Virginia, Abstr. 81.
Campbell R.G. & A.C. Dunkin, 1983. The effects of energy intake and dietary protein on nitrogen retention, growth performance, body composition and some aspects of energy metabolism of baby pigs. Br. J. Nutr. 49: 221-230
Chen, S.Y., J.P.F. D'Mello, F.W.H. Elsley & A.G. Taylor, 1978. Effect of dietary lysine levels on performance, nitrogen metabolism and plasma amino acid concentrations of lactating sows. Anim. Prod. 27:331-334.
Dourmad J.Y., M. Etienne & J. Noblet, 1991. Contribution à l'étude des besoins en acides aminés de la truie en lactation J. Rech. Porcine en France 23:61-68.
Duee, P.H. & J. Jung, 1973. Amino acid composition of sow's milk Ann. Zootech. 22:243-247.
Elliott, R.F., G.W. Vander Noot, R.L, Gilbreath & H. Fisher, 1971. Effect of dietary protein level on composition changes in sow colostrum and milk J. Anim Sci. 32:1128-1137.
Etienne M., J. Noblet & B. Desmoulin, 1985. Mobilisation des reserves corporelles chez la truie primipare en lactation Reprod. Nutr. Develop. 25:341-343.
Etienne M., J. Noblet, J.Y. Dourmad, & H. Fortune, 1989. Etude du besoin en lysine des truies en lactation J. Rech. Porcine en France 21:101-108.
Everts, H., 1994. Nitrogen and energy metabolism of sows during several reproductive cycles in relation to nitrogen intake. PhD Thesis, Wageningen Agricultural University, The Netherlands.
Everts H & R.A. Dekker, 1994. Effect of nitrogen supply on nitrogen and energy metabolism in lactating sows Anim. Prod. 59:445-454.
Johnston L.J., J.E. Pettigrew & J.W. Rust, 1991. Response of maternal line sows to dietary protein concentration during lactation. J. Anim. Sci. 69(Suppl 1) 188 Abstr
King, R.H., & A.C. Dunkin, 1986. The effects of nutrition on the reproductive performance of first-litter sows. 4. The response to graded increases in food intake during lactation. Anim Prod. 42:119-125.
King, R.H., C.J. Rayner & M. Kerr, 1993a. A note on the composition of sow's milk Anim. Prod. 57:500- 502.
King, R.H., M.S. Toner, H. Dove, C.S. Atwood, & W.G. Brown, 1993b. The response of first-litter sows to dietary protein during lactation. J. Anim. Sci. 71:2457-2463.
Lewis, A.J. & V.C. Speer, 1973. Lysine requirement of the lactating sow. J. Anim. Sci. 37:104-110.
Linzell J.L., T.B. Mepham, E.F. Annison, & C.E. West, 1969. Mammary metabolism in lactating sows: arteriovenous differences of milk precursors and the mammary metabolism of [^{14}C] glucose and [^{14}C] acetate. Br J. Nutr. 23:319-332.

Monegue H.J., G.L. Cromwell, R.D. Coffey, S.D. Carter & M. Cervantes, 1993. Elevated dietary lysine levels for sows nursing large litters. J. Anim. Sci 71:(Suppl 1) 67 (Abstr)

National Research Council, 1988. Nutrient Requirements of Swine (9th Ed.). National Academy Press, Washington, D.C.

O'Grady, J.F. & T.J. Hanrahan, 1975. Influence of protein level and amino-acid supplementation of diets fed in lactation on the performance of sows and their litters 1. Sow and litter performance Ir. J. Agric. Res. 14:127-135.

Pettigrew, J.E, 1993. Amino acid nutrition of gestating and lactating sows. 'Biokyowa Technical Review-5' (Nutri-Quest Inc: St Louis, USA).

Pettigrew, J.E., M. Gill, J. France & W.H. Close, 1992. A mathematical integration of energy and amino acid metabolism of lactating sows. J. Anim. Sci. 70:3742-3761.

Pettigrew, J.E., J.P. NcNamara, M.D. Tokach, R.H. King & B.A. Crooker, 1993. Metabolic connections between nutrient intake and lactational performance in the sow. Livest. Prod. Sci. 35:137- 152.

Ranford J.L., D.K. Revell, B.P. Mullan, I.H. Williams & J.K. Toussaint, 1994. Milk yield, but not milk composition, may be influenced by body fatness in primiparous sows. J. Anim. Sci. 72 (Suppl 1) 389 Abstr.

Richert, B.T., R.D. Goodband. M.D. Tokach & J.L. Nelssen, 1995. Valine and lysine independently improve sow productivity during lactation. J. Anim. Sci. 73(Suppl. 1):85.

Rousselow D.L., V.C. Speer & D.G. Haught, 1979. Leucine requirement of the lactating sow. J. Anim. Sci. 49:498-506

Sauber T.E., T.S. Stahly, R.C. Ewan & N.H. Williams, 1993. Interactive effects of sow genotype and dietary amino acid uptake on lactational performance of sows nursing large litters. J. Anim. Sci. 71 (Suppl 1) 66 (Abstr)

Speer, V., 1990. Partitioning nitrogen and amino acids for pregnancy and lactation in swine: A Review. J. Anim. Sci. 68:553-561

Spincer, J., J.A.F. Rook & K.G. Towers, 1969. The uptake of plasma constituents by the mammary gland of the sow. Biochem. J. 111:727-732.

Stahly T.S., G.L. Cromwell & H.J. Monegue, 1990. Lactational responses of sows nursing large litters to dietary lysine levels J. Anim. Sci. 68 (Suppl 1):369 Abstr.

Tokach, M.D., R.G. Goodband, J.L. Nelssen & L.J. Kats, 1993. Valine - a deficient amino acid in high lysine diets for the lactating sow. J. Anim. Sci. 71 (Suppl 1):68.

Tokach, M.D., J.E. Pettigrew, B.A. Crooker, G.D. Dial & A.F. Sower, 1992. Quantitative influence of lysine and energy intake on yield of milk components in the primiparous sows. J. Anim. Sci. 70:1864-1872.

Tritton, S.M., R.H. King, R.G. Campbell, A.C. Edwards, & P.E. Hughes, 1996. The effects of dietary protein and energy levels of diets offered during lactation on the lactational and subsequent reproductive performance of first-litter sows. Anim. Sci. 62:573-579.

Trottier, N., 1994. Protein metabolism in the lactating sow. PhD Thesis, University of Ilinois, Urbana- Champaign, U.S.A.

Whittemore, C., 1993. 'The Science and Practice of Pig Production.' (Longman Scientific and Technical:Essex).

8 Dietary fat and milk production

L. Babinszky

8.1 Introduction

An issue arising repeatedly in sow nutrition is whether the primary energy source in mixed diets should be fat or carbohydrate (starch). This debate has not, as yet, been settled. Whether the major energy source in mixed diets is carbohydrate or fat (animal fat or vegetable oil) in a given country is influenced by the climate, and the crops produced, as well as such factors as tradition and culture. The technical standard and level of development of the feed industry in the particular country is also important. From this it is apparent that the above issue cannot be solved exclusively on the basis of biology or digestive physiology. In countries where the climate is suitable for maize production, for example, and where there is a great tradition of this, there is evidence that in mixed diets the primary carbohydrate energy source tends to be maize. In such countries there is no widespread tradition of using added fats. A similarly important aspect is whether the feed industry of the country concerned has suitable equipment available and possesses technology appropriate for the production of dietary fats of high and constant quality and for mixing such fats into diets. While the use of carbohydrate (starch) provides an energy source of relatively constant quality, where dietary fats are concerned, the problem of variation in quality between batches frequently arises in the course of the production process.

There are major implications with respect to product quality and economic efficiency. In addition biochemical, physiological and biological factors associated with fat utilisation need to be considered.
This chapter illustrates how, when dietary fat is used in diet formulation, the chemical composition of sow's milk and primarily its fat content, changes, and also what effect the quantity of fat provided exerts on milk production in sows. Both factors play a major role in determining the economic efficiency of piglet rearing.

8.2 Role of dietary fat in sow nutrition

Fats (animal fat and vegetable oil) are of special importance as energy supplies. Animals obtain energy from nutrients by oxidising carbon and hydrogen. These elements are in a more reduced state in fats than in carbohydrates or proteins, so there is the potential for more oxidation and therefore a greater yield of energy (Pettigrew and Moser, 1991).
In general there are three separate reasons for the use of supplemental fat in sow diets. Firstly, the adding of fat to the diet during late gestation may improve

piglet survival. Secondly, several authors have suggested that supplemental fat during lactation may ameliorate loss of body tissue caused by the large nutrient demands for milk production. Thirdly, it has also been suggested that adding fat to the sow's diet prior to and after farrowing increases the fat content of the colostrum and milk. However, only limited information is available on the effect of dietary fat on milk production.

Many researchers (Moser and Lewis, 1980; Pettigrew, 1981; Drochner, 1989 and Babinszky, 1992) have studied the effects on lactation performance of adding fat to the sow's diet. Fat supplementation of pig diets is not a new idea. Moser and Lewis (1980) reported that in 1950 Hillier found that growing pigs can efficiently utilize diets containing a high fat level efficiently. This was reflected in an improvement in daily weight gain and feed conversion efficiency. Similar observations were made in poultry. Many researchers have demonstrated that the addition of fat to poultry diets improves feed conversion efficiency more than would be expected on the basis of the increased energy density (Vermeersch and Vanschoubroek, 1968; Jensen *et al.*, 1970). This effect has been referred to as an 'extracaloric' effect of fat. A large number of studies has shown that the effects of fat addition to the sow's diet are not consistent. This can be related to differences in fat composition, to differences in experimental design, and to different conditions in the experiments.

8.2.1 Some factors affecting fat utilisation by pigs

Composition and digestion of dietary fat

The major site of fat digestion in the gastrointestinal tract of the pig is the duodenum. Fat digestion involves emulsification of dietary fat by conjugated bile salts, followed by hydrolysis of triglycerides into mixtures consisting essentially of monoglycerides and free fatty acids (Wiseman, 1989).

Specific polyunsaturated fatty acids should be provided in the diet because they are required in the synthesis of prostaglandins and phospholipids. There is metabolic capacity for the interconversion of fatty acids, but with limitations. In particular, swine have no mechanism to form double bonds fewer than six carbon atoms away from the methyl end of a fatty acid. Some of the fatty acids required in pigs contain double bonds in this area; because these cannot be produced in the tissues they must be provided in the diet, and are thus referred to as essential fatty acids (Pettigrew and Moser, 1991).

In pigs, saturated fatty acids are absorbed less efficiently than unsaturated fatty acids (Freeman *et al.*, 1968). The micellar formation potential, and absorption of saturated fatty acids is increased in the presence of unsaturated fatty acids or monoglycerides, as reviewed by Stahly (1984). Therefore, the digestibility of a particular supplemental fat source in pigs is dependent on the fatty acid composition (ratio of unsaturated to saturated fatty acids) of the total diet. The digestibility of fat from diets which have a ratio higher than 1.5 of unsaturated to saturated (U/S) fatty acids is high (85-92%) compared to that of diets with a lower ratio (Stahly, 1984).

Pettigrew *et al.* (1989) concluded from their study and from the literature that nursing piglets can utilise medium-chain triglycerides more efficiently than traditional fat sources rich in long-chain triglycerides.
Moser and Lewis (1980), on the other hand, concluded from published data that the type of dietary fat seems to be of minor importance with respect to litter performance. Vegetable oil may have some advantages in terms of ease of handling, but animal fats are usually less expensive (Moser and Lewis, 1980).

The amount of dietary fat
The amount of fat in the sow's diet may play an important role in the performance of lactating sows and suckling piglets. Fat levels of between 7.5 and 15% have been used in most experiments.

The results of various studies show that the increase in weaning weight is more favourable if the dietary fat concentration in the sow's diet is at least 8% and is used throughout both late gestation and the lactation period (Pettigrew, 1981).

Duration and timing of supplementation
The duration of providing fat-supplemented diets is another variable which may influence the performance of piglets. In terms of the number of pigs weaned per litter, it seems to be more beneficial to add fat either in late gestation or in the lactation period, rather than in both periods (Moser and Lewis, 1980). In terms of the survival of piglets, the addition of fat to the sow's diet during gestation alone or during gestation and lactation gives the best response (Moser, 1983; Table 8.1).

Table 8.1. Effect of the period of feeding fat to sows on survival of the piglets[1] (Moser, 1983)

Parameter	Feeding fat to sows		
	Gestation only	Lactation only	Gestation + lactation
Pigs weaned/litter	+ 0.7 (3)[2]	+ 0.7 (2)	0.0 (17)
Survival (%)	+ 4.7 (4)	+ 1.2 (3)	+ 34 (22)

[1] Values show the difference between diets with added fat and the control treatments.
[2] No. of experimental comparisons.

Interactions between dietary fat and other nutrients
Stahly (1984) and Freeman (1984) concluded from their reviews that the digestibility of dietary fat is influenced by those factors which depress the absorption of nutrients in the small intestine. Altering the rate of passage of the digesta or insolubilization of the dietary fat are both important. Carbohydrate sources (e.g.

barley straw or potato starch) which depress the absorption of nutrients in the small intestine and stimulate fermentation in the hind gut have been shown to reduce fat digestibility in pigs (Stahly, 1984). Dietary fibre has also been shown to depress fat digestibility in the chick and laying hen (Scheele, 1981).

In a study performed by Bakker *et al.* (1995) animal fat was added incrementally (0, 35, 70 and 105 g/kg) to maize starch or to two sources of fermentable carbohydrates (260 g purified cellulose or 270 g soya-bean hulls per kg). A total of ninety-six castrated males received the 12 experimental diets. Results indicated that the fermentable carbohydrates significantly reduced the apparent digestibility of crude fat in growing and finishing pigs (30-105 kg).
High levels of dietary minerals (Ca, Mg) may also reduce the digestibility of long-chain fatty acids in rats. The intensity of this relationship in pigs, however, has not been clearly defined.
Pallauf and Huter (1993) found that calcium formate as an energy-providing mineral compound in a weaned piglet's diet (15.0 g/kg) had a negative effect on feed intake, daily gain and feed conversion efficiency, when the diet already met calcium requirements. In their study, the digestibility of fat in particular was significantly reduced. They concluded that for this reason total Ca should not exceed the optimum level when calcium formate is added to the piglets' diet.
Cunnane (1984) in his excellent review summarised the most important factors affecting essential fatty acid metabolism in pigs (Table 8.2).

Table 8.2. Factors affecting essential fatty acid metabolism (Cunnane, 1984)

Stimulatory	a) minerals	zinc
		selenium
	b) vitamins	vitamin B_6
		vitamin C
		vitamin E
Inhibitory	a) minerals	copper
		calcium
	b) other	mono-unsaturated fatty acids
		saturated fatty acids
		age
		corticosteroids

However, it should be noted, that the results of studies reported on the interactions are not consequent. Further experiments must elucidate such effects of other nutrients on the fat utilisation in pigs.

8.2.2 Dietary fat and the performance of lactating sows and their piglets

Energy status of piglets

Seerley *et al.* (1974) were the first to suggest that supplemental fat in the sow's diet in late pregnancy could improve the pre-weaning survival of the offspring by improving their energy reserves. Pigs are born with very low lipid energy reserves. They have large energy reserves in the form of glycogen, but much of this glycogen is depleted during the first 2 days after birth. Supplemental dietary fat for the sow before farrowing, increases the fat content of the pigs at birth, but this increase is so small that it is likely to be of only limited practical importance (Pettigrew 1981). However, such supplementation does increase the fat content of colostrum and milk.

Live weight of sows and piglets

Cox *et al.* (1983) reported that *ad libitium* fed sows given a control diet (no additional fat) or diets supplemented with 10% fat *ad libitum* lost weight during lactation on both diets. During the summer period no differences were found between the control and the treatment group. However, in the winter, sows fed the fat-supplemented diet lost more weight than control animals. Schoenherr *et al.* (1989) found that weight change in the *ad libitum* fed sow during a 22-day lactation period was not affected by diets containing starch or fat in either a thermoneutral (20 °C) or a hot (32 °C) environment.
Seerley *et al.* (1981) reported that sows fed a diet *ad libitum* without fat supplementation did not consume extra feed and did not show greater weight loss than sows receiving 10% added corn oil or 10% added animal fat in their diet. Control animals, which showed greater weight loss, generally had a lower energy intake. Nelssen *et al.* (1985) found that sows fed at a restricted level with a tallow-supplemented diet from gestation throughout lactation lost more weight during lactation than animals fed a diet with corn starch. They concluded that the short (6-day) period of adaptation to the diet containing animal fat may have resulted in a poor digestion of the fat. Restricted energy intake during lactation, lower digestion of dietary fat and higher energy content in the milk may result in extra weight loss in sows.

Data from the literature show that, overall, dietary fat has only a minor effect, or no effect, on piglet weight at either birth or weaning (Moser and Lewis, 1980). Pettigrew (1981) reviewed 16 trials (in which no creep feed was given during suckling) of which 9 trials showed a positive effect on the weaning weight of piglets when fat was added to the sow's diet and 7 trials showed no effect or a small negative effect. He concluded that the mean piglet weight at weaning appears to increase if the dietary fat concentration is at least 8%. Coffey *et al.* (1982) and Nelssen *et al.* (1985) reported no significant difference in average piglet weight during the suckling period if the sow's diet was supplemented with fat.
However, in another study performed by Coffey *et al.* (1994) it was found that

increasing lactation energy intake by adding 9 % fat resulted in greater pig weight gains up to 21 days of age (P <0.01).
Many studies have been conducted to determine the effect of dietary fat on weight change in sows and their piglets, but the results are inconsistent.
The results of these experiments indicate that supplemental fat during lactation may provide two benefits: a reduction in weight loss in sows and increased weaning weight of the litter. However, neither response is substantial and the cost of the fat supplement may not be justified (Pettigrew *et al.*, 1989).

Survival of piglets
Pre-weaning mortality is a major source of animal losses. During the suckling period the mortality of piglets is approximately 14 % (Baltussen, 1988). Many pre-weaning piglet deaths may result from a shortage of dietary energy (Pettigrew *et al.*, 1989). Addition of fat to the sow's diet in late gestation, therefore, might increase the fat content of the colostrum and milk, and this may increase the total amount of energy transferred to the piglets via the mammary glands of the sow (Pettigrew *et al.*, 1989). Reviews on the subject (Moser and Lewis, 1980; Pettigrew, 1981; Seerley, 1981; Drochner, 1989) suggest that this increased transfer of energy to the piglets improves their survival rate.

Most of the studies from the gestation group showed an improvement in piglet survival rate. However, when fat was added after farrowing, little effect was observed (Seerley, 1984).

Moser (1983) summarized the effect of dietary fat level in the sow's diet on survival of the piglets (Table 8.3).

Table 8.3. Effect of level of fat added to the diet of sows on the survival of the piglets[1] (Moser, 1983)

Parameter	Level of fat added (%)		
	< 7.5	7.5 to 15	>15
Pigs weaned/litter	- 0.1 (5)[2]	+ 0.2 (15)	+ 0.5 (4)
Survival (%)	+ 2.0 (10)	+ 3.8 (16)	+ 1.5 (5)

[1] Values show the difference between diets with added fat and the control treatments.
[2] No. of experimental comparisons.

He concluded that a minimum of 7.5 % fat should be added, and that there is little advantage of using levels greater than 15 %. Thus according to limited data available in the literature this range gives the best response in terms of the survival of piglets.

It should be noted that when pre-weaning survival is at an acceptable level, it is not improved by additional fat. With low pre-weaning survival, however, supplemental dietary fat can be beneficial, but there are probably more effective means of improving survival (Pettigrew *et al.*, 1989). Drochner (1989) also concluded from data in the literature that the positive effect of survival from providing additional dietary fat is predominant when birth weights are low and for large litters where low survival rates are involved.

8.3 Effect of dietary fat on the chemical composition of milk and on milk production

Before discussing the effect of dietary fat on the composition of milk and the amount of milk it is important to review information on obtaining milk samples and the techniques for measuring milk production.
The problem is, that both, milk sampling and the measuring of milk yield are difficult because of the physiological and anatomical characteristics of pigs.

8.3.1 Milk sampling

Sampling of milk for chemical analyses is mostly achieved by hand milking, using oxytocin injection and sometimes from milk obtained by machine milking. Den Hartog *et al.* (1987) demonstrated, that the amount of oxytocin can influence the chemical composition of milk (Table 8.4).

Table 8.4. Composition of sow milk sampled by manual stimulation or injections of 1 ml or 2 ml oxytocin (den Hartog et al., 1987)

	Manual stimulation	1 ml oxytocin	2 ml oxytocin	CV*
Dry matter (%)	19.7[1]	19.0[1,2]	18.3[2]	7.3
Ash (%)	0.8	0.8	0.8	5.5
Fat (%)	8.4[1]	7.7[1,2]	7.1[2]	15.7
Protein (%)	5.2	5.3	5.1	7.4
Lactose (%)	5.3[1]	5.2[12]	5.1[2]	5.2
Energy (J/g)	5312 [1]	5086 [1,2]	4779 [2]	11.2

*CV = Coefficient of variation calculated as (residual standard deviation/mean) x100
[1,2] Means in the same row with different letters differ P ≤ 0.05.

Data from Table 4 show that the dry matter, fat, lactose and energy contents of the milk sampled after 2 ml oxytocin injection were significantly lower than in milk sampled after manual stimulation ($P < 0.05$) while the contents in milk sampled after usage of 1 ml oxytocin were intermediate.
On the basis of these results it can be stated that one should be very careful in comparing milk data form experiments where milk is sampled by different methods or after the administration of different amounts of oxytocin.

8.3.2 Effect of supplementary dietary fat on the chemical composition of milk

The effect of dietary fat on the composition of milk (particularly its fat content) has been widely investigated. Fatty acids in the milk are derived from two sources. Firstly, they may originate from the blood lipids, which include both endogenous and dietary fatty acids. Secondly, fatty acids may be derived from *de novo* synthesis in the mammary glands (Hartmann and Holmes, 1989). This means that the concentration of fat in colostrum and milk can be increased by increasing the fat level in the sow's diet, as has been found in numerous studies (Miller *et al.*, 1971; Friend, 1974, Seerley *et al.*, 1974, 1978a,b; Boyd *et al.*,1978; Coffey *et al.*, 1982, Drochner, 1989, Shurson and Irvin, 1992).
Pettigrew (1981) found an apparent increase in milk fat concentration. The increase in total milk production was not statistically significant, but total milk fat increased ($P<0.001$). However, milk production was determined at about one week postpartum, considerably before peak production (Table 8.5).

In a study conducted by Babinszky *et al.* (1992a) a total of 63 primiparous hybrid

Table 8.5. Percentage milk fat, daily milk production and daily milk fat production as affected by fat in the sow's diet[1] (Pettigrew, 1981)

	Control	Animal fat	Corn oil	Fat minus control	Corn oil minus animal fat
Milk fat, %	6.50	6.78	7.88	0.83±0.40[3]	1.10±0.75[3]
Daily milk production, kg[4]	4.47	4.91	5.58	0,78±0.40	0.67±0.42
Daily milk fat production, g	283	328	445	103±14***	117±61

[a] A total of five replicates (54 sows).
[b] Measured approximately 7 days postpartum.
[c] Mean ± standard error for five replicates, weighted by harmonic mean number of litters per treatment.
[d] Measured approximately 8 days postpartum.
*** $P \leq 0.001$.

sows were used in two experiments to study the effect of different dietary fat levels (low, moderate and high) on the chemical composition of milk. It was concluded that the high level of dietary fat(125 g/kg DM in experiment 2) increased the dry matter, fat and energy content of milk (Table 8.6).

Table 8.6. Effect of dietary fat level on the chemical composition of sow's milk at 14 and 27 days of lactation[1](Babinszky et al., 1992a)

	Experiment 1			Experiment 2		
	Dietary fat level		RMSE[3]	Dietary fat level		RMSE
	L[2]	M		L	H	
Day 14:n (sows)	13	16		16	16	
Dry matter, g/kg	198	201	17	201 [4]	215 [5]	17
Protein, g/kg	51	51	4	52	52	3
Fat, g/kg	88	91	17	90 [4]	105 [5]	17
Energy, kJ/g	5.47	5.58	0.66	5.58[4]	6.14[5]	0.67
Day 27: n(sows)	15	14		16	16	
Dry matter, g/kg	189	194	11	195 [4]	210 [5]	12
Protein, g/kg	51	52	4	56	57	4
Fat, g/kg	79	80	10	80 [4]	96 [5]	12
Energy, kJ/g	5.12	5.21	0.40	5.26[4]	5.88[5]	0.48

[1] Milk samples were takes after an intravenous injection of 2 ml oxytocin.
[2] Fat content of diets: Exp. 1: L (low):43 g/kg DM, M (moderate):75 g/kg DM,
Exp. 2: L(low):37 g/kg DM, H (high):125 g/kg DM.
[3] Root mean square error.
[4,5] Different superscripts in the same line indicate significant differences among energy groups in exp.2. ($P \leq 0.05$).

Results from other studies (Coffey *et al.*, 1982; Drochner, 1989) show that protein, lactose and total solid content were not affected by the fat level in the sow's diet.

8.3.3 Techniques used for measuring milk production and their evaluation

Different methods are available for measuring the milk production of sows:

1. Rate of gain in piglets as an indication of milk production. Results from different studies have indicated that only 34 % of the variation in gain is associated with variation in milk intake.

2. Change in weight of the sows during nursing. This method may cause a substantial error, since milk yield is only a small part of the total weight of the nursing sow.
3. Determination of milk production by weighing piglets before and after suckling (weigh - suckle - weigh: WSW method).
4. Using the isotope dilution (ID) technique.

At present the latter two methods are used in most studies. However, it should be noted, that there is no universally accepted method.
The weigh-suckle-weigh (WSW) method described by several authors, including Lewis *et al.* (1978), den Hartog et al. (1984) and Babinszky *et al.* (1992b), is a widely accepted approach to estimating the milk consumption of piglets and, therefore, the milk production of sows.
The WSW method is based on the weight of piglets immediately before and after nursing by the sow. The WSW sequence is repeated several times during a day, and the sum of the weight gains of the piglets is taken as the amount of milk consumed. Between nursing bouts, the piglets are not allowed access to the sow and the time interval between nursings is determined by the investigator, not by the piglets or the sow. According to Pettigrew *et al.* (1985) this method has several disadvantages. It disrupts the social interaction between the sow and the litter and imposes an arbitrary nursing interval. The other problem is that the weight of the piglets is much greater, perhaps by a hundredfold, than the weight increment during a single nursing. Thus, a relatively small error in weighing the piglet can cause a relatively large error in measurement of the amount of milk consumed. Finally, loss of weight through defaecation, urination, metabolism and salivation during the nursing bout can cause serious underestimation of consumption if not corrected for.
The isotope dilution (ID) method for estimating milk consumption has been used with several species, including pigs (McDougall, 1977).
The ID method uses an isotope of hydrogen as a tracer to estimate body water turnover (water intake) in piglets. Assuming that milk or colostrum is the piglet's only source of water, one can calculate the amount of milk consumed if the composition of the milk is known. A major advantage of this method is that is does not disrupt the normal maternal-offspring relationship during the measurement period.

However, this method also entails some technical difficulties. Although in a study performed by Pettigrew *et al.* (1985) the results indicated that the ID method estimates milk consumption more accurately than does the WSW method, the accuracy of the ID method should be improved upon. In this study (Table 8.7) the ID estimates of milk consumption were 11.9 % lower than weigh-suckle-weigh estimates.

Table 8.7. Estimates of the daily milk consumption of piglets by the isotope dilution and weigh-suckle-weigh methods (n=42) (Pettigrew et al., 1985)

Day	Milk consumption (g)			
	Weigh-suckle-weigh		Isotope dilution	
	Mean	SD	Mean	SD
1	–	–	743	286
2	712	216	702*	341
3	–	–	851	373

* Less than mean of day 1 and day 3 estimates (P≤0.05).

8.3.4 Effect of dietary fat levels on milk production

The effect of dietary fat on the milk yield of sows as demonstrated in various studies is given in Table 8.8. The data highlight that comparison of results between different studies is difficult because data relating to the daily food and/or ME intake of sows during lactation are not always available.

Reference	Fat in diet	Feeding during lactation	Fat effect on feed or ME intake	Fat effect on milk yield
Pettigrew (1981)[1]	animal fat or corn oil	no data	no data	slightly increased
Boyd *et al.* (1982)[2]	tallow	*ad libitum*	isocaloric	slightly increased
Coffey *et al.* (1982)[2]	animal fat	rationed	isocaloric	positive
Lellis and Speer (1983)[2]	tallow	rationed	isocaloric	no effect
Shurson *et al.* (1986)[2]	animal fat	*ad libitum*	increased	positive
Schoenherr *et al.* (1987)[2]	choice white grease	*ad libitum*	increased	no effect

[1] Review and own results.

[2] Own experimental results.

Also, different techniques for the estimation of milk yield were used. These may influence the magnitude of milk production. Furthermore, in most studies multiparous sows were used or there was no information about the effects of parity. In another study performed by Babinszky *et al.* (1992a) it was also concluded that the daily milk yield was not influenced by different dietary fat levels. However, the energy efficiency of milk production from ME above maintenance was significantly improved by the high level (125 g/kg DM) of dietary fat (Babinszky *et al.*, 1991). These data are summarised in Table 8.9.

Table 8.9. Effect of dietary fat level on the efficiency of milk production from feed (Babinszky et al., 1991)

	Experiment 1			Experiment 2		
	Dietary fat level			Dietary fat level		
	L[1]	M	RMSE[2]	L	H	RMSE[2]
n (sows)	15	16		16	16	
Efficiency[3]	0.71	0.72	0.01[6]	0.70[4]	0.73[5]	0.01[6]

[1] Treatments are defined in Table 8.6.
[2] Root mean square error.
[3] The daily maintenance requirement of sows was fixed at 420 kJ/ ME/kg$^{0.75}$ for all treatment groups.
[4,5] Different superscripts in the same row indicate significant differences between treatment groups in exp. 2 ($P \leq 0.05$).
[6] For statistical analysis n=4 per treatment.

Seerley (1984) reported that milk production increased by approximately 30 % due to the addition of fat to sow diets. If isocaloric diets provided 10 % dietary fat from day 109 of gestation to farrowing and were also used in lactation, the feeding of fat prior to farrowing only, or throughout lactation, was equally effective in increasing milk yield on day 14 of lactation. Increased milk production due to the feeding of fat to sows has been reported by several authors, as reviewed by Seerley (1984). In Table 8.10 it can be seen that the percentage increase ranged from 8 % to 18 % in these studies.

From the results of the different studies presented here, it may be concluded that the addition of fat to the sow's lactation diet has only a slightly positive effect on the milk production of sows, if any effect at all.

Table 8.10. Effect of dietary fat on milk production (kg/day) (after Seerley, 1984)

Reference	Control sows	Fat-fed sows	Increase (%)
Kruse *et al.*, 1977	4.60	5.32	16
Pettigrew, 1978	3.82	4.48	18
Boyd, 1979	8.73	9.45	8
Coffey and Seerley, 1981	5.45	7.18	31
			$\bar{x}$18

8.4 Conclusions

High levels of fat in the lactation diet can increase the fat and energy contents of milk. This could exert a positive influence on the profitability of pig production.
In most experiments reviewed here, dietary fat levels from 7.5 to 15 % were used. This range gives the best response in terms of the survival of piglets.
With respect to the number of piglets weaned per litter, it seems to be more beneficial to add fat either in late gestation or during lactation, rather than in both periods.
Data from the literature indicate that the milk production of sows is only slightly affected by the addition of fat to the gestation and/or lactation diet.
However, by feeding a high level of dietary fat, the energy efficiency of milk production from feed ME can be improved.

8.5 References

Babinszky, L., M.W.A. Verstegen, L.A. den Hartog, W. van der Hel, T. Zandstra & J.T.P. Dam, 1991. Effect of dietary carbohydrate and fat on energy and nitrogen balances and milk production of lactating sows. In: C. Wenk and M. Boessinger (Eds), Energy Metabolism of Farm Animals, EAAP Publications. pp. 268-271. ETH-Zürich, Switzerland.

Babinszky, L., 1992. Energy metabolism and lactation performance of primiparous sows as affected by dietary fat and vitamin E. PhD thesis. Agricultural University Wageningen, The Netherlands.

Babinszky, L., M.W.A. Verstegen, L.A. den Hartog, T. Zandstra, P.L. van der Togt & J.T.P. van Dam, 1992a. Effect of dietary fat and I-tocopherol level in the lactation diet on the performance of primiparous sows and their piglets. Anim.Prod. 55,233-240.

Babinszky, L., D.J. Langhout, M.W.A. Verstegen, L.A. den Hartog, T. Zandstra, P.L.G. Bakker & J.A.M. Verstegen, 1992b. Dietary vitamin E and fat source and lactating performance of primiparous sows and their piglets. Livest. Prod. Sci. 30, 155-168.

Baltussen, W.H.M., 1988. Verschillen tussen praktijkbedrijven in voeding van zeugen en biggen. Proefstation voor de Varkenshouderij, Landbouw Economisch Instituut, Rosmalen. Proefverslag nummer P 1.28. pp. 29.

Bekker, G.C.M., R. Jongbloed, M.W.A. Verstegen, A.W. Jongbloed & M.W. Bosch, 1995. Nutrient apparent digestibility and the performance of growing fattening pigs as affected by incremental additions of faat to starch or non-starch polysaccharides. Anim.Sci. 60, 325-335.

Boyd, R.D., B.D. Moser, E.R. Peo Jr. & P.J. Cunningham, 1978. Effect of energy source prior to parturition and during lactation on piglet survival and growth and on milk lipids. J. Anim. Sci. 47, 883-892.

Boyd, R.D., B.D. Moser, E.R. Peo Jr., A.J. Lewis & R.K. Johnson, 1982. Effect of tallow and choline chloride addition to the diet of sows on milk composition, milk yield and preweaning pig performance. J. Anim. Sci. 54, 1-7.

Coffey, M.T., R.W. Seerley & J.W. Mabry, 1982. The effect of source of supplemental dietary energy on sow milk yield, milk composition and litter performance. J. Anim. Sci. 55, 1388-1394.

Coffey, M.T., B.G. Diggs, D.L. Handlin, D.A. Knabe, C.V. Maxwell Jr., P.R. Noland, T.J. Prince & G.L. Cromwell, 1994. Effects of dietary energy during gestation and lactation on reproductive performance of sows: A cooperative study. J.Anim.Sci. 72, 4-9.

Cox, N.M., J.H. Britt, W.D. Armstrong & H.D. Alhusen, 1983. Effect of feeding fat and altering weaning schedule on rebreeding in primiparous sows. J. Anim. Sci. 56, 21-29.

Cunnane, S., 1984. Essential fatty-acid/mineral interactions with reference to the pig. In: J.Wiseman (Ed) Fats in Animal Nutrition. pp. 167-183. Butterworths, London.

Drochner, W., 1989. Einflüsse von Fettzulagen an Sauen auf Aufzuchtleistung und Fruchtbarkeit [in German]. Übers. Tierernähr. 17, 99-138.

Freeman, C.P., 1984. The digestion, absorption and transport of fats. Non-ruminants. In: J. Wiseman (ed.). Fats in Animal Nutrition. pp. 105-122. Butterworths, London.

Freeman, C.P., D.W. Holme & E.F. Annison, 1968. The determination of the true digestibilities of interesterified fats in young pigs. Brt. J. Nutr. 22, 651-660.

Friend, D.W., 1974. Effect on the performance of pigs from birth to market weight of adding fat to the lactation diet of their dams. J. Anim. Sci. 39, 1073-1081.

Hartmann, P.E. & M.A. Holmes, 1989. Sow lactation. In: J.L. Barnett & D.P. Hennessy (Eds) Manipulating Pig Production II. pp. 72-97. Australasian Pig Science Association. Werribee, Victoria, Australia.

Hartog, L.A. den, M.W.A. Verstegen, H.A.T.M. Hermans, G.J. Noordewier & G.J.M. van Kempen, 1984. Some factors associated with determination of milk production in sows by weighing of piglets. J.Anim.Phys.Anim.Nutr. 51, 148-157.

Hartog, ,L.A. den, H. Boer, M.W. Bosch, G.J. Klaassen & H.A.M. van der Steen, 1987. The effect of feeding level, stage of lactation and method of milk sampling on the composition of milk (fat) in sows. J.Anim.Phys.Anim.Nutr. 58, 253-261.

Jensen, L.S., G.W. Schumaier & J.D. Latshaw, 1970. 'Extra caloric' effect of dietary fat for developing turkeys as influenced by calorie-protein ratio. Poul. Sci. 49, 1697-1704.

Lellis, W.A. & V.C. Speer, 1983. Nutrient balance of lactating sows fed supplemental tallow. J. Anim. Sci. 56, 1334-1339.

Lewis, A.J., V.C. Speer & D.G. Haught, 1978, Relationship between yield and composition of sows' milk and weight gains of nursing pigs. J.Anim.Sci. 47, 634-638.

McDougall, I.A., 1977. Dietary protein and amino-acid requirements for the lactating sow. PhD thesis. University of Aberdeen, Scotland.

Miller, G.M., J.H. Conrad & R.B. Harrington, 1971. Effect of dietary unsaturated fatty acids and stage of lactation on milk composition and adipose tissue in swine. J. Anim. Sci. 32, 79-83.

Moser, B.D., 1983. The use of fat in sow diets. In: Haresign, W. (ed.). Recent Advances in Animal Nutrition. pp. 71-80. Butterworths, London.

Moser, B.D. & A.J. Lewis, 1980. Adding fat to sow diets. An update. Feedstuffs 52, 36-62.
Nelssen, J.L., A.J. Lewis, E.R. Peo, Jr. & B.D. Moser, 1985. Effect of source of dietary energy and energy restriction during lactation on sow and litter performance. J. Anim. Sci. 60, 171-178.
Pallauf, J. & J. Huter, 1993. Studies on the influence of calcium formate on growth, digestibility of crude nutrients, nitrogen balance and calcium retention in weaned piglets. Anim.Feed.Sci.Techn. 43, 65-76.
Pettigrew, J.E. Jr, 1981. Supplemental dietary fat for peripartal sows: a review. J. Anim. Sci. 53, 107-117.
Pettigrew, J.E. Jr., A.F.Sower, S.G. Cornelius & R.L. Moser, 1985. A comparison of isotope dilution and weigh-suckle-weigh methods for estimating milk intake by pigs. Can.J.Anim.sci. 65, 989-992.
Pettigrew, J.E. Jr., M.D. Tokach, M. Overland & R.L. Moser, 1989. Use of supplemental fat in swine diets explored. Feedstuffs 61, 18-28.
Pettigrew, J.E. Jr. & R.L. Moser, 1991. Fat in swine nutrition. In: E.R.Miller, D.E. Ullrey & A.J.Lewis (Eds) Swine Nutrition. pp. 133-146. Butterworth-Heinemann.
Scheele, C.W., 1981, Mengvoeder samenstelling en mengvoeder benutting [in Dutch]. Plumveehouderij 36, 20-21.
Schoenherr, W.D., T.S. Stahly & G.L. Cromwell, 1987. The effects of dietary fat and fiber addition on yield and composition of milk from sows housed in a warm or hot environment. J. Anim. Sci. 65, 318. (Abstract).
Schoenherr, W.D., T.S. Stahly & G.L. Cromwell, 1989. The effects of dietary fat or fiber addition on yield and composition of milk from sows housed in a warm or hot environment. J. Anim. Sci. 67, 482-495.
Seerley, R.W., 1981. High fat rations for sows can benefit piglets. Feedstuffs 53, 34-41.
Seerley, R.W., 1984. The use of fat in sow diets. In: J. Wiseman (Ed) *Fats in Animal Nutrition*. pp. 333-352. Butterworths, London.
Seerley, R.W., F.M. Griffin & H.C. McCampbell, 1978a. Effect of sow's dietary energy source on sow's milk and piglet carcass composition. J. Anim. Sci. 46, 1009-1017.
Seerley, R.W., J.S. Maxwell & H.C. McCampbell, 1978b. A comparison of energy sources for sows and subsequent effect on piglets. J. Anim. Sci. 47, 1114-1120.
Seerley, R.W., T.A. Pace, C.W. Foley & R.D. Scarth, 1974. Effect of energy intake prior to parturition on milk lipids and survival rate, thermostability and carcass composition of piglets. J. Anim. Sci. 38, 64-70.
Seerley, R.W., R.A. Snyder & H.C. McCampbell, 1981. The influence of sow dietary lipids and choline on piglet survival, milk and carcass composition. J. Anim. Sci. 52, 542-550.
Shurson, G.C., M.G. Hogberg, N. DeFever, S.V. Radecki & E.R. Miller, 1986. Effects of adding fat to the sow lactation diet on lactation and rebreeding performance. J. Anim. Sci. 62, 672-680.
Shurson, G.C. & K.M. Irvin, 1992. Effects of genetic line and supplemental dietary fat on lactation performance of Duroc & Landrace sows. J.Anim.Sci. 70, 2942-2949.
Stahly, T.S., 1984. Use of fats in diets for growing pigs. In: J. Wiseman (Ed) Fats in Animal Nutrition. pp. 313-331. Butterworths, London.
Vermeersch, G. & F. Vanschoubroek, 1968. The quantification of the effect of increasing levels of various fats on body weight gain, efficiency of food conversion and food intake of growing chicks. Brt. Poul. Sci. 9, 13-30.
Wiseman, J., 1989. Fatty acids in pig nutrition. In: Fatty Acids in Animal Nutrition. Proc. Am. Soybean Ass. 41-56.

9 Nutritional effects during lactation and during the interval from weaning to oestrus

I. H. Williams

9.1 Introduction

Reducing the interval from weaning to oestrus is probably the single most important challenge that remains to improve the reproductive efficiency of domestic animals, including pigs (Robinson, 1990). Sows are usually anoestrous during lactation but generally return to oestrus within 10 days of weaning. Because this interval represents a relatively small fraction of the 150-day reproductive cycle (which includes both pregnancy and lactation), its importance is often over looked. Why then is the interval from weaning to oestrus so important? Can its effect on reproductive efficiency be adequately quantified? Does nutrition control this interval in any way and, if so, by what means? This review will focus on these important questions and attempt to resolve them. It will also explore ways to manipulate the weaning-to-oestrous interval particularly by nutritional management during lactation.

9.2 How important is the interval from weaning to oestrus?

The major objective in managing the breeding herd is to maximise the number of pigs weaned per litter and the number of litters produced per sow per year. It is the latter that is strongly influenced by the interval from weaning to oestrus through its effects on the so called 'non-productive days'. Non-productive days are those days when the sow is neither pregnant nor lactating and they include, i) the interval from weaning to effective service between successive litters, ii) the time from when the gilt enters the herd until she becomes pregnant, and iii) the time when the sow is weaned of her last litter until the day she is culled and removed from the herd.

What impact can a change in the interval from weaning to oestrus have on the productivity of a piggery? Using the computer simulation model, AUSPIG, Black *et al.* (1996) estimated that a reduction in the interval from weaning to oestrus from 10 down to 5 days would increase the profit of a 250-sow piggery by some 6%.

But the AUSPIG model is not yet sophisticated enough to take account of all of the effects that accompany a change in the interval from weaning to oestrus. As the interval becomes longer, the conception rate is likely to fall and there is an increase in the number of sows that fail to exhibit oestrus. This leads to an increase in the number of culled sows and an increase in replacement rate which in turn has a large effect on the number of non-productive days. For example, the herd target in a well-managed piggery might be 20 non-productive days per sow. Half this (10 days) is due to gilt entry into the herd, that is, the time from herd entry until the time she becomes pregnant. A quarter (5 days) might be made up of the interval from weaning to mating and the balance (5 days) might accrue because of conception failure (1.9 days), abortions (0.6 days), sows that do not farrow (1.1 days) and sow deaths (1.2 days). Hence, an increase in the weaning-to-oestrous interval affects the number of non-productive days not only because the farrowing interval is increased, but also because of a reduced conception and an increased replacement rate. Thus the profit increase calculated by Black *et al.* (1996) for reducing the interval from weaning to oestrus by five days might have been considerably more, perhaps double, if all the associated changes listed above had been considered. Vesseur *et al.* (1996) have highlighted these associated effects and have suggested that concentrating on this one factor, interval from weaning to oestrus, might lead to an overall improvement in reproductive performance. As they have so rightly pointed out the expected gain from keeping a primiparous sow is always higher than the expected gain from a replacement gilt.

9.3 Historical perspective

In the early 1980s, post-weaning anoestrus became recognised as a major problem in pig herds in Europe (Karlberg, 1980), North America (Hurtgen *et al.*, 1980) and Australia (King *et al.*, 1982). These studies showed that 20% of multiparous sows failed to exhibit oestrus within a week of weaning, but worse, the figure for first-litter sows often approached 50%. At first, nutrition was not considered to be a cause because earlier work by Elsley *et al, (*1969) and O'Grady *et al.* (1973) had shown that nutrition was not a factor in delayed return to oestrus after weaning. However, Fahmy (1981) later suggested that feeding and management of sows during lactation was important in determining the length of the post-weaning anoestrus, particularly in young sows.

The North Americans were among the first to demonstrate that nutrition played a major role in the interval from weaning to oestrus. In three experiments Reese *et al.* (1982) manipulated the food intake of sows during lactation and demonstrated that restriction of food intake during lactation extended the interval from weaning to oestrus. They offered first-litter sows high levels of energy (71 MJ DE per day) during lactation and consistently found that a high proportion of sows returned to oestrus within 7 days (94, 96 and 96% in experiments 1, 2 and 3). When energy intake was halved (35 MJ DE per d) the proportion of sows returning was only 50, 71 and 65%. High intakes of energy were associated with maintenance or only minor losses of liveweight and back fat while sows whose energy was restricted to half (35 MJ DE per day) lost large amounts of bodyweight and back fat (Table 9.1).

Table 9.1. The effect of energy intake in lactation on the changes in liveweight and back fat during lactation and the proportion of first-litter sows in oestrus after weaning

		Low	Medium	High
Energy intake (MJ of DE/day)		34.8		70.5
Experiment 1				
Lactation change	liveweight (kg)	-20.8		-0.6
	backfat (mm)	-7.5		-1.6
Sows in oestrus within 7 days of weaning (%)		50		94
Experiment 2				
Lactation change	liveweight (kg)	-18.0		0.6
	backfat (mm)	-4.4		-0.5
Sows in oestrus within 7 days of weaning (%)		71		96
Experiment 3				
Lactation change	liveweight (kg)	-25.7	-13.3	-3.3
	backfat (mm)	-8.4	-4.6	-1.8
Sows in oestrus within 7 days of weaning (%)		65	91	96

Studies in Australia paralleled the North American work and it was concluded that, if food intake was restricted during lactation, sows remained anoestrus after weaning for longer. King (1987) reviewed this work and used regression analysis to quantify the influence of several nutritional parameters on post-partum anoestrus. Parameters included the intake of protein and energy during lactation, the losses of liveweight, protein or fat during lactation, and the absolute bodyweight and mass of protein or mass of fat at weaning. He concluded that the reserves of body protein (as indicated by either the absolute amount of protein at weaning shown in Figure 9.1(a), or the protein loss during lactation shown in Figure 9.1(b)) were the best indicators of the length of the interval from weaning to oestrus in first-litter sows. The corollary of this is that if a first-litter sow loses no more that one kilogram of protein during lactation and has between 19 to 20 kg of body protein at weaning, she will return early, that is she will exhibit oestrus within 10 to 15 days of weaning. Other parameters such as fat or body weight loss, or live weight or fat weight at weaning were of lesser importance than measures of protein reserves, in predicting the interval.

Workers in the United Kingdom (Yang *et al.*, 1989) also reached similar conclusions to the North Americans and Australians. They fed sows to different target bodyweights and different levels of fat at the start of lactation, and then offered different amounts of feed during lactation. They also developed prediction equations, which were similar to those of King (1987), for the interval from

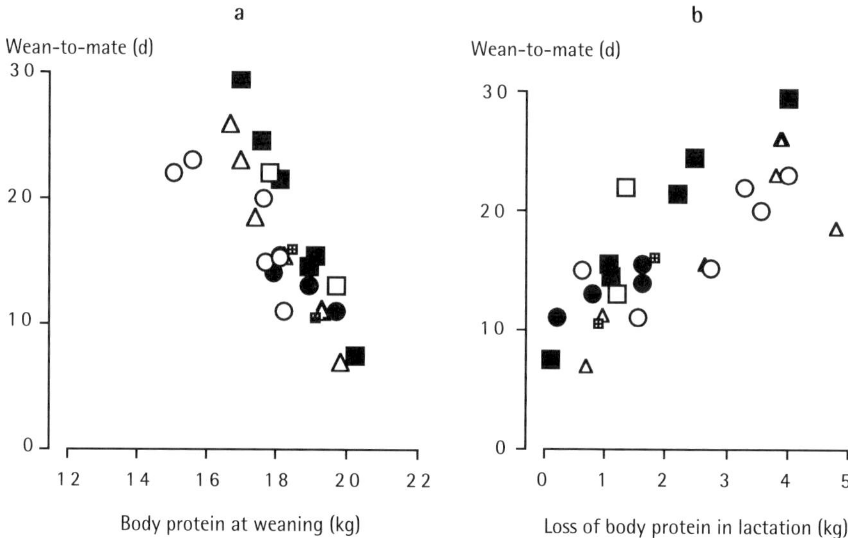

Figure 9.1. Body protein at weaning (a) and loss of body protein during lactation (b) verses the interval from weaning to oestrus in first-litter sows. Data compiled from King and Williams (1984a) (Δ), (1984b) (▲), King et al (1984) (⊞), King and Dunkin (1986a) (■) (1986b) (□), King and Dunkin (1986) (unpublished) (●), Mullan and Williams (1989) (○).

weaning to oestrus based on liveweight and back fat at weaning, and food intake during lactation.

In summary, post-weaning anoestrus particularly in first-litter sows became recognised as a major problem throughout the world in the early 1980s and, by the end of the decade, there was unequivocal evidence that nutrition during lactation had a major influence. This raised two major questions. First, why did post-weaning anoestrus become a problem of worldwide interest in the early 1980s? Second, why was nutrition implicated as a major cause when previous experiments conducted in the sixties and seventies rarely implicated nutrition as a major factor? The main reason is that the genotype of the animal has changed in the last 20 years but that management, particularly nutrition, which is appropriate for these newer hybrids has lagged behind (Whittemore, 1996). These questions will be addressed below.

9.4 Modern genotypes

Current genotypes differ from those of 20 years ago because quantitative genetics has been applied by large breeding companies to achieve lean pigs. While the conclusions in the early literature (Elsley *et al.*, 1969; O'Grady *et al.*, 1973) were unequivocal that nutrition played no role in reproduction, it is now accepted that nutrition plays a major role in reproduction. The effects of nutrition are most obvious in sows in their first reproductive cycle but are still evident although much reduced in the second cycle (Vesseur *et al.*, 1996). Mature sows show little response in reproduction traits to nutrition (Hughes, 1993).

The 1970s was a period of rapid change in the pig industry with consumers in many countries demanding less fat and more lean in meat. The pig industry responded by selecting its breeding animals for low backfat and thus the genotype of animals changed. By the early 1980s sow herds in many countries had been upgraded with improved hybrids that had been selected primarily for reduced back fat.

Selection for lower back fat probably changed animals in at least two ways. First, animals that were selected for lower back fat became bigger. If animals of larger mature body size are compared at the same live weight with smaller animals, they will be leaner simply because they are at a lower proportion of their mature body size and, hence, are physiologically younger than the smaller animals. Accordingly, they will have less fat.

The second and perhaps more subtle response to selection was that voluntary food intake (VFI) of selected animals may have been reduced. Many of the older genotypes consumed excess energy, well above that required for maximum protein synthesis. Hodge (1974), working with an old genotype in Australia, showed that pigs were capable of consuming very large amounts of energy even when they were young. For example, he showed that pigs that were 8 weeks of age and weighed 32 kg liveweight would consume approximately 20% more energy than was required for maximum protein deposition. This extra energy would be deposited as fat. So, any reduction in food intake of these animals would have a significant impact on reducing body fat. There is little doubt that selection for leanness (reduced back fat) can reduce the appetite of pigs (Smith & Fowler, 1978; Ellis *et al.*, 1979; Ellis *et al.*, 1983; Smith *et al.*, 1991). The reduction in VFI in response to a selection index for growth performance and back fat thickness under *ad libitum* feeding has been most clearly demonstrated by Smith *et al.* (1991) who, over an 11-year selection period, showed a reduced VFI for both boars and gilts over the live weight range of 30 to 90 kg. The VFI of 'selected' gilts was similar to that of control boars at 30 kg but then began to diverge so that by 90 kg, they consumed 13% less than the control boars.

Returning to the second question as to why nutrition is implicated as a major cause of delayed return to oestrus after weaning, this is because these newer hybrids are more prone to nutritional stress particularly during lactation. They are more prone than the earlier genotypes because, i) they begin lactation with less body reserves, ii) they have higher maintenance requirements, iii) they probably produce more milk and, iv) they eat less food. These newer hybrids are bigger animals and if they are mated at a similar body weight to their smaller, traditional counterparts they begin their reproductive life when they are physiologically younger. This means that they have less fat and more lean. When the proportion of lean increases, their maintenance requirements are also increased (Campbell & Taverner, 1988; McCracken, 1993). The energy needed for maintenance is proportional to protein turnover which, in turn, is proportional to the weight of protein at any given body weight (Emmans & Kyriazakis, 1989). Therefore, compared to traditional genotypes that are closer to their mature body size, these younger animals have i) higher maintenance requirements because they are leaner, ii) higher growth requirements because they are at a lower proportion of their mature body size, and iii) less of their own body reserves to channel away from their own maternal growth to support reproduction. Hence these new hybrids are more prone to nutritional stress than their traditional counterparts and it is the younger animals, the first-litter sows, that are most susceptable to undernutrition.

In parallel with the changes in genotypes driven by a demand for leaner meat were the attempts to increase reproductive efficiency by the stimulation of gilts to exhibit puberty early (Brooks & Cole 1974; Hughes, 1975). Whittemore (1996) highlighted the irony of inducing early puberty in these modern hybrids thus compounding the nutritional problem of animals beginning their reproductive life too early. He went further and suggested that research aimed at determining the nutrient requirements of these newer hybrids was progressing too slowly because it was often conducted on genotypes that were no longer relevant to industry. Whittemore himself overcame the problem by studying hybrid gilts (see Yang *et al.*, 1989). F.X. Aherne at the University of Alberta began an arrangement with a breeding company in the early 1980s to provide all the University Farm's replacement gilts and many others around the world have followed this lead as a means of keeping their experimental genotypes up to date.

In summary, modern genotypes are physiologically younger when they begin to breed, they enter lactation with less body reserves (fat and protein), they produce more milk and have a lower feed intake than their counterparts of 25 years ago.

9.5 Voluntary food intake in lactation

Any increase in voluntary food intake (VFI) during lactation is likely to reduce the interval between weaning and oestrus particularly for young sows that are suckling their first litter. This is a corollary of the close relationship between the interval from weaning to oestrus and weight loss in lactation (Figure 9.2) and the direct influence that food intake has on weight loss; the more the sow eats in lactation the less weight she is likely to lose.

Many factors influence VFI during lactation. They can be grouped for convenience under three main headings although some of them are interactive because they regulate food intake through similar mechanisms.

i) Animal factors:
- genetics
- parity, litter size, length and stage of lactation
- body weight and body composition

ii) Environmental:
- thermal (temperature, stock density, wind speed, humidity, insulation, radiation, evaporative cooling)
- photoperiod and disease

iii) Dietary factors:
- digestibility and energy density
- protein and amino acid balance
- physical characteristics (particle size, mash, pellets)
- feeder design, feeding frequency

Some of these factors can be manipulated by pig producers to increase VFI. For example, it is well established that VFI during lactation will be reduced if feed intake and live weight gains during pregnancy are high or if the protein content of the diets offered during either pregnancy or lactation is low. Other dietary factors can also be used to increase VFI during lactation, for example, increasing the energy density of diets and altering the form of the diets (wet versus dry, and pellets versus mash). Since many of these factors have been well covered in other reviews (O'Grady *et al.* 1985; Moser, 1985; Cole, 1990; Lynch, 1989) this review will only concentrate on areas which have received less attention or where there is newer information.

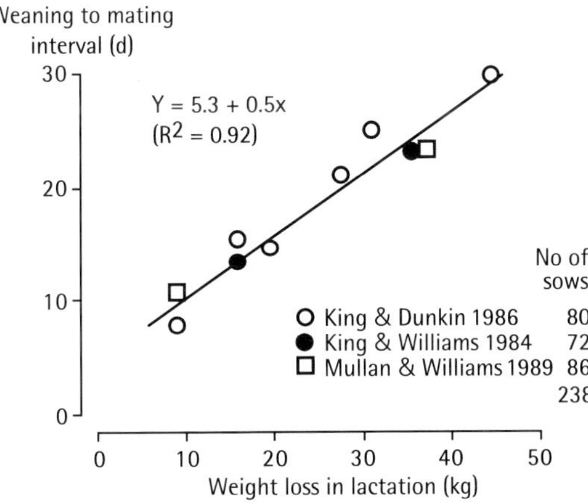

Figure 9.2. Interval from weaning to mating and weight loss in lactation for first-litter sows

9.5.1 Ambient temperature and voluntary food intake

Temperature has a large effect on food intake with low temperatures stimulating food intake and high temperatures reducing food intake. The response of animals to changes in ambient temperature is now well understood through the work of several people (L.E. Mount, C.W. Holmes, M.W.A. Verstegen, W.H. Close, L.R. Giles, B.P. Mullan and J.L. Black) but it is an area that many pig producers do not appreciate and hence the principles that are now well established are not always applied.

When ambient temperature falls below the zone of thermal comfort (i.e. below the lower critical temperature) the animal has to increase its heat production to maintain body temperature. As it does so, its food intake increases but the increase is generally insufficient to balance the extra heat lost so that the energy available for production is decreased. When air temperature rises above the lower critical temperature the animal maintains its body temperature and increases its heat loss by simple mechanisms (it stops huddling, it changes its posture to allow more contact with cooler surfaces, its peripheral blood supply is increased) that require little effort. With further increases in air temperature above the evaporative critical temperature, the pig can only control its body temperature by increasing heat loss through evaporation, mainly through the lungs, or by reducing its heat production by eating less (Figure 9.3). Reductions in VFI in response

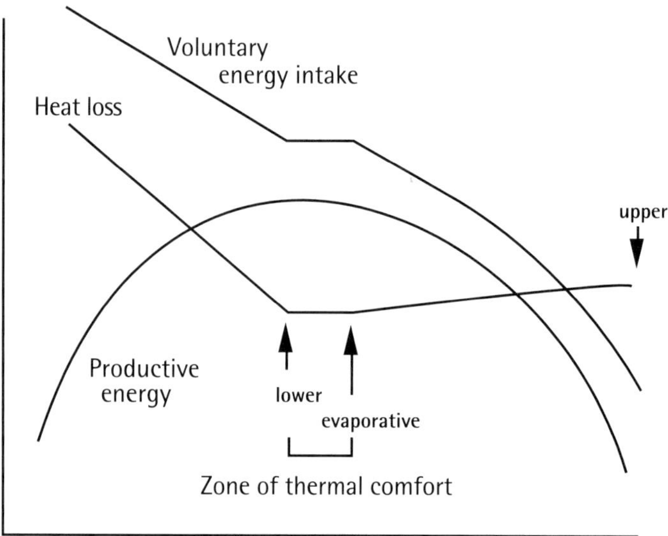

Figure 9.3. The influence of ambient (air) temperature on heat loss, voluntary energy intake and productive energy. (critical temperatures are shown in bold)

to heat stress can be very significant. For example, Giles & Black (1991) reduced the VFI of sows from 2.8 down to 0.9 kg/day when they increased ambient temperature from 22.7° to 31.4°C in pigs weighing 90 kg. In lactating sows, raising the air temperature from 18° to 28°C reduced voluntary food intake by 40% and milk output by 25% (Black *et al.*, 1993). For the most efficient production (i.e. maximum productive energy), the pig must be kept within its zone of thermal comfort somewhere between the lower and evaporative critical temperatures. The lower critical temperature and zone of thermal comfort are not constant but vary with a host of factors including skin wetness, air movement, relative humidity and the amount and composition of the diet all of which interact with ambient temperature to determine the extent of heat loss.

What is often not appreciated is that the zone of thermal comfort for sows in lactation may be a relatively narrow band of air temperatures (the ranges may be around 3° to 4°C), which indicates that the air temperature in the farrowing house must be closely controlled if the sow's productive energy is to be at a maximum. Another principle that is poorly understood is the very different needs of the sow and her piglets; the zone of thermal comfort for the piglets is often at least 10°C higher than that for the sow. The design of many modern farrowing houses with open creep areas often fails to accommodate the needs of both the sow and piglets and this often results in cold stress for the piglets while the sow suffers heat stress. This was demonstrated recently by Ranford and Mullan (personal communication) who measured the food intake of sows and growth rates of piglets in a commercial piggery without covered creeps. The animals were moved to a controlled environment where air temperature for the sow was maintained below 25°C and piglets were given fully-insulated creep boxes with curtains (30-35°C). The food intake of the sows increased by 1 kg in the second week of lactation (5.8 to 6.7 kg) and by an average of 0.6 kg over the whole of a three-week lactation and piglet growth increased by 30% from 178 to 228 g/d.

Controlled environments are often expensive to run and there are other ways, often less successful, of coping with heat stress in the sow and increasing her VFI. The animal's heat production can be decreased by decreasing the fibre and/or increasing the fat content of diets. Alternatively, the animal's heat loss can be increased and VFI stimulated by allowing the sow to increase the area of wet skin and, thereby, increase evaporative heat loss (McGlone *et al.*, 1988).

High air temperatures above the evaporative critical temperature not only reduce food intake but also reduce milk output. This reduction in milk output is more than would be expected from an equivalent decline in food intake for sows kept within the zone of thermal comfort (Black *et al.*, 1993). Why is this so? It seems that a heat stress induces blood to flow away from tissues like the mammary gland towards the skin.

Thus the effect of high temperature is both a reduction in food intake which will lead to a greater weight loss and a reduction in subsequent fertility. Coupled with this reduction in energy intake is an even greater reduction in the energy which ends up in milk.

9.5.2 Prior nutrition and body composition

It is now well established that the more a sow eats in pregnancy, the less she will eat in lactation. The data from Mullan & Williams (1989) presented below (Figure 9.4a) show this relationship. In their experiment they began with gilts of the same body weight and age at mating and fed them different amounts of food during pregnancy. They offered a high-protein diet ad libitum during lactation and found that VFI in lactation was depressed with high food intakes in pregnancy; a relationship that has been previously demonstrated. Why it happens is not known but there are several possibilities that may be linked to body reserves of fat and protein.

The gilts which eat more in pregnancy grow faster and are both heavier and fatter at the start of lactation. The importance of body weight and body fat at parturition on VFI in lactation has been studied by Williams and Smits (1991) who manipulated the rates of fat and lean gain during pregnancy by altering the dietary intakes of protein and energy. Some gilts weighed either 150 or 160 kg immediately after farrowing and, within each of these body weights, there were animals which differed in body composition. Body weight had a very small effect on food intake but the amount of body fat had a large effect. The conclusion made was that high body fat at farrowing is associated with low VFI during lactation (Figure 9.4b).

It is worth considering the mechanisms that might explain why fat animals eat less than lean ones. If control points could then be identified, it might be possible to manipulate these mechanisms to increase the VFI of sows during lactation. Firstly, the sow may use the rate of fat metabolism to monitor and regulate its energy status and hence VFI. The greater the amount of fat in the body the higher its turnover and the greater the release of fatty acids and glycerol into the blood stream. The concentration of these substrates or their extent of oxidation may act as signals that could be read by the liver and sent to the brain via vagal nerves. For example, Scharrer & Langhans (1986) increased the VFI of rats by inhibiting fatty acid oxidation in the liver and Wirtshafter & Davis (1977) reduced VFI by infusing glycerol into the blood stream. However, more recently Revell and Williams (1995, unpublished data) have recently infused glycerol into growing pigs without any effect on VFI.

An alternative mechanism which also involves measuring the animal's energy status may involve the hormone insulin. The suggestion here is that animals on

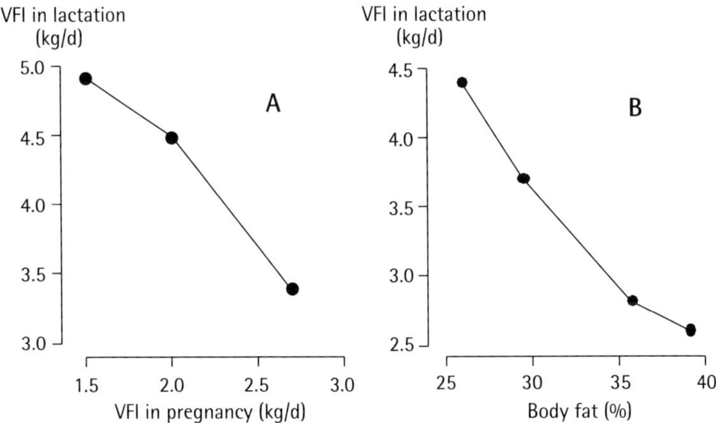

Figure 9.4 a. Voluntary food intake (VFI) in pregnancy and lactation for first-litter sows (from Mullan and Williams, 1989)
Figure 9.4 b. Body fat at parturition and voluntary food intake (VFI) during lactation for first-litter sows (from Williams and Smits, 1991)

higher food intakes (and hence ultimately fatter animals) have higher average levels of insulin in plasma. Higher levels of insulin in plasma would lead to higher levels in cerebral spinal fluid and this may act as a measure of accumulated energy intake. This is a difficult suggestion to support experimentally but there is some evidence that infusion of insulin into the brain reduces food intake. At present there is little scope to alter VFI through manipulation of insulin but controlling the oxidation of fatty acids by the liver may be a possibility.

The discovery of the hormone leptin provides another possible mechanism through which body fat might control food intake. Leptin is a protein that circulates in the blood stream and acts directly on the central nervous system to control food intake (Pelleymounter *et al.*, 1995). It is produced by the *obese* gene which itself is expressed only in fat tissue. The current hypothesis is that the more fat a sow accumulates the greater the expression of the *obese* gene in fat tissue and the greater the amount of circulating leptin, which in turn will act on the central nervous system to reduce food intake. Recently, pig leptin has been shown to be a potent inhibitor of food intake in gilts. Ramsay *et al.* (1997) administered pig leptin directly into the brain of gilts via an intracerebroventricular injection cannula and found that a single injection depressed food intake for 44 hours.

Another reason why fat sows eat less than lean sows is that they have a lower capacity to secrete energy in milk because they have fewer seceretory cells with which to make milk. The lowered capacity to use energy for milk production subsequently reduces VFI. Evidence for this comes from the slaughter of fat and lean (36 and 25 mm back fat) gilts at parturition where it has been demonstrated that, although fat animals have the same weight of mammary tissue, they have only half the number of milk secretory cells as the lean gilts (see Table 9.2).

Table 9.2. Number of secretory (alveolar) cells at 112 days of gestation in fat and lean gilts (from Head et al., 1991)

	Lean	Fat
Back fat (mm)	25	36
Mammary tissue (%)[1]		
Alveolar wall	39	40
Alveolar lumen	32	37
Adipose tissue	15	13
Connective tissue	14	10
Number of secretory cells (million/g mammary tissue)	141	70

[1] Proportional volumes of different tissues determined by counting cells.

Supply of endogenous substrates is another possibility as to why fatter animals may eat less than lean ones and, as with the previously discussed mechanism, this is linked to milk output and energy excretion. Fatter animals may have less body reserves, in particular protein, to supply endogenous substrates for milk production. If milk output is limited by the supply of endogenous amino acids then the capacity of the animal to use energy is limited and this, in turn, would limit food intake. Mahan & Mangan (1975) fed gilts during pregnancy on diets containing either 9, 13, or 18% crude protein and, provided they offered plenty of dietary protein (18% crude protein) during lactation and relied mostly on dietary amino acids to supply milk protein, found no effect of the pregnancy treatments on VFI. However, when the dietary supply of protein during lactation was limited by offering a diet with only 12% crude protein, then protein supply in pregnancy had a large effect on VFI in lactation (Figure 9.5). One interpretation of this interaction is that low protein in pregnancy limits the maternal gain of protein which in turn limits the protein reserves of the gilt at farrowing and, hence, her capacity to supply endogenous amino acids for milk.

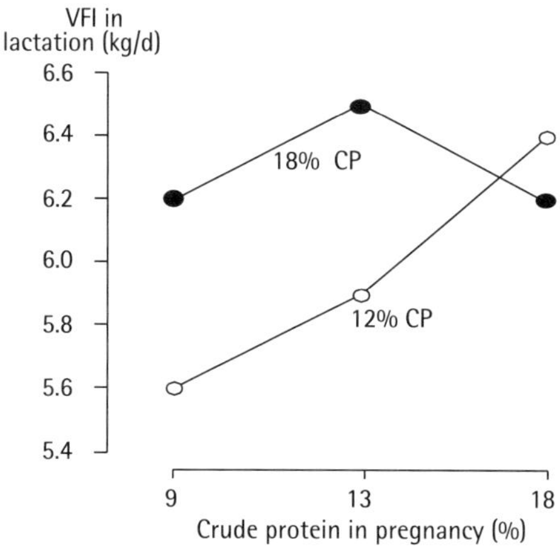

Figure 9.5. Voluntary food intake (VFI) of lactating sows fed either 12 or 18% crude protein after they received either 9, 13 or 17% crude protein during pregnancy (Mahan and Mangan, 1975)

9.5.3 Frequency of feeding and pattern of food intake

There is a commonly held opinion that animals, particularly lactating sows, will eat more if offered food more frequently than once each day. In a coordinated trial conducted at four research stations in the United States (NCR-89 1990) lactating sows ate the same amount of food irrespective of whether they were fed once or three times each day (Figure 9.6).

Weaver & Aherne (1993) have pointed out that offering food to sows two or three times each day does not mimic a free-choice situation and that sows may want to feed much more frequently. They fed lactating sows 24 times per day and compared this to feeding twice each day. Surprisingly, frequent feeding reduced daily food intake by 15% (7.2 versus 6.1 kg/day) but their data suggest that there is a diurnal pattern in food intake and that sows prefer to eat more at certain times of the day. If prevented from eating at these 'high-intake' times, which seem to be in the morning and the late afternoon, sows will not compensate by eating more at other times even when food is freely available. There is a need to identify exactly when these 'high-intake' times occur and what controls them so that feeding regimens can be designed which will maximise VFI.

9.5.4 Pattern of VFI thoughout lactation and interval from weaning to oestrus

As already pointed there is now unequivocal evidence that modern genotypes are prone to nutritional stress. The discussion above has focused on ways to increase the average VFI throughout the whole of lactation. However it is worth considering whether there might be specific times in lactation where food intake might have the greatest effect on reproductive performance. Most people, as Quesnel & Prunier (1995) have done, hypothesise that the nutritional deficit becomes relatively more important during the third and fourth weeks of lactation. It follows, that nutrition later in lactation is likely to have more influence on the interval from weaning to oestrus than nutrition earlier in lactation. Recent work by Zak *et al.* (1997) would support this suggestion. LH secretion was completely suppressed by restricting the food intake of sows for the first 21 days of lactation and then normal levels resumed with *ad libitum* feeding during the fourth week. Other work suggests that nutrition earlier in lactation is just as important as nutrition later in lactation. Koketsu *et al.* (1996) manipulated feeding level in each week of a 3-week lactation and found that if food intake was restricted in any week, oestrus after weaning was delayed. Tokach *et al.* (1992) divided sows into those that returned early and those that returned late and found that there were differences in LH secretion as early as two weeks into lactation and differences in insulin at day 7 of lactation. This also supports the view that nutrition early in lactation may be just as important as nutrition later in lactation. Catabolism of maternal tissues often starts not just at the beginning of lactation but at day 90 or 100 of gestation depending on the level of food intake during gestation. Millar (1996) reasoned that if gilts were fed sufficient to prevent catabolism in late gestation they might be coaxed to eat higher amounts of energy in early lactation and thereby improve subsequent reproduction. But despite increasing the feed intake of gilts from 2.3 to 3.9 kg/day from day 100 of gestation until farrowing she was unable to demonstrate any effects on feed intake during lactation or interval from weaning to oestrus.

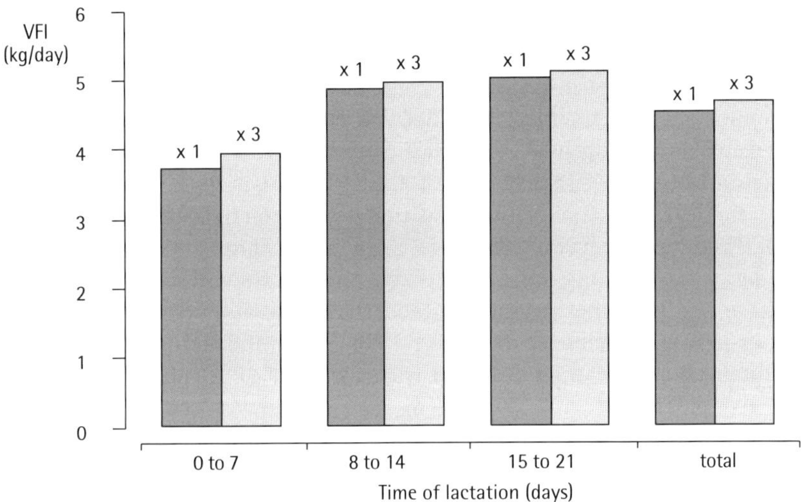

Figure 9.6. Voluntary food intake (VFI) of lactating sows fed either once (x1) or three times (x 3) per day. Adapted from (NCR-89 1990)

9.6 Nutritional control of reproduction

Nutrition during lactation has a major effect on reproduction particularly in young sows in their first reproductive cycle and the literature is full of experiments that support this view. However, most of these experiments are of an empirical nature, that is, nutrition has been altered in some way and the reproductive response measured either in terms of an outcome such as the interval from weaning to oestrus or some metabolite or hormone thought to be involved in the process. While empirical experiments are a necessary first step they need to be followed by investigations of the physiological mechanisms involved because, unless the underlying physiology is understood, reliable intervention and manipulation is generally unsuccessful.

9.6.1 Endocrinology and follicular growth

If a sow is to return to oestrus after weaning and commence another reproductive cycle she must have an ovary that is capable of both receiving and responding to the stimulus from the brain that will control the release of eggs for subsequent fertilisation. Hence there are two systems that must be competent and capable of communication with each other. Hormones are the means of communication; the ovary produces steroids and the hypothalamus induces the pituitary to produce and release gonadotrophins, luteinizing hormone (LH) and follicle stimulating hormone (FSH).

To produce eggs the ovary has to have follicles at the right stage of development, the pre-ovulatory stage, that can respond to the surge of LH that will lead to the release of eggs. However, follicles have to grow from the primordial stage to the pre-ovulatory stage and this development takes time and its control is complex. The most rapid stage of growth of the follicle is from antrum formation to the pre-ovulatory stage which for the pig is about 19 days (Morbeck *et al.*, 1992). Initial growth depends on gonadotrophins but this is followed by a stage when the growth of the follicle is responsive to, but not necessarily dependent on, gonadotrophins. There are many growth factors produced by the ovary itself that by paracrine and autocrine control seem more important than the gonadotrophins in determining whether the follicles reach the pre-ovulatory stage. Hunter *et al.* (1992) have discussed the roles that these growth factors might play in follicular growth. Epidermal growth factor and fibroblast growth factor are required together initially for growth of the antral follicle, followed by a need for follicle regulatory protein. As follicles continue to develop, insulin-like growth factor -1 (IGF-1) becomes important and might play a central role in determining which follicles remain dominant and subsequently produce an egg and which become atretic and die. Not only are these local growth factors important by themselves but it seems that they interact with oestradiol and FSH to control growth further. In sheep, when follicles change from being responsive to dependent on gonadotrophin and continue to grow larger than about 2.5 mm in diameter there is an absolute dependence on FSH which is higher than that in either the responsive stage or the pre-ovulatory stage (Scaramuzzi *et al.*, 1993). It is likely that this is the same in the pig. Luteinizing hormone is also required to produce the substrate that will form oestradiol. When luteolysis begins, FSH begins to decrease in concentration and LH becomes progressively more important. It builds up in concentration over several days until sufficient levels are reached to stimulate oestradiol production which, by positive feedback, induces the LH surge that causes ovulation.

As alluded to above the primary control of follicular growth is by the gonadotrophins, LH and FSH and the normal sequence of events for a sow in late pregnancy, early and late lactation and the period after weaning is as follows (Quesnel & Prunier, 1995). During pregnancy, progesterone from the ovary (the corpora lutea) and placenta depresses the output of gonadotrophin releasing hormone (GnRH), the hormone that stimulates the release of LH and FSH. LH is secreted in pulses from the pituitary gland in response to pulses of GnRH from the hypothalamus and, during late pregnancy, these pulses are very infrequent. However just after farrowing there is a burst of activity and the pulses of LH become very frequent so that the basal concentration of LH rises. Three or four days into lactation the release of LH is once again depressed and its concentration continues to decrease until day 14. Suckling stimulus is the main cause of this depression. The output of GnRH is suppressed by opioids released in response to suckling of the litter. Sucking stimulus decreases by the beginning of the third week and this allows the sow to begin to escape from this inhibition and so LH secretion increases. Pulses become more frequent and their amplitude increases. At weaning there is an increase in basal concentration of LH and pulses increase in frequency but may reduce in amplitude. For example Mullan *et al.* (1991) have shown that within 12 hours of weaning the number of LH pulses doubles (3 to 6 per 12 hours) and basal concentrations of LH more than doubles (0.2 to 0.5 ng/mL). This increase in LH continues for several days until there is sufficient LH to stimulate the ovary to release oestradiol which acts by positive feedback and stimulates the pituitary to release a massive surge of LH, the pre-ovulatory surge, which causes follicles to release eggs. Like LH, FSH is also controlled by GnRH but its release is continuous and not pulsatile (Scaramuzzi *et al.*, 1993).

9.6.2 Endocrinology of normal and prolonged intervals from weaning to oestrus

At parturition the sow has a population of healthy follicles which will die because the gonadotrophins that stimulate follicular growth are inhibited by the opioids released during suckling. As lactation proceeds, and the sow escapes from this inhibition, there is limited follicular growth but, while suckling continues, the sow remains anoestrus. Weaning allows an immediate increase in gonadotrophin output and, provided the ovary can produce oestradiol, the LH surge will cause ovulation. Therefore, oestrus after weaning might be prolonged either because of inadequate secretion of gonadotrophins or because follicular growth has been retarded for reasons connected to the ovary itself.

Whatever the reason for prolonged return to oestrus after weaning the secretion of LH in these sows is lower during lactation than in sows that return in the normal time (Quesnel & Prunier, 1995). LH rises after weaning whether or not sows have delayed returns to oestrus but the concentration of LH and its pulsatility are lower in those sows with delayed returns. For example, King & Martin (1989) prolonged the interval from weaning to oestrus from 7 to 19 days by restricting the protein intake of sows during lactation and found that the mean concentration of LH was reduced from 0.54 to 0.38 ng/mL for the 20 hours before weaning. Pulse frequency of LH was also less in the low-protein sows (0.8 verses 1.4 per 12 hours). After weaning LH concentration in the protein-adequate sows increased to 0.94 ng/mL (from 0.54). Levels in the sows fed low protein also increased but only to 0.74 ng/mL and the difference of 0.2 g/mL was still evident 7 days after weaning. Pulse frequency doubled (1.4 to 3.2 pulses/12 hours) after weaning in the protein-adequate sows and there was a similar increase in the sows fed low protein. As Quesnel & Prunier (1995) have pointed out it is often difficult to show significant differences. King & Martin (1989) used 6 sows per treatment. Mullan *et al.* (1991) used 7 sows per treatment and extended the interval between weaning and oestrus from 9 to 19 days by restricting food intake during lactation from *ad libitum* to 3 kg/day. The number of pulses per 12 hours before weaning was 1.7 for the restricted sows and 2.7 for the sows fed *ad libitum* and after weaning the pulses had increased to 3.2 and 6.1. None of these differences were statistically significant.

Besides reduced secretion of gonadotrophins in sows with extended intervals between weaning and mating, follicular growth may also be retarded such that the follicles do not respond properly to gonadotrophin. For example, Kirkwood *et al.* (1987) found low levels of oestradiol just after weaning in sows with extended intervals suggesting an abnormal response of follicles to LH stimulation. However, it is extremely difficult to distinguish whether delayed returns to oestrus are primarily due to a dysfunction at the hypothalamic or ovarian level or both. Scaramuzzi *et al.* (1993) have postulated that follicular growth might be dysfunctional in at least two ways. First, through increased exposure of follicles to FSH and, second, a direct effect whereby the follicles increase their sensitivity to gonadotrophins.

9.6.3 Nutritional cues for reproduction

Food intake

Luteinizing hormone is extremely responsive to food intake irrespective of whether animals are lactating or not; it is depressed by low intake and stimulated by high intake. Cosgrove *et al.* (1991) suppressed LH secretion in pre-pubertal gilts with a short period of maintenance feeding and then showed that it returned rapidly to normal levels on realimentation. Booth *et al.* (1996) have confirmed these findings. In lactating sows Koketsu *et al.* (1996) demonstrated reduced LH secretion (lower pulsatility) in first-litter sows that were restricted in any week of a 3-week lactation. Zak *et al.* (1997) suppressed LH secretion completely when they restricted the feed in gilts during the first 3 weeks of lactation but secretion was restored when the gilts were offered food ad libitum during the fourth week.

The same cannot be said for FSH because there is no consistent pattern between food intake and FSH levels in the blood (Quesnel & Prunier, 1995). In fact, Mullan *et al.* (1991) found that the highest levels of FSH both before and after weaning were in the sows which had the longest intervals from weaning to mating. Prunier *et al.* (1993) also found a negative relationship between levels of FSH before weaning and delayed oestrus after weaning. This does not necessarily mean that FSH is unimportant in the relationship between nutrition and reproduction but rather that the feedback relationships between follicular secretion and pituitary FSH are extremely dynamic (Scaramuzzi *et al.*, 1993)

From the relationships between nutrition and the gonadotrophins it is clear that the sow's food intake is monitored in some way and that the incoming nutrients (glucose, fatty acids, amino acids) are integrated with the body reserves. This information is then matched against the requirements for maintenance and growth, and reproduction is altered accordingly. There are two questions. First, are there certain metabolites and hormones that are crucial and, second, can they be manipulated to improve reproduction?

Components of the metabolic state

There have been several studies through which attempts have been made to relate the concentrations of metabolites and hormones during lactation to subsequent reproductive performance (Armstrong *et al.*, 1986; Mullan & Close, 1991; Tokach *et al.*, 1992; Prunier *et al.*, 1993; Zak *et al.*, 1997). One of the major problems is knowing when to take measurements of metabolites relative to the time of feeding. For example, as Quesnel & Prunier (1995) have shown the concentration of free fatty acids was about 1300 mmol/L just before feeding and 70 minutes later it was down to 200 mmol/L. Similar fluctuations were shown for glucose which was 3.5 mmol/L immediately before feeding but had doubled to 7.0 mmol/L 40 minutes later.

Tokach *et al.* (1992) overcame this obstacle by feeding first-litter sows every hour throughout a 28-day lactation. They separated their sows into two groups, those that returned early to oestrus after weaning (within 8 days) and those that returned late (after 15 days). In contrast to most of the other studies they could find no differences between the early and late returners in any of the plasma metabolites (glucose, triglycerides, non-esterified fatty acids, lysine, branch-chain amino acids and urea), at any stage of lactation. But they did find that the concentration of plasma insulin was elevated in the sows that returned to oestrus early. Following these and other studies Pettigrew & Tokach (1993) concluded that insulin and IGF-1 were the most likely candidates to connect nutrient intake to reproduction. They based this on correlations between the plasma concentration of the hormone or metabolite and the number of pulses of LH but they were also careful to point that their correlations were associations and not causal relationships. Mullan & Close (1991) also concluded that insulin might be the key player in the link between nutrition and reproduction after they manipulated the interval from weaning to oestrus by altering both nutrition and suckling stimulus. They induced first-litter sows to return early or late (11 versus 19 days) by changing both the energy intake of the sow (62 or 35 MJ ME/d) and/or the suckling stimulus with litters of either 6 or 12 piglets. Plasma insulin on day 10 and 17 of lactation in the early returners, that is, sows fed high energy (62 MJ ME/day) and with low suckling stimulus, was double that of the late returners which were restricted to a low-energy intake and a high intensity of suckling.

Glucose has been extensively studied as a candidate to link nutrition to reproduction because of its central role in metabolism and therefore energy balance. Mullan & Close (1991) found lower levels of glucose in first-litter sows with a delayed return to oestrus but the lower levels were only statistically significant at day 10 and not later in lactation. Prunier *et al.* (1993) found the opposite, sows returning later had the highest levels of glucose. Tokach *et al.* (1992) infused sows on day 18 of lactation with glucose and increased its concentration three fold but could not restore the frequency of LH pulses in those animals that had been restricted in energy. Glucose has been infused into sheep and successfully elevated the peripheral concentrations of both glucose and insulin but without any effect on LH concentrations (Boukhliq *et al.*, 1996). Cosgrove *et al.* (1997) has suggested that peripheral blood concentrations of glucose may be of limited relevance to the environment in the hypothalamus where the cells responsible for GnRH reside.

Other metabolites closely involved with energy balance are the free-fatty acids. They are the opposite to glucose in concentration and are high during lactation because they reflect tissue mobilisation (Quesnel & Prunier, 1995). As with glucose, loose associations can be shown between the level of free-fatty acids and delayed return to oestrus. Blood urea nitrogen can also be correlated with extended returns to oestrus (Brendemuhl *et al.*, 1987) but is it difficult to see this as anything but a marker for perhaps protein catabolism. However, Cosgrove *et al.* (1997) have suggested that if protein balance is a prime mediator of reproductive status individual amino acids might modulate GnRH and gonadotrophin secretion. They have listed a number of hypothetical pathways whereby amino acids could play a role and have suggested that such mechanisms should receive more research particularly as attention is focusing on the question of protein status of the sow and her reproduction.

As already discussed, sows must in some way monitor the dietary inputs and integrate them with body reserves to establish their energy balance. Animals do not possess receptors to measure energy *per se* (Jequier 1992) but controls for the balance of protein, carbohydrate and fat are known to exist (Flatt, 1988; Friedman *et al.,* 1986). Bray (1991) has suggested the following concepts for a regulatory system for nutrient balance; i) each major nutrient is regulated separately, ii) net oxidation of each nutrient is in proportion to the amount of nutrient in the diet, and iii) the regulation of nutrient stores is subject to positive and negative feedback signals that operate through the central nervous system. If these concepts are accepted is it difficult to see how a single metabolite can control reproduction.

Current consensus seems to be that circulating levels of energy metabolites have little direct role in regulating reproduction. Attention has now turned towards several metabolic hormones as the key players in the regulation of reproduction. Insulin reduces milk production (Goldobin 1976) and might improve energy balance. Exogenous insulin increases the pulse frequency of LH (Cox *et al.,* 1987). Most of the evidence is circumstantial and is derived from association. For example, Mullan & Close (1991) and Zak *et al.* (1997) found reduced insulin in sows that were restricted in food intake during lactation and showed a delayed return to oestrus. Other evidence in support of metabolic hormones playing a key role in reproduction come from *in vitro* studies and in two recent reviews by Pettigrew & Tokach (1993) and Cosgrove *et al.* (1997) a number of possibilities have been put forward. These include the presence of insulin receptors in the hypothalamus, the pituitary and the ovary. Insulin increases LH and FSH output and, in the ovary, it increases the binding of IGF-1, increases the uptake of amino acids, and promotes steroid metabolism. Likewise, there are receptors for IGF-1 in the hypothalamus, pituitary and ovary. In the ovary IGF-1 seems important but its role in the hypothalamus for secretion of GnRH is completely unknown. Cosgrove *et al.* (1997) have pointed out that IGF-1 responds much more slowly than either insulin or LH to changes in feeding.

In summary it seems that the metabolic hormones, insulin and IGF-1, are the most likely candidates for key roles in the regulation of reproduction and that the metabolites themselves are very much secondary. However direct evidence is limited.

9.7 References

Armstrong, J.D., Britt, J.H. & Kraeling, R.R., 1986. Effect of restriction of energy during lactation on body condition, energy metabolism, endocrine changes and reproductive performance in primiparous sows J. Anim. Sci. 63: 1915-1925.

Black, J.L., Davies, G.T. & Bradley, L.R., 1994. Future Needs in Swine Research. In Livestock Production for the 21 st Century: Priorities and Research Needs. pp. 229-249. (Ed. P.A. Thacker). Saskatoon, University of Saskatchewan.

Black, J.L., Mullan, B.P., Lorschy, M.L. & Giles, L.R., 1993. Lactation in sows during heat stress Livestock Prod. Sci. 35: 153-170.
Booth, P.J., Cosgrove, J.R. & Foxcroft, G.R., 1996. Endocrine and metabolic responses to realimentation in feed-restricted prepubertal gilts: Associations among gonadotrophins, metabolic hormones, glucose and uteroovarian development. J. Anim. Sci. 74: 840-848.
Boukhliq, R., Millar, D.W. & Martin, G.B., 1996. Effect of nutrition on the balance of production of ovarian and pituitary hormones in ewes Anim. Reprod. Sci. 41: 201-214.
Bray, G.A., 1991. Treatment for obesity: a nutrient balance/nutrient partition approach Nutr. Rev. 49: 33-45.
Brendemuhl, J.H., Lewis, A.J. & Peo, E.R., 1987. Effect of protein and energy intake by primiparous sows during lactation on sow and litter performance and sow serum thyroxine and urea concentrations J. Anim. Sci. 64: 1060-1069.
Brooks, P.H. & Cole, D.J.A., 1974. The effect of nutrition during the growing period and the oestrus cycle on the reproductive performance of the pig Livestock Prod. Sci. 1: 7-20.
Campbell, R.G. & Taverner, M.R., 1988. Genotype and sex effects on the relationship between energy intake and protein deposition in growing pigs J. Anim. Sci. 66: 676-686.
Cole, D.J.A., 1990. Nutritional strategies to optimize reproduction in pigs J. Reprod. Fert. 40: 67-82.
Cosgrove, J.R., Booth, P.J. & Foxcroft, G.R., 1991. Opioidergic control of gonadotrophin secretion in the prepubertal gilt during restricted feeding and realimentation J. Reprod. Fert. 98: 293-300.
Cosgrove, J.R., Kirkwood, R.N., Aherne, F.X., Clowes, E.J., Foxcroft, G.R. & Zak, L.J., 1997. A review - Management and nutrition of the early weaned weaned sow. Manipulating Pig Production VI Australasian Pig Science Association, Werribee. 33 - 56
Cox, N.M., Stuart, M.J., Althen, T.G., Bennett, W.A. & Millar, H.M., 1987. Enhancement of ovulation rate in gilts by increasing dietary energy and administering insulin during follicular growth J. Anim. Sci. 64:
Ellis, M., Smith, W.C., Henderson, R., Whittemore, C.T., Laird, R. & Phillips, P., 1983. Comparative performance and body composition of control and selection line Large White pigs. 3. Three low feeding scales for a fixed time Anim. Prod. 37: 253-258.
Ellis, M., Smith, W.C. & Laird, R., 1979. Correlated responses in feed intake to selection for economy of production and carcass lean content in Large White pigs Anim. Prod. 28: 424.
Elsley, F.W.H., Bannerman, M., Bathurst, E.V.J., Bracewell, A.G., Cunningham, J.M.M., Dodsworth, T.L., Dodds, P.A., Forbes, T.J. & Laird, R., 1969. The effect of level of feed intake in pregnancy and in lactation upon the productivity of sows Anim. Prod. 11: 225-241.
Emmans, G.C. & Kyriazakis, I., 1989. The prediction of the rate of food intake in growing pigs. In The Voluntary Food Intake of Pigs, pp. 110. Eds Forbes, J.M. *et al.,*. British Society of Animal Production, 110.
Fahmy, M.H., 1981. Factors influencing the weaning to oestrus interval in swine: A review World Review of Animal Production XV11: 15-28.
Flatt, J.P., 1988. Importance of nutrient balance in body weight regulation Diabetes/Metabolism Reviews 4: 571-581.
Friedman, M.I., Tordoff, M.G. & Ramirez, I., 1986. Integrated metabolic control of food intake Brain Res. Bull. 17: 855-859.
Giles, L.R. & Black, J.L., 1991. Voluntary food intake in growing pigs at ambient temperatures above the zone of thermal comfort. In Manipulating pig production III, pp. 162-166. Eds Batterham, E.S. Australian Pig Science Association, Victoria. 162-166.

Goldobin, M.I., 1976.The effect of hyperinsulinism on milk secretion and composition in sows Anim. Breed. Abstr. 44: 425.
Head, R.H., Bruce, N.W. & Williams, I.H., 1991. More cells might lead to more milk. Manipulating pig production 111 (Melbourne) Australasian Pig Science Association: Attwood. 76
Hodge, R.W., 1974. Efficiency of food conversion and body composition of the preruminant lamb and the young pig Br. J. Nutr. 32: 113-126.
Hughes, P.E., 1993. The effects of food level during lactation and early gestation on the reproductive performance of mature sows Anim. Prod. 35: 273-280.
Hunter, M.G., Biggs, C., Faillace, L.S. & Picton, H.M., 1992. Current concepts of folliculogenesis in monovular and polyovular farm species Journal of Reproduction & Fertility. Supplement 45: 21-38.
Jequier, E., 1992. Calorie balance versus nutrient balance. In Energy Metabolism: Tissue Determinants and Cellular Corollaries, pp. 123-137. Eds Kinney, J.M. & Tucker, H.N. Raven Press, New York. 123- 137.
King, R.H., 1987. Nutritional anoestrus in young sows Pig News Info 8: 15-22.
King, R.H. & Martin, G.B., 1989. Relationships between protein intake during lactat, LH levels and oestrous activity in first-litter sows Anim. Reprod. Sci. 19: 283-292.
Kirkwood, R.N., Baidoo, S.K., Aherne, F.X. & Sather, A.P., 1987. The influence of feeding level during actation on the occurrence and endocrinology of the postweaning oestrus in sows Can. J. Anim. Sci. 67: 405-415.
Koketsu, Y., Dial, G.D., Pettigrew, J.E., Marsh, W.E. & King, V.L., 1996. Influence of imposed feed intake patterns during lactation on reproductive performance and on circulation levels of glucose, insulin, and luteinising hormones in primiparous sows J. Anim. Sci. 74: 1036-1046.
Lynch, P.B., 1989. Voluntary food intake of sows and gilts, British Society of Animal Production, Edinburgh. 71-77
Mahan, D.C. & Mangan, L.T., 1975. Evaluation of various protein sequences on the nutritional carry-over from gestation to lactation with first-litter sows J. Nutr. 105: 1291-1298.
McCracken, K.J., 1993. High lean content or high lean growth rate - implications for nutrition. In Recent Advances in Animal Nutrition in Australia 1993, pp. 223-232. Eds Farrell, D.J. Department of Biochemistry, Microbiology and Nutrition, University of New England, Armidale, NSW. 223-232.
McGlone, J.J., Stansbury, W.F. & Tribble, L.F., 1988. Management of lactating sows during heat stress: Effects of water drip, snout coolers, floor type and a high-energy diet. J. Anim. Sci. 66: 885-891.
Millar, H., 1996. Nutrition of the periparturient sow. PhD thesis, University of Alberta.
Morbeck, D.E., Esbenshade, K.L., Flowers, W.L. & Britt, J.H., 1992. Kinetics of follicle growth in the prepubertal gilt Biol. Reprod. 47: 485-491.
Moser, R.L., 1985. Lactation feed intake management. In Misset International: Pigs, 26-29.
Mullan, B.P. & Close, W.H., 1991. Metabolic and endocrine changes during the reproductive cucle of the sow. In Manipulating Pig Production III, pp. 32. Eds Batterham, E.S. Australasian Pig Science Association, Werribee, Australia. 32.
Mullan, B.P., Close, W.H. & Foxcroft, G.R., 1991. Metabolic state of the lactating sow influences plasma LH and FSH before and after weaning. Manipulating pig production III Australasian Pig Science Association, Attwood, Victoria. 31
Mullan, B.P. & Williams, I.H., 1989. The effect of body reserves at farrowing on the reproductive performance of first-litter sows Anim. Prod. 48: 449-457.
NCR-89, 1990. Feeding frequency and the addition of sugar to the diet for the lactating sow J. Anim. Sci. 68: 3498-3501.

O'Grady, J.F., Elsley, F.W.H., MacPherson, R.M. & McDonald, I., 1973. The response of lactating sows and their litters to different dietary energy allowances. 1. Milk yield and composition, reproductive performance of sows and growth rate of litters Anim. Prod. 17: 65-74.
O'Grady, J.F., Lynch, P.B. & Kearney, P.E., 1985. Voluntary feed intake of lactating sows Livestock Prod. Sci. 12: 355-365.
Pettigrew, J.E. & Tokach, M.D., 1993. Metabolic influences on sow reproduction Pig News and Infromation 14: 69N-72N.
Prunier, A., Dourmad, J.Y. & Etienne, M., 1993. Feeding level, metabolic parameters and reproductive performance of primiparous sows Livestock Prod. Sci. 37: 185-196.
Quesnel, H. & Prunier, A., 1995. Endocrine basis of lactational anoestrus in the sow Reprod. Nut. Dévelop. 35: 395-414.
Ramsay, T.G., Yan, X., Barrett, J.B., Azain, M.J. & Barb, C.R., 1997. Recombinant porcine leptin reduces feed intake in swine J. Anim. Sci. 75 (supplement 1): 167.
Reese, D.E., Moser, B.D., Peo, E.R., Jr., Lewis, A.J., Zimmerman, D.R., Kinder, J.E. & Stroup, W.W., 1982. Influence of energy intake during lactation on the interval from weaning to first oestrus in sows J. Anim. Sci. 55: 590-598.
Robinson, J.J., 1990. Nutrition in the reproduction of farm animals Nutr. Res. Rev. 3: 253-276.
Scaramuzzi, R.J., Adams, N.R., Baird, D.T., Campbell, B.K., Downing, J.A., Findlay, J.K., Henderson, K.M., Martin, G.B., McNatty, K.P., McNeilly, A.S. & Tsonis, C.G., 1993. A model for follicule selection and determination of ovulation rate in the ewe Reprod. Fertil. Develop. 5: 459- 478.
Scharrer, E. & Langhans, W., 1986. Control of food intake by fatty acid oxidation Am. J. Physiol. 250: R1003-R1006.
Smith, C. & Fowler, V.R., 1978. The importance of selection criteria and feeding regimes in the selection and improvement of pigs Livestock Prod. Sci. 5: 415-423.
Smith, W.C., Ellis, M., Chadwick, J.P. & Laird, R., 1991. The influence of index selection for improved growth and carcass characteristics on appetite in a population of large white pigs Anim. Prod. 52: 193- 199.
Tokach, M.D., Pettigrew, J.E., Dial, G.D., Wheaton, J.E., Crooker, B.A. & Johnston, L.J., 1992. Characterization of luteinizing hormone secretion in the primiparous, lactating sow: relationship to blood metabolites and return-to-oestrous interval J. Anim. Sci. 70: 2195-2201.
Vesseur, P.C., Kemp, B. & Den Hartog, L.A., 1996. Reproductive performance of the primiparous sow - the key to improve farm production Pig News Info 17: 35N-40N.
Weaver, S. & Aherne, F.X., 1993. Lactating sows have a preference for when they are fed, University of Alberta, 60-61
Whittemore, C.T., 1996. Nutrition reproduction interactions in primiparous sows Livestock Prod. Sci. 46: 65- 83.
Wirtshafter, D. & Davis, J.D., 1977. Body weight: reduction by long-term glycerol treatment Science 198: 1271-1274.
Yang, H., Eastham, P.R., Phillips, P. & Whittemore, C.T., 1989. Reproductive performance, body weight, and condition of breeding sows with differing body fatness at parturition, differing nutrition during lactation, and differing litter size Anim. Prod. 48: 181-201.
Zak, L.J., Cosgrove, J.R., Aherne, F.X. & Foxcroft, G.R., 1997. Pattern of feed intake, and associated metabolic and endocrine changes, differentially affect post-weaning fertility in the primiparous sow. J. Anim. Sci. 75: 208-216.

10 Influence of pregnancy feeding on lactation performance

C.T. Whittemore

10.1 Introduction

The commitment to lactation is initiated not at parturition but at conception. Pregnancy is the profound prerequisite for lactation. Nutritionists have wrongly used the convenience of dividing the breeding cycle into phases: lactation; weaning to conception; pregnancy. Although the physiological processes interacting with nutrient supply differ substantially between these three phases, provision of nutrients solely for immediate requirements merely ensures sub-optimal reproductive performance overall. This fails to account for the animal's own cognisance of the inter-relationships between pregnancy and subsequent lactation, and between lactation and subsequent pregnancy.

The cycle of fatty tissue gains in pregnancy followed by fatty tissue losses in support of lactation is physiologically normal in the mammal, and in following this pattern the pig is no exception. The drive towards pregnancy weight gains in excess of those required for maternal growth, products of conception, and mammary development, follows from the expectation that lactational feed intake will be unable to supply, from exogenous sources, all of the nutrient requirements of lactation. There will be an absolute need to draw on endogenous body reserves to resource the deficit. That there are carry-over effects of pregnancy feeding upon lactation is a fundamental assumption of mammalian physiology and eating behaviour. Pregnancy feeding regimens for breeding pigs must therefore target the demands of lactation equally as much as the demands of the foetal load. These latter are, in any event, relatively small and not greatly influenced by immediate levels of nutrient intake; and maternal body tissue provides a ready buffer for foetal nutrition by giving way, through catabolism, to foetal demand.

10.2 Background

Earlier findings that severe nutritional insult in pregnancy had little influence upon reproductive performance have had to be reassessed, and nutrient recommendations revised, as a result of a number of factors including radical changes in pig genotype. Over the past two decades sow mature size has increased by some 30%, while backfat depth in slaughter pigs has decreased by at least a similar proportion (Whittemore, 1996; MLC, 1975; MLC, 1995). Kerr & Cameron (1996a) found gilts selected over 7 generations for lean food conversion had only

11.3mm P2 backfat depth compared to 20.3 mm for pigs selected for daily feed intake. There is evidence that selection pressure against backfat depth has been counter-productive for sow productivity, and national statistics (MLC, 1975) would tend to suggest that the benefits of cross-breeding and of selection for litter size may have done little more than arrest what would otherwise have been a decline in sow prolificacy. It is nonetheless evident that, due to a combination of genetic selection and improved peri-parturient management, the contemporary breeding sow is suckling a substantially larger litter, with potentially greater total litter weight gains than was the case previously. But Kerr & Cameron (1995) and Kerr & Cameron (1996b) have shown that selection for leanness during growth is both genetically and physiologically negatively correlated with subsequent reproductive performance.

Whittemore *et al.* (1980) described substantial genotypic differences in sow fatness between breeding companies; P2 backfat depth at first mating ranging from 13.8-18.7 mm. A pregnancy feeding level of 2.3 kg of a diet of 12.8 MJ DE, 154g CP, and 7g lysine/kg was found to be inadequate to replenish lactation fatty tissue losses, achieving P2 backfat gains of only 3.9 mm in pregnancy following lactation losses of 6.9 mm. The same authors raised the spectre that genetically lean strains of pigs may have inadequate body fat content to optimise reproductive performance, and this has been amply demonstrated by many others since then. Most recently, Kerr & Cameron (1996a) found that live weight and backfat depth at mating is an accurate predictor of genetic merit for reproductive traits. Selection strategies for low feed intake and reduced backfat depth (both consequences of selection against carcass fatness) were found by Kerr & Cameron (1996c) to result in pig strains with reduced fat depth at farrowing and reduced performance of sucking piglets.

10.3 Nutrient requirements of pregnancy

The pregnant sow requires food to supply the nutrient demands of her maintenance, the growth of the products of conception in the uterus, and the growth of mammary tissue to resource the impending lactation. To this long-standing convention must now be added the substantial requirements for growth necessitated by the modern large-maturing genotypes conceiving at only 50% (or less) of their mature size, and therefore under impulsion simultaneously to grow and reproduce. As lactation is essentially the catabolic phase of the reproductive cycle, it follows that if maternal body growth is to occur, it must occur during pregnancy. Given the expectation of lipid and protein catabolism from the sow's body tissue to furnish the shortfall in nutrients for milk synthesis during lactation, pregnancy nutrient allowances must further accommodate the deposition of these reserves by laying down lipid (especially) and protein tissues over and above all the aforementioned requirements.

10.3.1 Maintenance

Little has been published to amend the views of ARC (1981) and NRC (1988) that the daily energy requirements for maintenance may be safely estimated at 0.44 MJ ME.W(kg)$^{0.75}$. Noblet & Etienne (1987a, b) suggest a similar value of 0.43 MJ ME.W$^{0.75}$, while Whittemore & Yang (1989) suggest 0.48 MJ ME. W$^{0.75}$. The possibility of an increase in maintenance requirement with advancing pregnancy was not confirmed either by Close (1987) or Noblet & Etienne (1985, 1987a).

Estimated protein requirements for maintenance during pregnancy range from 0.94W$^{0.75}$ (Carr *et al.*, 1977) to 2.50W$^{0.75}$ g/day (Beyer *et al.*, 1988).

Sow live weight through advancing parities is highly dependent on genotype (ultimate mature size), feeding regimen, and the environment. The acceptably fed sows of Yang *et al.* (1989) had average pregnancy weights (W) of 157, 199, 233 and 245 kg for parities 1-4 respectively. Sow weight at first conception was 123 kg.

10.3.2 Pregnancy gains of conception products

Some 84 MJ of energy and 2.7 kg protein are deposited in the total gravid uterus between conception and term (Black *et al.*, 1986; Noblet *et al.*, 1985), or an average of 0.7 MJ and 24g nett daily. A k value of 0.72 (Close *et al.*, 1985) for energy, and a material efficiency of 0.5 for protein calculates to an average daily ME and CP requirement of 1 MJ ME and 48g protein. Noblet *et al.* (1985) measured a total deposition in the developing mammary gland during pregnancy of 48 MJ and 547g protein, or a daily average over pregnancy of 0.6 MJ ME and 9.5g CP. Average total requirements for products of conception therefore total 1.6 MJ ME and 58g CP daily during pregnancy.

Much has been made of the curvilinear increase in growth accretion, and therefore in nutrient demand, of foetal, uterine and mammary tissues as pregnancy advances (see review of Whittemore & Morgan, 1990); and it is self-evident that the demands at the end of pregnancy for these purposes are greater than at the beginning. Noblet *et al.* (1985) present net daily energy and protein estimates for depositions in the total gravid uterus of,

Energy MJ/day = $0.107e^{0.027t}$
Protein g/day = $3.606e^{0.026t}$

suggesting nett requirements for day (t) 110 to be 2.1 MJ and 63g protein, or 3 MJ ME and 126g CP as gross dietary requirements. As a proportion of the total daily energy and protein requirements these latter are relatively small, and there is likely to be little gained in practice from trying to increase short-term pregnancy nutrient supply by such relatively small amounts as the pregnancy approaches term. In any event, the predisposition of the pig in late pregnancy to become catabolic will ensure that, for animals with adequate body condition, there will be no short-term inadequacy of nutrients for foetal requirements (Whittemore *et al.*, 1980).

10.3.3 Pregnancy maternal growth

Sows grow from first conception at 120-150 kg live weight over four parities to double their size and achieve 300-350 kg final mature live weight (Williams *et al.*, 1985). Whittemore & Morgan (1990) forwarded the proposition,

$$Pt = A.e^{-e^{-0.005(t)}}$$

where Pt is the total protein mass, A is the mature weight approximating to a total protein mass of 45 kg, and t is the number of days from first conception. The value of 0.005 for the growth parameter is about half that found in the growing (non-pregnant) pig, while Pt approaches A at around $t = 500$ days between parities 3 and 4. Conception to conception gains of protein for the four parities approximate to 12, 8, 5 and 2 kg (see also Whittemore & Yang, 1989). Everts & Dekker (1995) suggested 8.5 kg maternal protein deposition in primiparous pregnancy. Everts (1994) fed up to 481g protein daily to pregnant sows and determined maternal body protein deposition rates of 84g/day. Although earlier pig genotypes usually contained a lipid mass (Lt) two or more times greater than the protein mass ($Lt>2Pt$; O'Grady *et al.*, 1975), Lt for the adequately fed sows of Yang *et al.* (1989) could be determined as the rather less,

$$Lt = 1.1\ Pt^{1.1}$$

with a value of $Lt<Pt$ identified as threatening reproductive failure. Conception to conception gains of lipid for four parities suggested by Whittemore & Morgan (1990), approximate to 17, 11, 7 and 3 kg. Everts & Dekker (1995) measured maternal lipid deposition rates of 20 kg in the primiparous pregnancy.

Energy requirements for maternal growth in pregnancy can be calculated using the assumption that the efficiencies of conversion (k) of dietary ME to retained lipid and protein are,

$$k_l \cong 0.74$$

and

$$k_p \cong 0.54$$

although the latter may be optimistic (Kielanowski, 1972).

Efficiency of use of dietary protein for protein deposition is highly feed-quality dependent but, given acceptable diets, a gross material efficiency of 0.50 may be taken as a likely upper value. Requirements of 300g of good quality dietary protein in early pregnancy and 375g daily in late pregnancy were determined by Etienne (1991) and Everts & Dekker (1994a).

10.3.4 Pregnancy deposition of lactational reserves

Conception to conception gains of protein for purposes of pregnancy maternal growth assume no change in protein mass during lactation, and imply that maternal gains comprise all the growth required to be achieved during pregnancy. This assumption is unlikely to be safe (King & Dunkin, 1986a and 1986b; King, 1987; Etienne *et al.*, 1985; Etienne *et al.*, 1989; Aherne *et al.*, 1995; Clowes *et al.*, 1995; Whittemore & Yang, 1989), and an allowance for further protein gain during each pregnancy is likely to be judicious to provide for subsequently expected rates of daily body protein catabolism during lactation which may range from 0 to some 100g daily, depending on the adequacy of lactational dietary protein supply.

Similarly, expectations for lipid losses catabolised from the maternal body in support of lactation require to be balanced *pro rata* by lipid gains during pregnancy in addition to those identified as a part of normal maternal growth. Lipid losses during lactation determined by Whittemore & Yang (1989) ranged from 0.24-0.52 kg daily, and those of Etienne *et al.* (1985) from 0.1-0.3 kg daily. Everts & Dekker (1994b) measured energy losses of 0.39 MJ/W(kg)$^{0.75}$. An allowance for 10 kg of catabolised lipid over the lactation is therefore well justified, and if the conception to conception gains of lipid identified earlier as a necessary part of maternal growth are to be made during pregnancy, then lactational lipid catabolism requires to be balanced by additional *pro rata* pregnancy gains.

10.4 Field Trials

10.4.1 Influence of pregnancy feeding level upon lactation feed intake

It has long been understood that there is an inverse relationship between pregnancy feeding level and sow appetite in lactation; almost certainly mediated through sow body fatness at parturition (Yang *et al.*, 1989). There is great variation, however, in the quantitative importance of this phenomenon. Williams & Smits (1991) found lactation food intake to fall from 4.4 kg daily to 2.7 kg daily as gilt body fatness rose from 25% to 35% lipid; both of these fatness levels being substantially higher than would be likely to be found in modern European hybrids. Mullan and Williams (1988, 1989) found a 1 mm decrease in P2 backfat depth at parturition to be worth only 0.1 kg increase in daily voluntary feed intake in lactation; while increased volume of food in late pregnancy may actually enhance lactation appetite (Matte *et al.*, 1994; Farmer *et al.*, 1996). The latter proposition was supported by the similar findings of Dourmad (1991) and Yang *et al.* (1989):

Food intake (kg/day) in lactation = 7.6 - 0.13 P2 (mm) back fat depth at parturition.

An even lower multiplier for P2 (0.08) was found by Miller (1996).

It may be concluded that for the modern genotype, which has little tendency to excessive body fatness in any event, the positive benefits of arriving at the point of parturition in good body condition, and carrying lipid reserves available to support lactation and to help attainment of acceptable fatness levels through to weaning, far outweigh the small negative effects that may exist consequent upon the undoubted, but slight, inverse relationship between pregnancy and lactation feed intakes.

10.4.2 Feeding level in late pregnancy

With regard to the influence of feeding in late and early pregnancy, it is as well to recall that in 1971 Elsley and co-workers (Elsley *et al.*, 1971) found no effect of pattern of intake during pregnancy on sow performance.

An increase in the rate of pregnancy feeding in the last trimester would be unlikely to increase litter size (Elsley, 1973; Henry & Etienne, 1978; Den Hartog & Van Kempen, 1980; Hillyer & Philips, 1980; ARC 1981; Whittemore *et al.*, 1984). But the proposition that late pregnancy feeding might increase piglet birth weight is unsurprising in view of the exponential growth being made by the foetal load at this time. Aherne & Kirkwood (1985) consider elevated feeding in the last trimester to be justified when the average birth weight is below 1 kg. There is evidence that catabolism of maternal body lipid stores can be initiated in late pregnancy without detriment, provided that adequate reserves are already available. Close *et al.* (1985) and Noblet *et al.* (1990) suggest that sows ingesting less than 25 MJ DE daily in the last quarter of pregnancy are likely to lose body fat at this time. Elevated levels of feeding at the end of pregnancy in response to increasingly rapid foetal gains may therefore be contra-indicated, and the utilisation of body lipid stores to support the final charge of foetal growth may be physiologically normal (Whittemore *et al.*, 1980; Cole, 1990). Hovell *et al.* (1977) found pregnancy feed intakes of 19.5, 25.8 and 32.1 MJ ME/day to result in individual birth weights of 1.08, 1.10 and 1.29 kg, rather supporting the contentions of Aherne & Kirkwood (1985), but showing that increase in birth weight can be just as readily achieved by increasing the amount of feeding throughout pregnancy as increasing it in the last trimester alone. Etienne (1991) also confirmed a linear response of piglet birth weight to energy intake in pregnancy. High level feeding at the end of pregnancy is thought to predispose to agalactia, mastitis, dystocia and metritis (Göransson, 1989), a contention supported by Head & Williams (1991) and Head *et al.* (1991). Aherne *et al.* (1995) nevertheless recommended an increase in feed supply of 1-2 kg from day 100 through to parturition, having found no negative effects of this practice, but benefit for herds with problems of low piglet birth weight. It is also relevant that the fat and lean gilts of Head and co workers were 36 mm and 25 mm P2 respectively, both of which levels of fatness are far in excess of that which might be expected in contemporary European hybrids. Swedish workers, with their penchant for debunking preconceptions, have shown high level feeding (*ad libitum*) before parturition to have no peri-parturient disadvantages, but a significant advantage in terms of enhancement of lactation feed intake and reduction in the rate of lactational mobilisation of fat reserves (Neil, 1996). Elevated dietary lipid intake toward the end of pregnancy can increase lipid levels marginally in both the foetus and colostral milk (Pettigrew, 1981). The present author's view is that the debate is largely academic as piglet birth weight should not be a problem in sows which are not suffering from reproductive disease, and which are adequately fed throughout pregnancy. Miller (1996), after comprehensive review of the literature, concludes that the major advantage of increasing sow feed intake in late gestation is in maintaining sow condition prior to lactation, rather than conferring any birth weight advantages on piglets. The solution to problems of low piglet birth weight are therefore unlikely to lie in quick fixes at the end of pregnancy, and more likely to lie in attention to veterinary matters and to nutrition throughout the whole of the pregnancy period.

10.4.3 Feeding level in early pregnancy

As has been discussed thus far, carry-over effects of pregnancy feeding on lactation yield are likely to be consequent on (1) provision of endogenous nutrient reserves for milk synthesis and, (2) the size of the piglets at birth and the litter size. The number of piglets in the litter is influenced not only by ovulation rate, but also during pregnancy consequent upon the relative success of embryonic implantation and survival. Sows which have been consistently well fed and are in good body condition will have higher ovulation rates (Kirkwood & Aherne, 1985; Beltranena *et al.*, 1991), and improved embryo survival. Whilst increased feed intake in early pregnancy has been previously associated with decreased embryo survival (Den Hartog & van Kempen, 1980), there is little contemporary evidence to support this contention. Increased feeding level in early pregnancy will increase the rate of maternal tissue deposition, and that was not found to adversely affect embryo survival by either Toplis *et al.* (1983) or Dyck (1991). Similarly, Pharazyn *et al.* (1991) showed that level of feeding in early gestation had no affect upon embryo survival rate in inherently fertile gilts. The view that low level feeding in early pregnancy may somehow be beneficial to subsequent litter size is therefore now largely discredited. Hughes (1993) found 3.5 kg feed per day in early pregnancy to have no negative effect on subsequent litter size compared to 1.75 kg. Kirkwood *et al.* (1990) compared 3.6 and 1.8 kg of food per day in the first trimester, finding no effect for sows fed adequately in lactation, but a positive benefit in embryo survival from the higher level of feeding (3.6 kg daily) when sows were inadequately fed (3 kg feed daily) in lactation. Recent work from the Swedish Pig Centre (Svalov, unpublished) also demonstrated a positive relationship between level of feeding in early gestation and subsequent reproductive performance in terms of litter size.

10.4.4 Influence of positive depositions of maternal body protein and lipid during pregnancy

Many of the studies deriving relationships between pregnancy feed intake and pregnancy gains used feed with levels of energy and protein density different from those used currently; reports of experimental findings couched in terms of food supplied (rather than nutrients supplied) should therefore be cautiously interpreted. With a diet of 13.2 MJ DE and 162g CP/kg, Yang *et al.* (1989) determined that an extra 0.24 kg of feed daily will add a 1 mm increment of P2 back fat depth and a 6 kg increment of live weight by the end of the pregnancy. The latter value being similar to that determined by Henry and Etienne (1978) and the former similar to that measured by Whittemore *et al.* (1988).

Sow live weight and fatness gains in pregnancy are the medium for positive carry-over effects into lactation. Whittemore *et al.* (1988) derived the positive relations:
- Number born alive per litter = 10.0 + 0.05 sow live weight change in pregnancy
- Total weight of live born (kg) = 12.8 + 0.08 sow live weight change in pregnancy

and further demonstrated the efficacious use of pregnancy gains in the support of lactation with the inverse relationships:
- sow back fat change in lactation = 1.9 - 0.25 back fat change in pregnancy
- sow maternal live weight change in lactation = 8.5 - 0.22 sow maternal live weight change in pregnancy

showing heavier fatter sows to lose more weight and fat in lactation.

Piglet birth weight is positively, but only slightly related to gestation energy intake up to levels as high as 40 MJ ME per day (Elsley *et al.*, 1969; Noblet *et al.*, 1985).

For parity 1 gilts, Yang *et al.* (1989) found the following positive influences of fatness, sow live weight and pregnancy food intake upon the weight of piglets at birth

Weight of piglets at birth (kg) = 1.01 + 0.021P2 at parturition (mm)
Weight of piglets at birth (kg) = 0.43 + 0.0053 live weight at parturition (kg)
Weight of piglets at birth (kg) = 0.89 + 0.0015 total pregnancy food intake (kg)

Yang *et al.* (1989) fed sows in pregnancy over 4 parities, to be thin (12.3 mm P2) or fat (19.3 mm P2) at the time of each parturition (achieved with average feed intakes of 2.8 and 3.5 kg daily), the thin sows gaining 1.9 mm in pregnancy and losing 2.5 mm in lactation, while the fat sows gained 5.7 mm in pregnancy and lost 5.0 mm in lactation. Respective weight changes were +40 and -13, and +60 and -26 kg. Carry-over effects of fatness at parturition extended beyond lactation to the weaning to oestrus interval in gilts (14.2 *v* 9.1 days), but not in the multiparous sows (6.7 *v* 7.3). Piglet growth rate from 0-21 days postpartum, indicating lactation yield, was positively influenced by sow fatness at parturition (193 *v* 205g/day). Fat sows at parturition also had one more piglet born per litter and weaned 10 kg more total litter weight at 28 days.

10.5 Nutrient requirements of lactation

The absolute requirement for pregnancy gains of lipid and protein to furnish the needs of milk synthesis in lactation is dependent upon (a) the level and composition of the milk yielded and (b) the level and composition of nutrients supplied daily during lactation.

10.5.1 Litter size and lactation yield

Lactation yield is in part a consequence of sucking intensity, which in pigs is dependent upon individual piglet weight and potential daily growth rate, and the number of piglets in the litter (Elsley, 1971; Noblet *et al.*, 1988). Miller (1996) confirmed a strong positive relationship between sow live weight and fat losses in lactation, and litter size and piglet weight. As has been reviewed above, there is an established relationship between feed level in the last trimester of pregnancy and piglet birth weight, and between feed level throughout pregnancy and litter size; the latter probably being mediated through positive maternal body condition effects on embryonic implantation and foetal survival. There also appears to be a positive influence of short-term pregnancy feeding in early pregnancy on the number of piglets born (Kirkwood *et al.*, 1990); although conventional wisdom implied the reverse (Den Hartog & van Kempen, 1980).

10.5.2 Nutrient demand and supply during lactation

Noblet and Etienne (1987b) found 3.7g of milk to result in 1g of piglet liveweight gain, while Whittemore & Morgan (1990) give the energy cost of piglet gain to be 22 MJ ME/kg and the energy value of milk as 5.4 MJ ME/kg, and it may therefore be computed:

Lactational demand (milk yield) = daily piglet gain x no. of piglets in litter x 4

a proposition also supported by the work of Noblet *et al.* (1988).

A weaning weight of 7 kg at 21 days following a birth weight of 1.2 kg indicates that a litter of 12 sucking piglets would require an average daily milk yield of 13.3 kg. For calculation purposes an average milk yield of 11 kg daily over a 21-28 day lactation is used.

From various authorities (Elsley, 1971; ARC, 1981; Burlacu *et al.*, 1983; Verstegen *et al.*, 1985; Noblet & Etienne, 1987b; Beyer *et al.*, 1988) it may be concluded that 7.7 MJ ME and 120g crude protein (assuming a material efficiency of 0.5) are required for the formation of 1 kg of milk, and the daily requirement for milk production is therefore 85 MJ ME and 1320g crude protein with an acceptable amino acid balance (0.7-0.8 ideal).

To the nutrient demands of milk synthesis should be added those of maintenance. Given a sow of 200 kg liveweight, these would amount to 23 MJ ME and 106g crude protein per day. Total lactation nutrient demands calculate to 108 MJ ME and 1426g crude protein per day.

Sow feed intakes over the lactation may vary from <3 to >8 kg daily (Lodge, 1962; Cox *et al.*, 1983; King *et al.*, 1984; Danielsen & Nielsen, 1984; Young & King, 1987) depending greatly upon the circumstances of environment and management. Only at the highest levels would a lactation sow diet with 14 MJ ME and 200g of acceptable quality protein per kg approach the supply of the full nutrient demand from ingested nutrients alone. It may be taken therefore that for litters of >10 sucking piglets aspiring to achieve an acceptable weaning weight of >6 kg at 21 days, a maternal feed intake of <8 kg (even of a high-quality diet) will unavoidably result in the catabolism and use of maternal body lipid and protein; body reserves which must necessarily have been accumulated during pregnancy.

Body lipid can be converted for milk synthesis with an efficiency of about 0.85 (ARC, 1981; Noblet & Etienne, 1987b; Beyer *et al.*, 1988), and the equivalent efficiency for body protein is likely to be similar (Beyer *et al.*, 1988). It will be assumed that the catastrophic possibility of degrading maternal body protein for the purposes of supplying energy will not occur.

Putative lactational losses of maternal body lipid and protein, required to have been provided in the form of tissue reserves at the point of parturition, are presented in Table 10.1.

Table 10.1. Calculated daily weights of body lipid & protein tissue usages[1] required to support lactation[2] at various lactational feed intakes

	Daily lactational feed intake[3] (kg)		
	4	6	8
Maternal body lipid usage (kg/day)	1.56	0.72	-0.074[4]
Maternal body protein usage (g/day)	736	265	-87
Maternal body lipid usage (kg/lactation)	32.8	15.1	-1.54[4]
Maternal body protein usage (kg/lactation)	15.5	5.6	-1.8

[1] these values may be in excess of determined live weight losses as some catabolised lipid may be replaced by water.
[2] 11 sucking piglets for 21 days.
[3] diet of 14MJ ME and 200g good quality CP/kg
[4] negative values indicate body tissue gains.

These calculated values can be scrutinised in the light of the findings of King & Williams (1984), Yang *et al.*, (1989), Kirkwood *et al.* (1990), Baidoo *et al.* (1992a, 1992b), and many others that P2 backfat losses in lactation of 6 mm or more are in no way exceptional, and Mullan & Williams (1990) found 1 mm change in P2 backfat depth to be associated with 3.3 kg of body lipid loss. Whittemore *et al.* (1980) measured P2 backfat losses in the course of a 35-day lactation to range between 4.6 and 8.4 mm, depending upon genotype; all genotypes being considered to be adequately fed. With regard to protein losses, Etienne *et al.* (1985) measured muscle losses in lactation of 11.3 kg (which would approximate to some 100g or more of body protein loss daily), while Etienne *et al.* (1989) measured a negative nitrogen balance of 10.3g nitrogen, or 64.4g protein daily. King & Dunkin (1986b) found protein losses during lactation ranging from 45g daily through to the highest level of 126g of maternal body protein loss daily during lactation. King & Dunkin (1986a) found that even well fed gilts lost during lactation 100g protein from their maternal bodies daily. The calculated values in Table 1 are therefore largely in accord with experimental findings, although the calculated losses might be somewhat higher than those found by some experimental workers. Whittemore & Yang (1989) found sows to lose, on average, 0.32 kg of lipid and 107g of protein daily during lactation, with equivalent values for animals fed only 3 kg daily in lactation being 0.6 kg lipid and 180g of protein. King (1987) indicates daily losses in lactation of 0.73 kg lipid and 150g protein daily, while Mullan (1987) demonstrated that 0.72 kg lipid and 220g protein could be lost daily from sows with low lactation feed intakes.

Table 10.1 illustrates the following points:

- in the absence of accumulated reserves of both lipid and protein laid down during pregnancy, lactational yield and piglet growth will be compromised, and the sow will also lose essential maternal body tissue to the detriment of subsequent reproductive performance - not least a lengthened weaning to oestrus interval and reduced subsequent litter size;
- larger litters or heavier weaning weights will require proportionately greater reserves;
- a zero nutrient requirement, accumulated in the course of the previous pregnancy, for lactation will only occur with an intake of 8 kg or more of a high nutrient density diet; substantial lipid and protein losses can be expected in lactation, and equivalent gains required in pregnancy, if sow lactational feed intakes of 6 kg prevail (as is common);
- solutions at feed intakes of <5 kg are unfeasible (i.e. daily required milk yields are unlikely to be forthcoming and piglet growth rates will be reduced as the daily rates of maternal body tissue catabolism required are physiologically unreasonable);
- lipid is likely to be lost at a greater rate than protein in normal circumstances;
- body lipid usage rates will be higher if the diet has an energy density of <14 MJ ME/kg
- body protein usage rates will be higher if the diet has a protein density of <200g/kg or if the protein were of a lower quality than would allow a material efficiency of protein use of 0.5

10.6 Calculation of nutrient requirements in pregnancy

Given the lactational losses presented in Table 10.1, and the axiomatic requirement that they be provisioned in the course of the previous pregnancy, then pregnancy nutrient allowances can be calculated as a sum of the requirements for maintenance, maternal growth, the products of conception, and the creation of lactational reserves. For the purpose of calculating the nutrient requirements of pregnancy, the allowance for building up lactational reserves is calculated on the assumption that the subsequent lactation feed intake will be an average of 6 kg daily of a diet of 14 MJ ME and 200g CP/kg. Table 10.2 shows that in the primiparous gilt maternal growth comprises a significant proportion of the total requirement of both energy and protein; as does the lactational reserve. Indeed, some authorities might suggest that for the first pregnancy such allowances as are calculated are unreasonable, representing 3 kg daily of a diet with 14 MJ ME and 150g CP/kg. However, it is most pertinent to note that Yang *et al.* (1989) were only able to achieve target backfat depths at farrowing of 20 mm P2 by feeding levels of similar magnitude (3.6 kg daily of a diet with 12.7 MJ ME). A lesser supply will, it is indicated, result in reduced maternal growth and reduced subsequent milk yield, with the often observed result of gilts being unable to wean large litters of acceptably-sized piglets, and finishing first lactation with depleted body reserves of both lipid and protein. Sows given less nutrients than indicated in Table 10.2 may, of course, counterbalance their position by consuming more than 6 kg of food in lactation, obviating the need for the deposition of a lactation reserve of lipid and protein in pregnancy.

Table 10.2. Factorial calculation of dietary energy and protein requirements in pregnancy

		Parity			
		1	2	3	4
Maintenance[1]	MJ ME/day	19.4	23.3	26.4	27.0
	g CP/day	88	106	120	124
Maternal growth[2]	MJ ME/day	12.4	8.1	5.1	2.2
	g CP/day	208	138	86	34
Products of conception	MJ ME/day	1.6	1.6	1.6	1.6
	g CP/day	58	58	58	58
Lactation reserve[3]	MJ ME/day	9.1	9.1	9.1	9.1
	g CP/day	97	97	97	97
Total	MJ ME/day	42.5	42.1	42.2	39.9
	g CP/day	451	399	361	313

[1] W = 157, 199, 233 and 245kg.
[2] Protein retained = 104, 69, 43 and 17g Lipid retained = 147, 96, 61 and 26g.
[3] From Table 1; 6kg feed intake.

10.7 Conclusion

The influence of pregnancy feeding on lactation performance (and subsequent re-breeding) can be profound. The direct effects through the influence of pregnancy feeding on sow body weight, litter size and piglet birth weight are arguably less important than the indirect effects upon milk yield, mediated through the need for a lactational reserve. Where lactation feed intakes are high (8 kg daily or above), and where the quality of the lactation diet is good (14 MJ ME and 200g/kg or above), there is unlikely to be a great need for lactational nutrient reserves, even for litters of 11-12 piglets achieving target 21-day weights of 6 kg or above. However, where feed intakes in lactation and/or diet specifications are less than this, then for adequate lactation yields to be supported the sow must draw upon body reserves of lipid and protein, both of which require to have been accumulated in the previous pregnancy. Pregnancy deposition of the necessary lipid and protein reserves may be calculated *pro rata* in accordance with the difference between required lactation yield and lactation nutrient supply. Given the prevailing position for achieved lactational nutrient intakes in most improved hybrid sows world-wide, it is suggested that pregnancy feeding regimens should provide more adequately for the sows' needs for both energy and protein during pregnancy, particularly in the first two parities.

This chapter has argued that short-term nutritional tactics at the beginning and end of pregnancy will be largely irrelevant for sows maintained in adequate body condition. Given this position, pregnancy feeding can be considered in an holistic and strategic way, targeting the following requirements:

- maintenance;
- products of conception (foetal load, uterine development, placenta and associated tissues, mammary development);
- maternal growth of body protein and lipid;
- deposition of protein and lipid reserves available to support the forthcoming lactation.

These requirements sum to feeding levels somewhat greater than is conventional in many contemporary production systems using improved hybrid breeding sows. Such requirements are not recommendations, but it must be accepted that if they are not met, then:

- lactation feeding levels must supply nutrients at rates in excess of those usually found in commercial practice (>8 kg of a high-quality nutrient-dense diet daily); and/or
- lactation yield will fail to reach potential with commensurate effects on potential piglet growth, and possibly also on subsequent re-breeding success; and/or
- maternal growth ambitions of the sow will be curtailed; and/or
- maximum litter size, piglet birth weight, and mammary development will not be achieved.

Alternatively, the high factorial estimates for nutrient requirements in pregnancy in comparison to field expectations might be taken to indicate a research need to examine the nature and efficiency of pregnancy tissue depositions.

10.8 References

Agriculture Research Council, 1981. The Nutrient Requirements of Pigs. Commonwealth Agricultural Bureaux, Slough, 307pp.

Aherne, F.X., & R.N. Kirkwood, 1985. Nutrition and sow prolificacy. J. Reprod. Fertil. Suppl. 33, 169-183.

Aherne, F.X., H. Miller, E. Clowes & L. Zak, 1995. Nutritional effects on sow reproduction. Proc. Minnesota Nutrition Conference.

Baidoo, S.K., E.S. Lithgoe, R.N. Kirkwood, F.X. Aherne & G.R. Foxcroft, 1992a. Effect of lactation feed intake on endocrine status and metabolite levels in sows. Canadian J. Anim. Sci. 72, 799-807.

Baidoo, S.K., F.X. Aherne, R.N. Kirkwood & G.R. Foxcroft, 1992b. Effect of feed intake during lactation and after weaning on sow reproductive performance. Canadian J. Anim. Sci. 72, 911-917.

Beltranena, E., G.R. Foxcroft, F.X. Aherne & R.N. Kirkwood, 1991. Endocrinology of nutritional flushing in gilts. Canadian J. Anim. Sci. 71, 1063-1071.

Beyer, M., L. Hoffman, R. Schiemann, W. Jentsch, G. Burlacu, M. Iliescu, E.C. Machajew, L. Babinszky, H. Gundel, L. Lassota, M. Walach-Janiak & L. Zeman, 1988. Biological basics for the factorial derivation of the energy and protein requirements for pregnant and lactating sows and suckling piglets. Fifth International Symposium on Protein Metabolism and Nutrition. E.A.A.P. Publication No. 35 Wissenschaftliche Zeitschrift der Wilhelm-Pieck-Universität Rostock, 37, 92-93.

Black, J.L., R.G. Campbell, I.H. Williams, K.J. James & G.T. Davies, 1986. Simulation of energy and amino acid utilisation in the pig. Res. Dev. Agric. 3, 121-145.

Burlacu, G., M. Iliescu & P. Caramida, 1983. Efficiency of food utilisation by pregnant and lactating sows. 1. The influence of diets with different concentrations of energy on pregnancy and lactation. Arch. Tierenäh, 33, 23-45.

Carr, J.R., K.N. Boorman & D.J.A. Cole, 1977. Nitrogen retention in the pig. Brit. J. Nutr. 37, 143-155.

Close, W.H., 1987. Some conclusions of the AFRC Working Party on the energy requirements of sows and boars. Anim. Prod. 44, 464.

Close, W.H., J. Noblet & R.P. Heavens, 1985. Studies on the energy metabolism of the pregnant sow. 2. The partition and utilisation of metabolisable energy intake in pregnant and non-pregnant animals. Brit. J. Nutr. 53, 267-279.

Clowes, E.J., I. Williams, J.R. Pluske, L. Zak & F.X. Aherne, 1995. Nutrient balance in restricted, *ad libitum* and superalimented sows. Proc. Canadian Soc. Anim. Sci., Ottawa, 591.

Cole, D.J.A., 1990. Nutritional strategies to optimise reproduction in pigs. J. Reprod. Fertil. Suppl. 40, 67-82.

Cox, N.M., H.H. Breitt, W.D. Armstrong & H.D. Alhusen, 1983. Effect of feeding fat and altering weaning schedule on rebreeding in primiparous sows. J. Anim. Sci. 56, 21-29.

Danielsen, N.V., & H.E. Nielsen, 1984. The influence of different feeding levels on the performance of lactating sows. Proceedings of the 35th Meeting of the E.A.A.P., The Hague.

Den Hartog, L.A., & G.J.M. van Kempen, 1980. Relation between nutrition and fertility in pigs. Neth. J. Agric. Sci. 28, 211-227.

Dourmad, J.Y., 1991. Effect of feeding level in the gilt during pregnancy on voluntary feed intake during lactation and changes in body composition during gestation and lactation. Livestock Prod. Sci. 27, 309-319.

Dyck, G.W., 1991. The effect of post-mating diet intake on embryonic and foetal survival, and litter size in gilts. Canadian J. Anim. Sci. 71, 675-681.

Elsley, F.W.H., 1971. Nutrition and lactation in the sow. In: I.R. Faulkner (Ed) Lactation, Butterworths, London, 393-411.
Elsley, F.W.H., 1973. Nutrition of the female pig during pregnancy and lactation. Paper presented to Pig Commission, E.A.A.P., Vienna.
Elsley, F.W.H., M. Bannerman, E.V.J. Bathurst, A.G. Bracewell, J.M.M. Cunningham, T.L. Dodsworth, P.A. Dodds, T.J. Forbes & R. Laird, 1969. The effect of feed intake in pregnancy and in lactation upon the productivity of sows. Anim. Prod. 11, 225-241.
Elsley, F.W.H., E.V.J. Bathurst, A.G. Bracewell, J.M.M. Cunningham, J.B. Dent, T.L. Dodsworth, R.M. MacPherson, & N. Walker, 1971. The effect of pattern of food intake in pregnancy upon sow productivity. Anim. Prod. 13, 257-270.
Etienne, M., 1991. Apports énergétiques de gestation et accrétion des protéines chez la truie nullipare. J. Recherches Porcines en France 23, 69-74.
Etienne, M., J. Noblet & B. Desmoulin, 1985. Mobilisation des réserves corporelles chez la truie primipare en lactation. Reprod. Nutr. Dévelop. 25, 341-344.
Etienne, M., J. Noblet, J.Y. Dourmad & H. Fortune, 1989. Études du besoin en lysine des truies en lactation. J. Recherches Porcines en France 21, 101-108.
Everts, H., 1994. Nitrogen and energy metabolism of sows during several reproductive cycles in relation to nitrogen intake. PhD Thesis, University of Wageningen, Netherlands.
Everts, H., & R.A. Dekker, 1994a. Effect of nitrogen supply on the retention and excretion of nitrogen and on energy metabolism of pregnant sows. Anim. Prod. 59, 293-302.
Everts, H., & R.A. Dekker, 1994b. Effect of nitrogen supply on nitrogen and energy metabolism in lactating sows. Anim. Prod. 59, 445-454
Everts, H., & R.A. Dekker, 1995. Effect of protein supply during pregnancy on body condition of gilts and their products of conception. Livest. Prod. Sci. 42, 27-36.
Farmer, C., S. Robert & J.J. Matte, 1996. Lactation performance of sows fed a bulky diet during gestation and receiving growth hormone releasing factor during lactation. J. Anim. Sci. 74, 1298-1306.
Göransson, L., 1989. The effect of feed allowance in late pregnancy on the occurrence of agalactia post partum in the sow. J. Vet. Med. A. 36, 505-513.
Head, R.H., & I.H. Williams, 1991. Mammogenesis is influenced by pregnancy nutrition. In: E.S. Batterham (Ed.) Manipulating Pig Production III. Australasian Pig Science Association, Victoria, 33.
Head, R.H., N.W. Bruce & I.H. Williams, 1991. More cells might lead to more milk. In: E.S. Batterham (Ed.) Manipulating Pig Production III. Australasian Pig Science Association, Victoria, 76.
Henry, Y., & M. Etienne, 1978. Alimentation énergétique du porc. J. Recherches Porcine en France 10, 119-166.
Hillyer, G.M., & P. Phillips, 1980. The effect of increasing feed level to sows and gilts in latge pregnancy on subsequent litter size, litter weight and maternal body weight change. Anim. Prod. 30, 469 (Abs).
Hovell, F.D. De. B., R.M. MacPherson, R.M.J. Crofts & K. Pennie, 1977. The effect of energy intake and mating weight on growth, carcass yield and litter size of female pigs. Anim. Prod. 25, 233-245.
Hughes, P.E., 1993. The effects of food level during lactation and early gestation on the reproductive performance of mature sows. Anim. Prod. 57, 437-446.
Kerr, J.C., & N.D. Cameron, 1995. Reproductive performance of pigs selected for components of efficient lean growth. Anim. Sci. 60, 281-290.
Kerr, J.C., & N.D. Cameron, 1996a. Responses in gilt traits measured during performance test at mating and at farrowing with selection for components of efficient lean growth rate. Anim. Sci. 63, 235-241.
Kerr, J.C., & N.D. Cameron, 1996b. Genetic and phenotypic relationships between performance test and reproduction traits in Large White pigs. Anim. Sci. 62, 531-540.

Kerr, J.C., & N.D. Cameron, 1996c. Responses in gilt post-farrowing traits and pre-weaning piglet growth to divergent selection for components of efficient lean growth rate. Anim. Sci. 63, 523-531.
Kielanowski, J., 1972. Energy requirements of the growing pig. In: D.J. Cole (Ed) Pig Production, Butterworths, London, 183-201.
King, R.H., 1987. Nutritional aneostrus in young sows. Pig News & Information 8,15-22.
King, R.N., & I.H. Williams, 1984. The effect of nutrition on the reproductive performance of first-litter sows. 1. Feeding level during lactation and between weaning and mating. Anim. Prod. 38, 241-247.
King, R.N., I.H. Williams & T. Barber, 1984. A note on the estimation of the chemical body composition of sows. Anim. Prod. 43, 167-170.
King, R.H., & A.C. Dunkin, 1986a. The effect of nutrition upon the reproductive performance of first litter sows. 3. The response to graded increases in feed intake during lactation. Anim. Prod. 42, 119-125.
King, R.H., & A.C. Dunkin, 1986b. The effect of nutrition on the performance of first-litter sows. 4. The relative effects of energy and protein intakes during lactation on performance of sows and their piglets. Anim. Prod. 43, 319-325.
Kirkwood, R.N., & F.X. Aherne, 1985. Energy intake, body composition and reproductive performance of the gilt. J. Anim. Sci.:60, 1518-1529.
Kirkwood, R.N., S.K. Baidoo & F.X. Aherne, 1990. The influence of feeding level during lactation and gestation on the endocrine status and reproductive performance of second parity sows. Canadian J. Anim. Sci. 70, 1119-1126.
Lodge, G.A., 1962. The nutrition of the lactating sow. In: J.T. Morgan & D. Lewis (Eds) Nutrition of Pigs and Poultry, Butterworths, London, 224-237.
Matte, J.J., S. Robert, C.L. Girard, C. Farmer & G.P. Martineu, 1994. Effect of bulky diets based on wheat bran or oat hulls on reproductive performance of sows during their first two parities. J. Anim. Sci. 72, 1754-1760.
Meat & Livestock Commission, 1975. Meat & Livestock Pig Yearbooks 1975 and following. Milton Keynes.
Meat & Livestock Commission, 1995. Pig Year Book 1995. Meat & Livestock Commission, Milton Keynes, 149pp.
Miller, H.M., 1996. Aspects of nutrition and metabolism in the peri-parturient sow. PhD Thesis, University of Alberta, Canada.
Mullan, B.P., 1987. Seeking sow know-how. Farmers Weekly, November 21, 45-56.
Mullan, B.P., & I.H. Williams, I.H., 1988. The effect of body reserves at farrowing on the performance of first-litter sows. Anim. Prod. 46, 494.
Mullan, B.P., I.H. Williams, 1989. The effect of body reserves at farrowing on the reproductive performance of first litter sows. Anim. Prod. 48, 449-457.
Mullan, B.P., & I.H. Williams, 1990. The chemical composition of sows during their first lactation. Anim. Prod. 51, 375-387.
National Research Council, 1988. Nutrient Requirements of Swine. National Academy Press, Washington, 9th Edn. 93pp.
Neil, M, 1996. *Ad libitum* lactation feeding of sows introduced immediately before, at, or after farrowing. Anim. Sci. 63, 497-505.
Noblet, J., & M. Etienne, 1985. Utilisation of energy during pregnancy and lactation in swine. Paper 73, 10th Symposium on Energy Metabolism, Airlie House, Virginia.
Noblet, J., W.H. Close & R.P. Heavens, 1985. Studies on the energy metabolism of the pregnant sow. 1. Uterus and mammary tissue development. Brit. J. Nutr. 53, 251-265.
Noblet, J., & M. Etienne, 1987a. Metabolic utilisation of energy and maintenance requirements in pregnant sows. Livest. Prod. Sci. 16, 243-257.
Noblet, J., & M. Etienne, 1987b. Metabolic utilisation of energy and maintenance requirements of lactating sows. J. Anim. Sci. 64, 774-781.

Noblet, J., M. Etienne & J.Y. Dourmad, J.Y., 1988. Besoins énergétiques de la truie allaitante: determination par la méthode factorielle. INRA Prod. Anim. 1, 355-358.
Noblet, J., J.Y. Dourmad & M. Etienne, 1990. Energy utilisation in pregnant and lactating sows: modelling of energy requirements. J. Anim. Sci. 68, 562-572.
O'Grady, J.F., F.W.H. Elsley, R.M. MacPherson & I. McDonald, 1975. The response of lactating sows and their litters to different dietary energy allowances. 2. Weight changes and carcass composition of sows. Anim. Prod. 20, 257-265.
Pettigrew, J.E., 1981. Supplemental dietary fat for peripartal sows: a review. J. Anim. Sci. 53, 107-117.
Pharazyn, A., L.A. Den Hartog, G.R. Foxcroft & F.X. Aherne, 1991. Dietary energy and protein intake, plasma progesterone and embryo survival in early pregnancy in the gilt. Canadian J. Anim. Sci. 71, 949-952.
Toplis, P., M.F.J. Ginesi & A.E. Wrathall, 1983. The influence of high food levels in early pregnancy on embryo survival in multiparous sows. Anim. Prod. 37, 45-48
Verstegen, M.W.A., J. Mesu, G.J.M. van Kempen & C. Geerse, 1985. Energy balances of lactating sows in relation to feeding level and stage of lactation. J. Anim. Sci. 60, 731-740.
Whittemore, C.T., 1996. Nutrition reproduction interactions in primiparous sows. Livest. Prod. Sci. 46, 65-83.
Whittemore, C.T., M.F. Franklin & B.S. Pearce, 1980. Fat changes in breeding sows. Anim. Prod. 31, 183-190.
Whittemore, C.T., A.G. Taylor, G.M. Hillyer, D. Wilson & C. Stamataris, 1984. Influence of body fat stores on reproductive performance of sows. Anim. Prod. 38, 527 (Abs).
Whittemore, C.T., W.C. Smith & P. Phillips, 1988. Fatness, live weight and performance response of sows to food level in pregnancy. Anim. Prod. 47, 123-130.
Whittemore, C.T., & H. Yang, 1989. Physical and chemical composition of the body of breeding sows with differing body subcutaneous fat depth at parturition, differing nutrition during lactation and differing litter size. Anim. Prod. 48, 203-212.
Whittemore, C.T., & C.A. Morgan, 1990. Model components for the determination of energy and protein requirements for breeding sows: a review. Livest. Prod. Sci. 26, 1-37.
Williams, I.H., W.H. Close. & D.J.A. Cole, 1985. Strategies for sow nutrition: predicting the response of pregnant animals to protein and energy intake. In: W. Haresign & D.J. Cole (Eds) Recent Advances in Animal Nutrition, Butterworths, London, 133-147.
Williams, I.H., & R.J. Smits, 1991. Body protein losses can be minimised during lactation. In: E.S. Batterham (ed) Manipulating Pig Production III. Australasian Pig Science Association, Victoria, 73.
Yang, H., P.R. Eastham, P. Phillips & C.T. Whittemore, 1989. Reproductive performance, body weight and body condition of breeding sows with differing body fatness at parturition, differing nutrition during lactation, and differing litter size. Anim. Prod. 48, 181-201.
Young, L.G., & G.J. King, 1987. Gestation energy levels for sows. Ontario Swine Res. Rev., 24-31.

11 Nitrogen intake and metabolism during pregnancy and lactation

H. Everts

11.1 Introduction

The number of weaned piglets per sow per year is an important financial parameter for the sow herd. Theoretically, a sow can produce at least 25 weaned piglets per year. Lower numbers of weaned piglets, as observed in practice, can be due to small litter sizes, high piglet mortality or low breeding frequency. The skill of the farmer, housing, breeding and nutrition all affect litter size, mortality and breeding frequency. For three reasons nutrition is often seen as one of the most important factors. Firstly, optimal nutrition is essential to enable the sow to express her potential productivity. Secondly, nutrition can be changed quantitatively and qualitatively rather easily without high investment costs, and thirdly, in terms of energy, nitrogen and minerals, nutrition is the most important input for the process of piglet production. Nowadays, the balance between input and output is seen as an important component of the sustainability of a production process. Criteria for sustainability are difficult to formulate (De Wit *et al.*, 1995), but it is clear that the gross efficiency of the utilisation of nutrients must be high.

Gross efficiency (retention/intake), depends on the size of inevitable nutrient losses and the actual nutrient retention and the relation between intake and retention. Figure 11.1 is an example of a linear-plateau relationship between intake and retention. The gross efficiency is highest where the plateau phase starts. At lower levels of nutrient intake the gross efficiency is negatively affected by the contribution from the inevitable losses and at higher levels by the decreasing partial efficiency. Figure 11.2 gives an example of a non-linear relationship between intake and retention. In this situation the highest gross efficiency is not observed at the highest level of retention, but at the point where the effect of the inevitable losses compensates the decreasing partial efficiency. From this example it is clear that maximisation of retention does not always guarantee the highest gross efficiency. Therefore, it is better to look for optimisation instead of maximisation. However, in the process of optimisation, the health and well-being of the sows and piglets must also be taken into account.

In the last decade, the negative impact of highly intensified pig production on the environment has been recognised as a serious problem. Especially in areas with a high density of pigs, the accumulation of minerals, ammonia volatilisation and nitrate in drinking water are an environmental threat (Jongbloed and Lenis, 1993). One of the major problems is the excretion of nitrogen with urine and faeces. The nitrogen excreted with urine and faeces originates, directly or indirectly, from the ingested dietary nitrogen.

When the growth of piglets until weaning is included but the rearing of the gilts up to 120 kg body weight is excluded, then for sows a gross efficiency of nitrogen utilisation of 0.18 can be calculated (Coppoolse *et al.*, 1990). This implies a high rate of excretion of nitrogen with faeces and urine by sows. To reduce the nitrogen excretion a better insight into the relationship between nitrogen intake and metabolism during pregnancy and lactation is required.

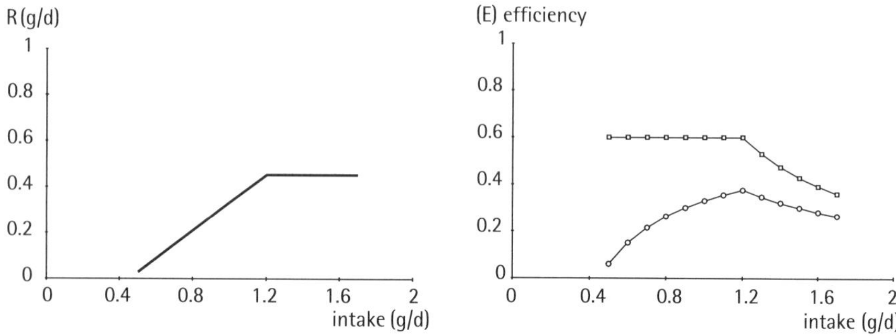

Figure 11.1. Relationship between intake and retention (R) and efficiency (E) according to a linear-plateau concept. Left: intake and retention. Right: intake and partial efficiency (□) and gross efficiency (○)

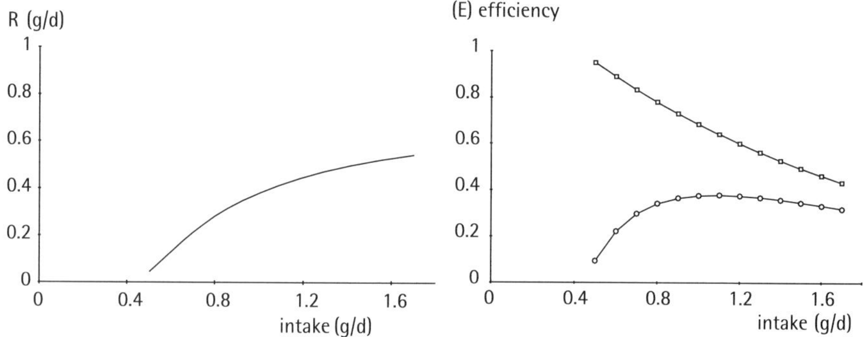

Figure 11.2 Relationship between nutrient intake and retention (R) and efficiency (E) according to a non linear concept. Left: intake and retention. Right: intake and partial efficiency (□) and gross efficiency (○)

11.2 Amino acids and the efficiency of nitrogen utilisation

Most of the nitrogen in normal diets is present as protein (6.25 x nitrogen). Protein supplies the sow with amino acids. The importance of the essential amino acids is underlined by the use of (ileal) digestible amino acids in the formulation of diets for pigs (CVB, 1996). Much emphasis is placed on the role of the most limiting amino acids such as lysine, methionine, cystine, threonine, tryptophan and isoleucine. The amounts of (ileal) digestible essential amino acids in a diet can be measured relatively easily, although there remains discussion concerning the importance of the endogenous losses and the real availability of amino acids to the animal. However, the major problem is how to calculate the animal's requirements for these essential amino acids. The amino acid requirements for pregnant sows can be considered in three parts: maintenance, protein gain in the products of conception and maternal protein gain. For lactating sows the situation is even more complicated: maintenance, milk protein production and maternal protein gain or mobilisation. The requirement for an amino acid can be calculated based on:

- the maintenance requirement for the amino acid (AA_m)
- nitrogen retention in the products of conception (NR_{pc}), maternal gain (NR_{mg}) and milk (NL)
- the amino acid content per g N in the products of conception (AA_{pc}), maternal gain (AA_{mat}) and milk (AA_l)
- the partial efficiencies for maintenance (e_m), gain in the products of conception (e_{pc}), maternal gain(e_{mat}), milk production (e_l) and mobilisation (e_r).
- the apparent ileal digestibility of the amino acid (D_{aa})

The figures for partial efficiencies can have a considerable effect on the calculated requirement for an amino acid and, especially for sows, knowledge about these partial efficiencies is very limited. The most simple concept, assuming the same partial efficiency for all processes, results in equation (1) for the pregnant sow, equation (2a) for the lactating sow with a positive nitrogen retention and equation (2b) for the lactating sow with a negative nitrogen retention. In this last equation an estimate of the partial efficiency of mobilising amino acids into milk amino acids is required. When the assumption of a single estimate of partial efficiency for all processes is rejected, then more complicated equations are needed (equation (3) and (4a,b)). The idea of different partial efficiencies for specific amino acids increases the number of equations even further.

$$\text{Required AA}_{preg.} = (AA_m + NR_{pc} \times AA_{pc} + NR_m \times AA_{mat})/e/D_{aa} \quad (1)$$

$$\text{Required AA}_{lact.} = (AA_m + NL \times AA_l + NR_m \times AA_{mat})/e/D_{aa} \quad (NR_m>0) \quad (2a)$$

$$= (AA_m + NL \times AA_l + NR_m \times AA_{mat} \times e_r)/e/D_{aa} \quad (NR_m<0) \quad (2b)$$

$$\text{Required AA}_{preg.} = (AA_m / e_m + NR_{pc} \times AA_{pc} / e_{pc} + NR_m \times AA_{mat} / e_{mat}) / D_{aa} \quad (3)$$

$$\text{Required AA}_{lact.} = (AA_m/e_m + NL \times AA_l/e_l + NR_m \times AA_{mat}/e_{mat})/D_{aa} \quad (NR_m>0) \quad (4a)$$

$$= \{AA_m/e_m + (NL \times AA_l + NR_m \times AA_{mat} \times e_r)/e_l\}/D_{aa} \quad (NR_m<0) \quad (4b)$$

Besides the uncertainty concerning selection of the partial efficiencies, there is a problem in calculating the amounts of amino acids retained in the different compartments. The total nitrogen retention of a pregnant sow is relatively easy to measure, but the partitioning over the different compartments can only be measured by comparative slaughter. The concept of an ideal protein relevant to the growing pig seems less suitable for application to pregnant and lactating sows. Table 11.1 gives the patterns relative to lysine for some essential amino acids related to maintenance, protein gain in foetuses, maternal body protein and milk protein. This information indicates that it is difficult to formulate an ideal protein for sows. For the calculation of an ideal protein, knowledge about the partitioning of the protein gain, in foetal and maternal protein, is needed. Moreover, the maintenance requirement has a larger impact on the amino acid composition of the protein for a sow then for a growing/finishing pig. This is due to the higher live weight of a sow and the relatively low rate of protein gain, especially in the first months of pregnancy. A wide range in estimated amino acids patterns (expressed as percentage of the lysine requirement) can be calculated for sows differing in live weight, maternal protein gain, protein gain in the products of conception and milk protein production.

Table 11.1. The patterns for some essential amino acids (expressed as a percentage of lysine (=100%)) and the amount of lysine per 16 g N

	Maintenance[1]	Conceptus[2]	Maternal body[3]	Milk[4]
Lysine	100	100	100	100
Methionine	25	24	29	26
Cystine	111	22	15	21
Threonine	147	56	53	59
Tryptophan	30	12	12	17
Isoleucine	44	49	55	55
g lysine/ 16 g N	-	5.9	6.6	7.5

[1] Growing pigs (Fuller *et al.*, 1989).
[2] Conceptus at d 109 of pregnancy (Everts and Dekker, 1995a).
[3] First and third parity sows (Everts and Dekker, 1995a,b).
[4] Mean value from King *et al.* (1993), Elliot *et al.* (1971), Duée and Jung (1973), Dourmad *et al.* (1991) and Helms (1978).

An additional problem is that a surplus of amino acids is catabolised regardless of the amino acids being balanced. The catabolism of amino acids results in a higher excretion of urea with the urine. The amount of urea depends on the

number of ammonia-groups present in the different amino acids.
As the uncertainty and the problems related to amino acid metabolism are considered, then it must be concluded that a study of nitrogen metabolism during pregnancy and lactation at the amino acid level is too complicated with present technology. A study at the level of nitrogen is easier and cheaper, especially for performing experiments and also for predicting nitrogen excretion. Such studies are only useful when an indication of the pattern of the most important dietary essential amino acids is given. In our own experiments discussed in this chapter, the supply of essential amino acids in relation to lysine was equal or higher than that suggested by Whittemore and Morgan (1990) (Table 11.2).

Table 11.2. The pattern of some essential amino acids expressed as a percentage of lysine (=100%)

	Experimental diets[1]	Whittemore and Morgan (1990)
Lysine	100	100
Threonine	74 - 77	64
Valine	100 -101	71
Isoleucine	73 - 84	57
Tyrosine + Phenylalanine	146 -157	100
Histidine	51 - 53	36
Cystine + Methionine	71 - 77	57
Tryptophan	20 - 22	20

[1] diets used in studies conducted by Everts and co-workers (Everts and Dekker, 1994a,b; Everts and Dekker, 1995a,b).

11.3 Nitrogen requirement during pregnancy

The nutrient supply for mature sows during pregnancy needs to meet the energy and nitrogen requirements for the maintenance of the sow and for the development of products of conception and those of the mammary glands. Younger sows also require additional nutrients to grow to maturity and older sows to compensate for losses during the previous lactation. Theoretical nitrogen requirements have been calculated by Vanschoubroek and van Spaendonck (1973), Speer (1990) and Everts and Dekker (1994a). Whittemore and Morgan (1990) and Williams *et al.* (1993) designed models to determine optimal protein requirements for pregnant sows.
Information about the requirement for nitrogen can also be derived from serial slaughter studies with gilts. In some studies the change in chemical body composition of pregnant gilts was compared with that of non-pregnant gilts (De Wilde ,

1980a,b; Hovell *et al.*, 1977; Lodge *et al.*, 1979; Shields and Mahan, 1983; Walach-Janiak *et al.*, 1986a). In other experiments the effect of different feeding levels on body composition of gilts (Hovel *et al.*, 1977; Walach-Janiak *et al.*, 1986b) and on the products of conception (Noblet *et al.*, 1985) was investigated. The effect of protein supply at a constant level of energy supply was studied in comparative slaughter experiments by Everts and Dekker (1995a) and Shields *et al.* (1985).
Differences in nutrient supply affected maternal body composition, but not the composition of the products of conception. The levels of protein were probably high enough to prevent an effect on the products of conception. The negative effect of a severe nitrogen restriction (2-6 g N per sow per day) on nutrient accretion in the products of conception is well known (Pond, 1973; Atinmo *et al.*, 1974; Hammell *et al.*, 1976; Leuillet *et al.*, 1979; Pond *et al.*, 1991). A more moderate nitrogen restriction (24 - 28 g N per sow per day) can tend to lead to lower piglet birth weights (Mahan, 1977, 1979). But at a nitrogen supply of about 30 g N per sow per day, foetal growth appears to be guaranteed (Duée, 1976). King and Brown (1993) presented a linear relation between nitrogen intake and nitrogen retention in gilts. At a daily nitrogen intake of about 30 g they measured a nitrogen retention of about 14 g, which equals the amount of nitrogen retained in the products of conception (Noblet *et al.*, 1985). When nitrogen supply exceeds about 30 g per day, then the supply seems to be related to maternal protein gain until the maximum level of maternal nitrogen retention is reached. This maximum rate of maternal nitrogen retention depends on the level of energy supply (King and Brown, 1993; Hovell *et al.*, 1977; Kemm, 1974) and probably also on parity number or age of the sow (Carr *et al.*, 1977; Everts and Dekker, 1994a).
From the literature an estimate of the nitrogen requirement for a sufficient development of the products of conception can be derived (30 g N/d). An estimate of the nitrogen requirement for the maternal body stores is more elusive, because information about an ideal development of the body composition of a sow during successive parities is lacking.

11.4 Nitrogen efficiency and excretion during pregnancy

Instead of optimum requirements for pregnant sows, minimum nitrogen requirements are needed, if the aim is to reduce nitrogen excretion. The highest reduction in nitrogen excretion can be realised, when the efficiency of dietary nitrogen utilisation is maximised. But such aspects as acceptable litter sizes and piglet birth weights should not be ignored. From nitrogen balance experiments conducted in mid and late pregnancy during three parities (Everts and Dekker, 1994a) it was concluded that nitrogen excretion decreases proportionately (35 to 40 %), when the daily dietary nitrogen supply decreases from 60 to 40 g N in mid pregnancy and from 75 to 50 g N in late pregnancy. The latter workers observed no effects on litter size nor on piglet birth weights, but the number of balance trials was too small to draw firm conclusions. Especially in late pregnancy the daily maternal nitrogen retention was 8 to 10 g lower with the restricted nitrogen supply. The gross efficiency of dietary nitrogen utilisation differed between the two levels of nitrogen supply only in mid pregnancy, but not in late pregnancy and a significant relationship between nitrogen intake and nitrogen retention could only be derived in late pregnancy, as shown in Figures 11.3 and 11.4. The derived relationship, expressed per kg metabolic body weight was :

$$NI = 0.46\ (\pm\ 0.08) + 1.66\ (\pm\ 0.21) \times NR\ (R^2_{adj} = 0.48)$$

This equation indicates a maintenance requirement of 0.46 g N per kg metabolic body weight and an efficiency of nitrogen utilisation above maintenance of 0.6. These values are fairly close to those reported by Beyer (1986), who observed a maintenance requirement of 0.5 and an efficiency above maintenance of 0.6 (assuming a digestibility coefficient for nitrogen of 0.8).
In the study, the results for which are given in Figure 11.3, the supply of nitrogen ranged between 0.7 and 1.5 g N per kg metabolic body weight. When a maintenance requirement of 0.45 g is taken into account, then with an efficiency of 0.6 the nitrogen retention can vary between 0.15 to 0.63 g nitrogen. However, the highest level of nitrogen retention observed was 0.4. This level of nitrogen retention is equal to a daily nitrogen retention of about 16 g and includes the nitrogen retained in the products of conception. At this stage of pregnancy the nitrogen retained in the products of conception is estimated to be about 2 g N per day (Noblet *et al.*, 1985). Thus the highest maternal nitrogen retention was about 14 g for this genotype of sows.

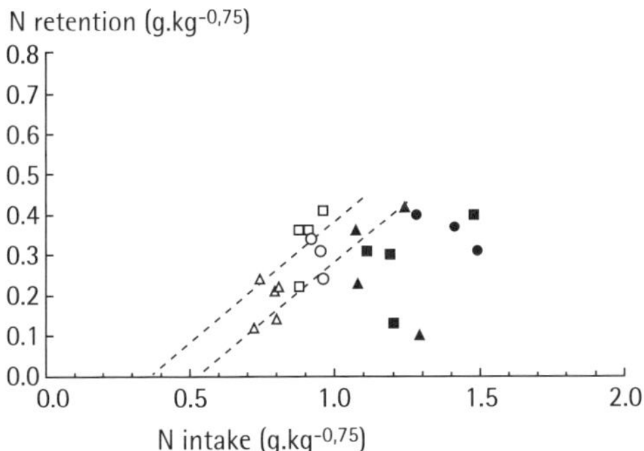

Figure 11.3. Relationship between nitrogen retention (NR) and nitrogen intake (NI) in g N per kg metabolic body weight during mid pregnancy. Parity numbers are indicated as : 1 = ○, 2 = □, 3 = Δ. Open symbols indicate the observations on a diet with 16 g N per kg and the closed symbols on a diet with 26 g N per kg. The lines indicate the theoretical relationship of NI = 0.45 + 1.66 x NR with a confidence interval of 2 times the standard deviation.

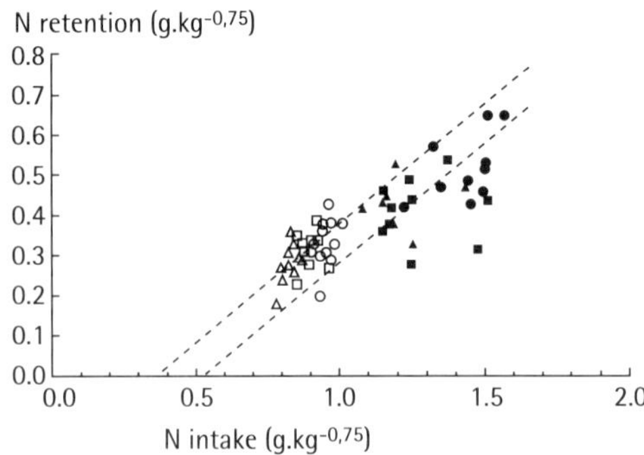

Figure 11.4. Relationship between nitrogen retention (NR) and nitrogen intake (NI) in g N per kg metabolic body weight during late pregnancy. Parity numbers are indicated as : 1 = ○, 2 = □, 3 = Δ. Open symbols indicate the observations on a diet with 16 g N per kg and the closed symbols on a diet with 26 g N per kg. The lines indicate the theoretical relationship of NI = 0.45 + 1.66 x NR with a confidence interval of 2 times the standard deviation.

From Figure 11.3 it can also be concluded that a dietary supply above 1.1 g N per kg metabolic body weight had no positive effect on nitrogen retention and can be seen as an oversupply of N to the sows in mid pregnancy.

In late pregnancy the supply of nitrogen ranged between 0.8 and 1.55 g N per kg metabolic body weight. With the same assumptions for maintenance and efficiency the expected nitrogen retention could vary between 0.2 and 0.66. The highest rate of nitrogen retention in late pregnancy was about 0.6. This is equal to a daily nitrogen retention of about 30 g. In late pregnancy, about 14 g nitrogen is retained in the products of conception (Noblet *et al.*, 1985). Thus the maximal maternal nitrogen retention was about 16 g per day. This level is close to that measured during mid pregnancy.

From these data it can be concluded that there are considerable possibilities to reduce nitrogen excretion, but that maternal nitrogen retention will be affected. This effect can be expected when nitrogen supply above maintenance is lower then 30 g (= (2+16)/0.6) in mid pregnancy and 50 g (=(14+16)/0.6) in late pregnancy. When the parity number increases, there is a tendency for maternal nitrogen retention to decrease (Everts and Dekker, 1994a, 1995b) and thus these figures can be reduced.

11.5 Nitrogen efficiency and excretion during lactation

The nitrogen requirement of the lactating sow is often expressed on the basis of lysine, because it is often the first limiting amino acid. There is a large variation in reported nitrogen and lysine requirements for lactation. For example, Pettigrew (1993) indicated that reported lysine requirements ranged between 20 and 53 g per day. This variation can be explained by differences in the number of suckling piglets, the ability of sows to produce milk and the growth potential of the suckling piglets. In most experiments with lactating sows the number of suckling piglets was rather low (Sohail *et al.*, 1978) or the mean daily piglet gain was close to or below 200 g per day (Beyer, 1986; Noblet and Etienne, 1986, 1987). The amount of milk consumed per piglet per day in the second to the fourth week of lactation has been estimated to be about 1 kg (Babinszky, 1992). With such a milk production a piglet gain of about 250 g per day can be expected, assuming that there is about 4 g milk needed for 1 g gain (Everts *et al.*, 1995). For a sow with 10 suckling piglets a milk production of about 10 kg per day seems a reasonable estimate. This is much higher than the 5 kg milk assumed by Speer (1990).

Everts and Dekker (1994b) observed that sows with a daily litter gain of about 2.65 kg supported a gross efficiency of dietary nitrogen utilisation of about 40 % and thus excreted around 60 % of their ingested nitrogen in the urine and faeces. From their studies it was also concluded that a higher dietary nitrogen and lysine supply decreased the mobilisation of the sow's body protein without affecting the daily litter gain, but it increased the fat mobilisation of the sows. This latter effect was also shown by Pettigrew *et al.* (1991). The dietary nitrogen requirement for a lactating sow was estimated to range between 162 and 185 g N per day, depending on the parity number and the amount of nitrogen retained by the piglets. This estimate is higher than those of Beyer (1986) and Speer (1990). The main reason for this discrepancy is the difference in estimated milk production and thus in piglet liveweight gain.

A theoretical calculation of the nitrogen requirement, assuming a maintenance requirement of 0.45 g N per kg metabolic body weight, a partial efficiency of ingested nitrogen into milk nitrogen of 0.6 and a partial efficiency of mobilised body nitrogen to milk nitrogen of 1.0, agrees fairly well with the observed values of Everts and Dekker (1994b) (see Figure 11.5). However, other values were used by King (see Chapter 7).

In relation to the pregnancy period, Everts and Dekker (1994b) concluded that the possibilities to reduce nitrogen excretion during lactation are limited. This is mainly due to the relatively short period of lactation compared to pregnancy and to the high output of nitrogen as milk protein compared to the maintenance requirement.

11.6 Nitrogen excretion per sow per year and the body composition of sows

From nitrogen balance trials during pregnancy and lactation and from comparative slaughter trials, Everts (1994) concluded that it is possible to reduce nitrogen excretion by about 25 %. In Table 11.3. it can be seen that the determined nitrogen excretion is higher with the method of comparative slaughter than with the balance technique. This may be due to the known overestimation of nitrogen retention in balance trials (Just *et al.*, 1982). The use of a diet with a higher nitrogen content

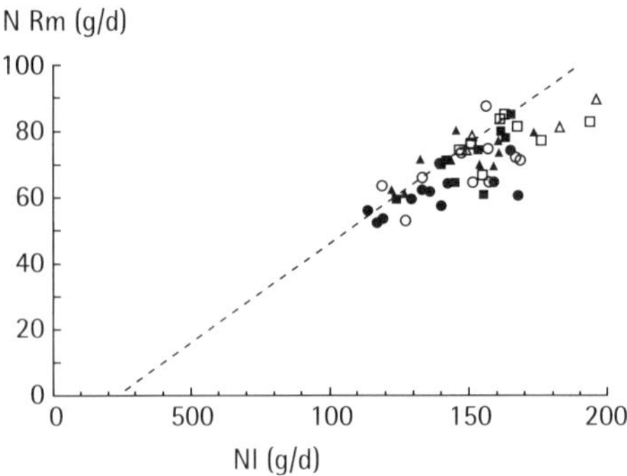

Figure 11.5. Relationship between corrected nitrogen milk production (NR_m) and nitrogen intake (NI) in g N. NR_m is calculated as NR_{litter} x 1.18 + NR_{sow}. Parity numbers are indicated as : 1 = ○, 2 = □, 3 = Δ. Open symbols indicate the observations on a diet with 32 g N per kg and the closed symbols on a diet with 26 g N per kg. The line indicates the theoretical relation of NI = 0.45 x metabolic live weight + 1.66 x NR_m for a sow of 195 kg live weight without nitrogen mobilisation.

Table 11.3. Nitrogen excretion per sow per year in kg, calculated from balance trials and comparative slaughter studies (between brackets = % of the treatment with 24.7 g N in the diet during pregnancy and lactation)

Nitrogen content of the diet		Balance		Comparative slaughter	
Pregnancy	Lactation				
24.7	24.7	20.3	(=100 %)	22.2	(=100 %)
24.7	28.5	20.7	(102 %)	23.4	(105 %)
16.7	24.7	14.5	(71 %)	16.0	(72 %)
16.7	28.5	15.2	(75 %)	17.3	(78 %)

(+ 15 %) during lactation increased the nitrogen excretion by only 2 to 6 %.
The effect of the nitrogen content of the diet during pregnancy and lactation on body composition (Table 11.4) indicates a significant effect of nitrogen supply during pregnancy on the nitrogen deposition in the first parity and suggests a decrease in nitrogen deposition with increasing parity number on the treatments with a relatively high nitrogen supply during pregnancy. Sows with a restricted nitrogen supply during pregnancy compensated their lower nitrogen retention in the first reproductive cycle, in the second and third reproductive cycles. The nitrogen supply during lactation hardly affected the nitrogen deposition during a reproductive cycle.

Table 11.4. Estimated nitrogen deposition (kg) in the sows during 3 reproductive cycles (Everts and Dekker, 1995b)

Nitrogen content of the diet		Reproductive cycle		
Pregnancy	Lactation	1.	2.	3.
24.7	24.7	0.70	0.53	0.33
24.7	28.5	0.72	0.70	0.08
16.7	24.7	0.36	0.78	0.38
16.7	28.5	0.36	0.53	0.51

When the protein body mass of sows is estimated with the model:

$$\text{Protein mass} = A + B \times \exp^{(-k \times \text{age})}$$

derived from the data of Everts and Dekker (1995b), then a maximum protein mass of about 42 kg was estimated for third parity sows at the highest levels of nitrogen supply. This value is fairly close to values observed by Whittemore and Yang (1989) for fourth parity sows. Based on these observations the following hypothesis can be developed. A breeding sow has a biological need to have a protein store of about 40 kg in her body and she is trying to realise this according to a certain pattern. This can be hampered by a limited nitrogen supply during pregnancy and/or a high mobilisation of protein during lactation. Compensation can be achieved by increasing protein gain during pregnancy, by increasing the efficiency of protein gain or by decreasing the mobilisation during lactation. When only small litters are reared, in combination with a high feeding level during lactation, the protein mass will increase towards a high level (Whittemore and Yang, 1989) and will then halt when the adult size is reached. However, information about the adult size of the protein mass of a sow is uncertain and probably also depends on the genotype of the sow.

In addition to the protein mass, there is a fat mass in the sow. This fat mass can be seen as an energy store which can be mobilised relatively easily compared to the protein mass. When there exists too large a discrepancy between the protein mass and the fat mass, problems with reproductive performance can be expected, especially in young sows (Everts and Sebek, 1992). There is little convincing evidence concerning the relationship between body stores and reproductive performance of sows. But in humans it is well known that a high protein mass and a small fat mass can prevent the start of the menstrual cycle in young girls or can stop the menstrual cycle in woman with excessive muscle development (Frisch, 1988). This is discussed further in Chapter 10.

11.7 Effect of reproductive characteristics on nitrogen excretion compared to nutritional measures

As shown in the first part of this chapter it is possible to reduce nitrogen excretion by nutritional manipulation. However, it is important to estimate the effect on nitrogen excretion of other factors, such as: increasing the litter size, improving the survival of piglets, increasing the farrowing index and lowering the replacement rate of sows.

At first sight it seems logical and attractive to express the excretion of nitrogen per sow per year. However, this way of expression is only valid when the production of weaned piglets per sow per year remains constant. When a measure affects both the excretion of nitrogen and the number of weaned piglets, then the expression of nitrogen excretion per sow per year can easily lead to incorrect conclusions. Therefore, it is better to express the nitrogen excretion per weaned piglet for breeding sows and per kg of edible meat for fattening pigs.

Everts (1994) used a theoretical model to calculate the effect on nitrogen excretion per weaned piglet of varying reproductive parameters. In these calculations the nitrogen required for the rearing of the gilts from a live weight of 8 kg was also included. The model predicted the same nitrogen intake and excretion as calculated by Coppoolse *et al.* (1990), when the contribution form the rearing of the sow was excluded, and fixed values for farrowing index (2.2), sow replacement rate (48 %), litter size (alive + stillborn) (11), piglet mortality (17 %) and nitrogen content of the diet fed during pregnancy (26 g N per kg) were used. Using these fixed values it was calculated that about 16 % of the ingested nitrogen per weaned piglet was needed for rearing, 60 % for pregnancy and 24 % for lactation. From the total retained nitrogen per weaned piglet about 29 % was retained in reared gilts, 12 % in the sow, 56 % in weaned piglets and 3 % in dead piglets. The model calculated a gross efficiency of dietary nitrogen utilisation of about 21 %. This efficiency is higher than that calculated by Coppoolse *et al.* (1990) due to the contribution of the rearing period of the sow.

Table 11.5. Linear relations between nitrogen excretion per weaned piglet in g N (Y) defined as NEX_p and some reproductive characteristics (X) (between brackets = tested range), according to the model $Y = C + \beta_1 \times X$. (Everts , 1994)

Y	C	β_1	X	(range)	R^2_{adj}	RSD
NEX_p	1067.8	+ 13.2	Piglet mortality in %	(5-20)	0.99	5.3
NEX_p	1170.6	+ 2.6	Yearly replacement rate sows in %	(20-50)	0.95	7.7
NEX_p	2431.9	- 97.0	Litter size (borne alive + stillborn)	(11-14)	0.99	10.7
NEX_p	2341.9	-499.6	Farrowing index	(2.0-2.4)	0.99	4.9
NEX_p	307.8	+ 38.3	N content pregnancy diet (g/kg)	(16-26)	1.00	0.0

Table 11.5 gives linear models for the effect of changes in the reproductive characteristics tested on nitrogen excretion (per weaned piglet).
A decrease in piglet mortality of 1 % causes a reduction in nitrogen excretion per weaned piglet of 13 g N. The three main reasons for piglet mortality are starvation, crushing by the sow and stillbirths (Dyck and Swierstra, 1989). Besides the feeding level in late pregnancy (Cromwell *et al.*, 1989), hygienic conditions at farrowing, the micro-climate for piglets, housing system and feeding during lactation are important factors influencing piglet mortality. It is possible to reduce piglet mortality, but the effect on nitrogen excretion is relatively small.
A reduction in replacement rate of sows in a herd has only a minor effect on the nitrogen excretion. This small effect is due to the accompanying decrease in nitrogen retention in reared gilts and sows. With a yearly replacement rate of 48%, about 148 g nitrogen per weaned piglet is retained in the rearing gilts and in the sows, but with a replacement rate of 20 % this amount of retained nitrogen dropped to 65 g. For herds with a low priority for genetic improvement, economic studies have indicated that a sow should produce at least 7 litters (Kroes and van Male, 1979; Scholman and Dijkhuizen, 1989). This is equivalent to a yearly replacement rate of less than 30 %. It is concluded that the level of yearly replacement is not important for the nitrogen excretion per weaned piglet, but that it is determined by the preferred level of selection and economic considerations.
In contrast to yearly replacement rate, litter size has a strong influence on the nitrogen excretion per weaned piglet. However, this effect holds only when piglet mortality does not increase at the same time. From the model it was clear that the effect of litter size on nitrogen excretion per weaned piglet is not linear: an increase in litter size from 11 to 12 has more effect on nitrogen excretion than an increase from 13 to 14 piglets. Litter size can be increased by genetic selection, however, the progress is relatively slow. Another way to increase litter size is the reduction of embryonic mortality. For gilts there are well-known effects of feeding level on embryonic mortality (Dyck and Strain, 1983), but for sows there is little evidence for such an effect.
An increase in farrowing index of 0.1 reduces the nitrogen excretion per weaned piglet by about 50 g. Increasing the farrowing index above 2.4 requires a shortening of the lactation period and the interval between weaning and next pregnancy. The lactation length can be reduced to about three weeks (Te Brake, 1978; Varley, 1982), but the interval between weaning and next pregnancy seems to depend on management (Fahmy *et al.*, 1979) or on the suckling intensity (Foxcroft, 1992).
Compared to the manipulation of the reproductive characteristics, reduction of the nitrogen content of the pregnancy diet seems to be a powerful and effective method for decreasing the nitrogen excretion per weaned piglet. However, the main assumptions for this measure are that neither the production level of the sow nor the sow's body composition change. As seen before it can be concluded that these assumptions are not completely valid. To achieve a nitrogen content below 16 g per kg often requires the use of synthetic amino acids. This is only

attractive when the price of synthetic amino acids is economic and the production process for these synthetic amino acids does not consume much energy nor cause pollution.
When all reproductive characteristics are improved to realistic levels (farrowing index 2.3, replacement rate 38 %, litter size 13, piglet mortality 10 %) in combination with a reduction in the nitrogen level of the pregnancy diet (from 26 to 16 g per kg), then the nitrogen excretion can be reduced from about 1300 to about 700 g per weaned piglet and the gross efficiency of nitrogen utilisation can be increased from 0.20 to 0.30. Even in such an ideal situation the excretion per weaned piglet still remains relatively high. However, for the production of pork weaned piglets are indispensable.

11.8 Possible feeding strategies for breeding sows with respect to nitrogen

Many possible feeding strategies can be designed for breeding sows, depending on preference for the development of body condition and liveweight of the sows during their productive life. With respect to longevity, Den Hartog (1984) proposed having a moderate growth rate during the rearing period. After the rearing period two completely different feeding strategies can be proposed.
The first strategy is based on the belief that sows have a biological drive to reach a certain protein mass in their body. To fulfil this drive sows must be fed (during the first parities) with a protein-rich diet during pregnancy and lactation. Such a high protein supply during pregnancy guarantees a maximal rate of maternal protein deposition. In addition, during lactation a high protein supply during lactation minimises protein mobilisation. The amount of fat can be regulated by varying dietary energy supply. The fat deposition can be regulated much more easily during pregnancy than during lactation due to the limited feed intake capacity of young sows in this phase of the reproductive cycle. If the ratio between lean mass and fat is considered to be important for reproductive performance of young sows as is indicated by observations in humans (Frisch, 1988), then special attention must be given to the required amount of body fat in the young sow.
When the sow has reached her adult protein mass, she can be fed according to the requirements for maintenance and during pregnancy for the development of the products of conception, and during lactation for milk production, without mobilising her body stores.
In such a feeding strategy, sows will have a high live weight and this means a high maintenance requirement for energy and protein. This affects the gross efficiency of the utilisation of protein in a negative way and thus environmental contamination increases. The only way to reduce environmental pollution in such a feeding strategy is to prevent an excessive supply of protein during the first parities. This last point can only be realised when there is enough information about the maximum protein mass of sows differing in genetic background.

Additional objections to this feeding strategy are the low mean age of sows in practice and the lack of knowledge concerning the regulation of feed intake during lactation in young sows.
The second feeding strategy is based on a slow development of the protein mass. When protein with a good pattern of amino acids is supplied at a level just below the required amounts to express the maximum capacity of protein retention, then the gross efficiency of utilisation of ingested protein can be maximised. For sows the growth performance is not as important as for fattening pigs. When such a feeding strategy results in a lower reproductive performance, this indicates that the restriction has been too severe.
An additional advantage of a slow development of protein mass is the relatively low liveweight of the sows compared to the first feeding strategy. Also, the amount of body fat required to reach a desired lean to fat ratio is reduced.
In such a feeding strategy, the restriction during pregnancy is relatively easy to apply, but during lactation it can be more complicated due to the limited feed intake of the young sows. To prevent an imbalance between protein and fat mobilisation during lactation, it is possible to feed lactating sows a diet with a protein (or amino acid) to energy ratio which is comparable to that in the body of the sow.

11.9 Conclusions

The required dietary nitrogen intake during pregnancy is heavily dependent upon the amino acid composition of the protein suplied and is a function of the desired maternal body nitrogen deposition in the sow. The calculation of the required amount of an essential amino acid for a pregnant sow is hampered by the lack of information about the partial efficiencies of utilisation for individual amino acids and for the different processes which require amino acids (maintenance, development of the products of conception and maternal protein gain). Besides the energy supply, the level of supply of an amino acid can also influence the partial efficiency (Helms, 1978).
Especially in the first month of pregnancy, the desired maternal nitrogen deposition of young sows has a large impact on the required nitrogen. There is a lot of information available about the effects of feeding strategy on body composition of gilts, but the effects of differences in body composition on their reproductive performance requires more study.
The effects of varying nitrogen and amino acid supply during lactation have mainly been tested in sows with a moderate capacity for milk production. Increased milk production requires a higher supply of nutrients, unless a higher mobilisation of body stores is acceptable. Also during lactation, there is uncertainty about the efficiency of conversion of dietary to milk protein and from the body stores into milk. The observed effects of amino acid supply (lysine) on the energy mobilisation warrant further investigation.
Nitrogen metabolism during pregnancy seems to interact with nitrogen meta-

bolism during lactation. This can be explained by the biological drive of the sow to reach her adult protein mass. When the development of body protein is on target, she may tolerate a higher nitrogen loss during lactation than when the development of the protein mass is retarded.
In the last decade, environmental pollution due to intensive animal production has become more recognised. This means that it is important to reduce the nitrogen excretion by sows. Besides improvements in reproductive characteristics, such as litter size and piglet mortality, reduction of the nitrogen content of the diet fed during pregnancy seems to be the most powerful tool. The effect of changing the nitrogen content of the diet fed during lactation is limited. The challenge for the near future seems to be in designing a feeding strategy which guarantees a supply of amino acids, but including the lowest amount of protein necessary for development of the body composition of the sows during their reproductive life, so that the reproductive performance remains at a high level. To achieve this, synthetic amino acids and highly digestible protein sources may be necessary. However, synthetic amino acids are only attractive when the price is reasonable and the production process of these synthetic amino acids does not causes pollution. The use of highly digestible protein sources is only acceptable when these products are unsuitable for human consumption.

11.10 References

Atinmo, T., W.G. Pond & R.H. Barnes, 1974, Effect of maternal energy vs. protein restriction on growth and development of progeny in swine. J. Anim. Sc. 39, 703-711.
Babinzsky, L., 1992, Energy metabolism and lactation performance of primiparous sows as affected by dietary fat and vitamin E. Thesis, Agricultural University Wageningen, The Netherlands, pp. 159
Beyer, M.,1986, Untersuchungen zum Energie- und Stoffumsatz von graviden und lactierende Sauen sowie Saugferkeln - eine Beitrag zur präzisierung des Energie- und Proteinsbedarfes. Promotionarbeit, Forschungszentrum für Tierproduction, Dummerstorf-Rostock, Germany, pp.234.
Brake, J.H.A. te,1978. An assessment of the most profitable length of lactation for producing piglets of 20 kg body weight. Livest. Prod. Sci. 5, 81-94.
Carr, J.R., K.N. Boorman & D.J.A. Cole, 1977, Nitrogen retention in the pig. Br. J. Nutr. 37, 143-155.
Coppoolse, J., A.M. van Vuuren, J. Huisman, W.M.M.A. Janssen, A.W. Jongbloed, N.P. Lenis & P.C.M. Simons, 1990, [Excretion of nitrogen, phosphorus and potassium by livestock, now and tomorrow]. D.L.O., Wageningen, The Netherlands, pp.131.
Cromwell, G.L., D.D. Hall, A.J. Clawson, G.E. Combs, D.A. Knabe, C.V. Maxwell, P.R. Nolan, D.E. Orr Jr. & T.J. Prince, 1989, Effects of additional feed during late gestation on reproductive performance of sows: a co-operative study. J. Anim. Sci. 67, 3-14.
Dourmad, J.Y., M. Etienne & J. Noblet, 1991, A contribution to the study of amino acid requirement for lactation in sows. J. Rech. Porc. France, 23, 61-68.
Duée, P.H.,1976, Chronologie de l'apport azote pendant le cycle de réproduction chez la truie. Ann. Zootechn. 24, 199-212.
Duée, P.H. & J. Jung, 1973, Amino acid composition of sow's milk. Ann. Zootechn. 22, 243-247.

CVB, 1996. Verkorte tabel. Voedernormen landbouwhuisdieren en voederwaarde veevoeders. CVB-reeks nr 20, augustus, 1996, Centraal Veevoederbureau, Lelystad.
Dyck , G.W. & J.H. Strain, 1983, Post mating feeding level effects on conception rate and embryonic survival in gilts. Can. J. Anim. Sci. 63, 579-585.
Dyck , G.W. & E.E. Swierstra, 1989, Causes of piglet death from birth to weaning. Can. J. Anim. Sci. 67, 543-547.
Elliot, R.F, G.W. van der Noot, R.L. Gilbreath & H. Fisher,1971, Effect of dietary protein level on composition changes in sow colostrum and milk. J. Anim. Sci. 32, 1128-1137.
Everts, H., 1994. Nitrogen and energy metabolism of sows during several reproductive cycles in relation to nitrogen intake. Thesis, Agricultural University Wageningen, The Netherlands. pp 156.
Everts, H. & L.B.J. Sebek, 1992. Effect of lysine supply during lactation on reproductive performance in sows. Proc. Int. Pig Vet. Soc., The Hague, The Netherlands (17-20 august), p. 611. (abstract).
Everts , H. & R.A. Dekker, 1994a, Effect of nitrogen supply on the retention and excretion of nitrogen and on energy metabolism of pregnant sows. Anim. Prod. 59, 293-301.
Everts, H. & R.A. Dekker, 1994b, Effect of nitrogen supply on nitrogen and energy metabolism in lactating sows. Anim. Prod. 59, 445-454.
Everts, H. & R.A. Dekker, 1995a, Effect of protein supply during pregnancy on body composition of gilts and their products of conception. Livest. Prod. Sci. 43, 27-36.
Everts, H. & R.A. Dekker, 1995b, Effect of protein supply during pregnancy and lactation on body composition of sows during three reproductive cycles. Livest. Prod. Sci. 43, 137-147.
Everts, H., M.C. Blok, B. Kemp, C.M.C. van der Peet-Schwering & C.H.M. Smits, 1995. Normen voor lacterende zeugen. Uitgangspunten en factoriële afleiding van de behoefte aan energie en darmverteerbare aminozuren voor lacterende zeugen. C.V.B.-documentatierapport nr. 13. Centraal Veevoeder Bureau, Lelystad, The Netherlands, pp. 45.
Fahmy, M.H., W.B Holtman & R.D. Baker, 1979. Failure to recycle after weaning, and weaning to oestrus interval in crossbred sows. Anim. Prod. 29, 193-202.
Foxcroft, G.R., 1992. Nutritional and lactational regulation of fertility in sows. J. Reprod. Fert. (Suppl.) 45, 113-125.
Frisch, A.,1988. Fatness and fertility. Scientific American 258, 70-77.
Fuller, M.F., R. MacWilliam, T.C. Wang & L.R. Giles, 1989. The optimum dietary amino acid pattern for growing pigs. 2. Requirements for maintenance and for tissue protein accretion. Br. J. Nutr. 62, 255-267
Hammell, D.L., D.D. Kratzer, G.I. Cromwell & V.W. Hays, 1976. Effect of protein malnutrition of the sow on reproductive performance and on postnatal learning and performance of the offspring. J. Anim. Sci. 43, 589-597.
Hartog , L.A. den, 1984, The effect of energy intake on development and reproduction of gilts and sows. Thesis, Agricultural University Wageningen, The Netherlands, pp. 117.
Helms, W., 1978. Zur Verwertung von Futterproteinen definierter Zusammensetzung und Ergänzung beim lactierenden Schwein. Thesis, Göttungen, Germany.
Hovell , F.D. DeB., R.M. MacPherson, R.M.J. Crofts & R.I. Smart, 1977. The effect of pregnancy, energy intake and mating weight on protein deposition and energy retention of female pigs. Anim. Prod. 25, 281-290.
Jongbloed, A.W. & N.P. Lenis, 1993, Excretion of nitrogen and some minerals by livestock. Nitrogen flow in pig production and environmental consequences. Ed. Verstegen, M.W.A., L.A. den Hartog, G.J.M. van Kempen & J.H.M. Metz. Pudoc ,Wageningen, E.A.A.P publication 69, 22-36.
Just, A., J.A. Fernandez & H. Jorgensen, 1982. Nitrogen balance studies and nitrogen retention. Digestive physiology in the pig. Ed. Laplace, J.P. & A.A. Rerat. Les colloques de l'Institute Nationale de la Recherceh Agronomique no. 12, 111-122.

Kemm, E.H., (1974). A study of the protein and energy requirements of the pregnant gilt (Sus scrofa domesticus). PhD Thesis, University of Stellenbosch, South Africa.
King, R.H. & W.G. Brown, 1993. Interrelationships between dietary protein level, energy intake and nitrogen retention in pregnant gilts. J. Anim. Sci. 71, 2450-2456.
King, R.H., C.J. Rayner & M. Kerr, 1993. A note on the amino acid composition of sow's milk. Animal Production 57, 500-502.
Kroes, Y. & J.P. van Male, 1979. Reproductive lifetime of sows in relation to economy of production. Livest. Prod. Sci. 6, 179-183.
Leuillet, M, M. Etienne & E. Salmon-Legagneur, 1979. Consequences d'une tres forte restriction azotée a differentes periodes de la gestation de la truie sur le développement des foetus. Ann. Biol. Anim. Biochem. Biophys, 19(B), 217-223.
Lodge, G.A., D.W. Friend & M.S. Wolynetz, 1979. Effect of pregnancy on body composition and energy balance of the gilt. Can. J. Anim. Sci. 59, 51-61.
Mahan, D.C.,1977. Effect of feeding various gestation and lactation dietary protein sequences on long term reproductive performance in swine. J. Anim. Sci. 45, 1061-1072.
Mahan, D.C. 1979, Effect of dietary protein sequence on long term sow reproductive performance. J. Anim. Sci. 49, 514-521.
Noblet , J., W.H. Close, R.P. Heavens & D. Brown, 1985. Studies on the energy metabolism of the pregnant sow. 1. Uterus and mammary tissue development. Br. J. Nutr. 53, 251-265.
Noblet, J. & M. Etienne, 1986. Effect of energy level in lactating sows on yield and composition of milk and nutrient balance of piglets. J. Anim. Sci. 63, 1888-1896.
Noblet , J. & M. Etienne, 1987. Body composition, metabolic rate and utilisation of milk nutrients in suckling piglets. Reprod. Nutr. Develop. 27, 829-839.
Pettigrew, J.E., M.D. Tokach, B.A. Crooker & A.F. Sower, 1991. Energy-protein interactions in the lactating sow: metabolites and milk synthesis. Energy Metabolism in Farm Animals. Ed. Wenk, C. & M. Boessinger. E.A.A.P. publication no. 58, 349-352.
Pettigrew, J.E., 1993. Amino acid nutrition of gestating and lactating sows. Biokyowa Techn. Review 5, 1-18.
Pond, W.G., 1973. Influence of maternal protein and energy nutrition during gestation on progeny performance in swine. J. Anim. Sci. 36, 175-181.
Pond , W.G., R.R. Maurer & J. klindt, 1991. Fetal organ response to maternal protein deprivation during pregnancy in swine. J. Nutr. 121, 504-509.
Scholman G.J & A.A. Dijkhuizen, 1989. Determination and analysis of the economic optimum culling strategy in swine breeding herds in Western Europe and the USA. Neth. J. Agric. Sci. 37, 71-74.
Shields Jr, R.G. & D.C. Mahan, 1983. Effects of pregnancy and lactation on the body composition of first litter female swine. J. Anim. Sci. 57, 594-603.
Shields Jr., R.G., D.C. Mahan & P.F. Maxson, 1985. Effect of dietary gestation and lactation protein levels on reproductive performance and body composition of first-litter female swine. J. Anim. Sci. 60, 179-189.
Sohail, M.A., D.J.A. Cole & D. Lewis, 1978. Amino acid requirement of the breeding sow. 2. Dietary lysine requirement of the lactating sow. Br. J. Nutr. 40, 369-376.
Speer , V.C., 1990. Partitioning nitrogen and amino acids for pregnancy and lactation in swine: a review. J. Anim. Sci. 68, 553-561.
Vanschoubroek, F & R. van Spaendonck , 1973. Faktorieller Aufbau des Protein- und Aminosaurenbedarfs tragender Sauen. Zeitscht. Tierphys. Tierern. und Futterm. 31, 71-91.
Varley, M.A., 1982. The time of weaning and its effects on reproductive function. Control of pig reproduction, Ed. Cole, D.J.A. & G.R. Foxcroft. Butterworth Scientific, London.
Walach-Janiak, M., St. Ray & H. Fandrejewski, 1986a. The effect of pregnancy on protein, water and fat deposition in the body of gilts. Livest. Prod. Sci. 15, 261-269.

Walach-Janiak, M., St. Ray & H. Fandrejewski, 1986b. Protein and energy balance in pregnant gilts. Livest. Prod. Sci. 15, 249-260.
Whittemore, C.T. & C.A. Morgan, 1990. Model components for the determination of energy and protein requirements for breeding sows: a review. Livest. Prod. Sci. 26, 1-37.
Whittemore, C.T. & H. Yang, 1989. Physical and chemical composition of the body of breeding sows with differing body subcutaneous fat depth at parturition, differing nutrition during lactation and differing litter size. Anim. Prod. 48, 203-212.
Wilde, R.O. de, 1980a, Protein and energy retention in pregnant and non-pregnant gilts. I. Protein retention. Livest. Prod. Sci. 7, 497-504.
Wilde, R.O. de, 1980b, Protein and energy retention in pregnant and non-pregnant gilts. II. Energy retention. Livest. Prod. Sci. 7, 505-510.
Williams, I.H., W.H. Close & D.J.A. Cole, 1993. Strategies for sow nutrition: predicting the response of pregnant animals to protein and energy intake. Recent Developments in Pig Nutrition 2. Ed. Cole, D.J.A., W. Haresign & P.C. Garnsworthy. Nottingham University Press. pp 317-331`.
Wit, J. de , J.K. Oldenbroek, H. van Keulen & D. Zwart, 1995, Criteria for sustainable livestock production: a proposal for implementation. Agriculture, Ecosystems and Environment 43, 219-229

12 Nutritional strategy and reproduction

C.M.C. van der Peet-Schwering, J.W.G.M. Swinkels, L.A. den Hartog

12.1 Introduction

The nutritional needs of lactating sows are substantial. The commercial objective concerning a lactating sow is to produce a high number of healthy piglets during her life at minimal cost. This means that two main aspects are important in a feeding strategy for the lactating sow: 1) optimal milk production (quantity and quality) for the piglets and 2) preventing reproductive failure. When the food intake of sows during lactation is too low to meet the requirements for maintenance and milk production, body reserves are mobilized. This may result in reproductive failure. In this review, an optimal nutrition (energy and protein) for lactating sows will be described. Secondly, the effects of under-nutrition on the reproduction of sows will be discussed. In the third part of this review, a physiological concept that explains the impact of nutrition on reproduction will be presented. Finally, the factors that may affect the food intake of the lactating sow and the aspects which are important in developing a feeding strategy for the lactating sow will be highlighted.

12.2 Factorial approach to determining energy and protein requirements

The energy and protein requirements for lactating sows can be estimated using a factorial approach (Everts *et al.*, 1995; see also Chapter 11). In this approach it is necessary to estimate the requirements for maintenance and milk production and to know the efficiencies of utilisation of dietary energy and protein as well as the efficiencies of utilisation of energy and protein from body reserves for milk production. Also, the ideal body composition of sows in relation to longevity should be known.

12.2.1 Development of body composition

Data concerning development of the ideal body composition in sows in relation to longevity have not been presented in the literature. Everts *et al.* (1994) arbitrarily proposed a standard sow (Table 12.1) based on the weight and backfat thickness of sows on six experimental farms in the Netherlands.

From parturition to conception, the average loss in weight is 17.5 to 25.0 kg. Between weaning and conception, the average loss in weight is 13.5 ± 5 kg (Everts and Dekker, 1991).

Table 12.1. Proposed development of body composition of sows (kg) (exclusive of intra-uterine contents)

Parity	1	2	3	4	5
Body composition at conception:					
bodyweight[2]	120.0	150.0	175.0	190.0	205.0
protein	18.4	23.4	27.8	30.7	33.1
fat	25.5	29.6	33.1	33.9	35.3
water[1]	62.6	79.6	94.6	104.4	112.5
Deposition during pregnancy:					
bodyweight	55.0	47.5	37.5	32.5	27.5
protein	8.0	6.9	5.4	4.4	3.3
fat	15.1	13.0	10.3	9.9	9.6
water[1]	27.2	23.5	18.4	15.0	11.2
Mobilisation from parturition to conception:					
bodyweight	25.0	22.5	22.5	17.5	17.5
protein	3.0	2.5	2.5	2.0	2.0
fat	11.0	9.5	9.5	8.5	8.5
water[1]	10.2	8.5	8.5	6.8	6.8

[1] Amount of water = amount of protein * 3.4 (Everts and Dekker, 1991) .
[2] Gut fill is assumed to be 6% of bodyweight.

12.2.2 Maintenance

The estimate of the energy requirement for maintenance in sows ranges from 0.420 MJ ME per kg $BW^{0.75}$ (BW = body weight) to 0.456 MJ ME per kg $BW^{0.75}$ (ARC, 1981; Close *et al.*, 1985; Noblet and Etienne, 1987a). In reviews by Noblet *et al.* (1990), Whittemore and Morgan (1990) and Everts *et al.* (1995) a value of 0.440 MJ ME per kg $BW^{0.75}$ was proposed.
The estimate of the protein requirement for maintenance ranges from 47 to 133 g/d for a sow of 200 kg (Carr *et al.*, 1977; Whittemore *et al.*, 1978; ARC, 1981; Beyer *et al.*, 1988). Everts *et al.* (1995) proposed a protein requirement for maintenance for a 200 kg sow of 2.1 g/d per kg $BW^{0.75}$ or 112 g/d. The choice for this protein requirement is debatable but it falls within the above mentioned range.

12.2.3 Milk production

Composition of the milk

The fat content of sow's milk ranges from 61 to 106 g/kg, the protein content from 46 to 57 g/kg and the lactose content from 52 to 59 g/kg (Helms, 1978; Goerke, 1979; Noblet and Etienne, 1986; Den Hartog *et al.*, 1987; Klobassa, 1987; Babinszky, 1992). Noblet and Etienne (1986) found that the milk composition changes during the first two weeks after farrowing. Thereafter, the milk composition remains fairly stable. According to Everts *et al.* (1995), the mean composition of sow's milk is 72 g fat, 52 g protein and 55 g lactose per kg of milk. This means an energy content of the milk of 5 MJ per kg.

Elliot *et al.* (1971), Duee and Jung (1973), Helms (1978), Dourmad *et al.* (1991) and King *et al.* (1993) determined amino acid concentrations in sow's milk (Table 12.2). There is good agreement in the amino acid concentration of sow's milk between these studies. Therefore Everts *et al.* (1995) used an overall mean value.

Table 12.2. Amino acid composition of sow's milk (g per 16 g nitrogen)

Amino Acid	Elliot *et al.* (1971)	Duee & Jung (1973)	Helms (1978)	Dourmad *et al.* (1991)	King *et al.* (1993)	Mean
Lysine	7.30	7.75	7.86	7.39	7.09	7.48
Methionine	1.80	2.10	1.88	2.00	1.97	1.95
Cystine	1.37	1.80	1.60	1.66	1.33	1.55
Tryptophan	1.37	-	-	1.10	1.33	1.27
Threonine	4.83	4.30	4.23	4.34	4.18	4.38
Leucine	8.87	8.90	8.58	8.69	8.09	8.63
Isoleucine	3.87	4.25	4.08	4.26	4.22	4.14
Valine	4.73	6.20	5.17	5.10	5.46	5.33
Histidine	3.53	2.70	2.94	3.91	2.84	3.18
Arginine	4.90	5.00	4.95	5.47	4.62	4.99
Phenylalanine	4.03	4.15	4.34	4.19	3.93	4.13
Tyrosine	5.00	4.15	4.22	4.11	3.90	4.28

Amount of milk

The milk production of the sow can be estimated from the piglet weight gain during the suckling period. Several authors (Salmon-Legagneur and Aumaitre, 1962; Goerke, 1979; Noblet and Etienne, 1986 and 1987c; Babinszky, 1992; Mullan *et al.*, 1993) determined the amount of milk needed per gram of growth for a suckling piglet. The estimates for the amount of milk per gram growth ranged from 3.82 to 4.95 g/g, with a mean of 4.2 g milk per g growth (and an energy content of the milk of 5 MJ per kg). The milk production can be calculated as follows: milk production (g/d) = piglet weight gain (g/d) x 4.2 x number of piglets.

Use of energy and protein for milk production
The efficiency of utilisation of dietary ME for energy in milk (k_l) and the efficiency of utilisation of energy from body reserves for milk production (k_{rl}) have been described by several researchers. Noblet *et al.* (1990) proposed a value of 0.72 for k_l and a value of 0.88 for k_{rl} (Table 12.3).

Table 12.3. Estimates for the efficiency of utilisation of dietary ME (kl) and energy from body reserves (krl) for energy in milk

Reference	k_l	k_{rl}
Burlacu *et al.* (1983)	0.712	
Verstegen *et al.* (1985)	0.68	
Beyer (1986)	0.79	0.88
Noblet and Etienne (1987[b])	0.715	0.886
Babinszky (1992)	0.70-0.73	
Noblet *et al.* (1990) (mean)	0.72	0.88

The efficiency of utilisation of dietary protein for milk protein production ranges from 0.61 (Beyer, 1986) to 0.71 (Burlacu *et al.*, 1985). For the factorial approach Beyer (1986) suggested a value of 0.70. The efficiency of utilisation of body protein to milk protein is 0.86 (Beyer, 1986). For the efficiency of utilisation of body amino acids to milk protein and for the efficiency of utilisation of dietary amino acids for milk protein, Everts *et al.* (1995) proposed values of 0.86 and 0.80, respectively.

12.2.4 Nutritional needs of the lactating sow

Using the factorial approach and the above mentioned assumptions, the energy and protein requirements of lactating sows can be calculated. The requirements for specific nutrients will not be considered.

Energy requirement
The energy requirement for lactating sows is dependent on litter size, growth of the piglets and lactation number of the sow. In Table 12.4, the calculated ME requirement per day, assuming no mobilisation of body reserves, is presented for sows nursing 10 piglets. The energy requirement of the sow is calculated, assu-

ming litter weight gains of 2000, 2200 and 2500 g/d. Besides, it is assumed that the sows with lactation number 1 to 5 weigh 175, 197.5, 212.5, 222.5 and 232.5 kg, respectively.

Table 12.4. ME-requirement (MJ per day) for sows nursing 10 piglets during a 28 day lactation period (based on Everts et al., 1995)

Litter weight gain (g/d)	Lactation number				
	1	2	3	4	5
2000	79.3	81.3	82.7	83.5	84.3
2200	84.6	86.6	88.0	88.8	89.6
2500	92.6	94.6	96.0	96.8	97.6

The energy requirement ranges from 79.3 to 97.6 MJ ME per day, this is 6.1 to 7.6 kg per day of a diet containing 12.9 MJ ME per kg.

Protein requirement

In Table 12.5, the estimated requirements, assuming no mobilisation of body reserves, for ileal digestible lysine, methionine, cystine, threonine, tryptophan and isoleucine are presented for a sow weighing 175 kg and nursing 10 piglets with a litter weight gain of 2000, 2200 and 2500 g/d.

Table 12.5. Requirement for ileal digestible amino acids (g/d) for a sow weighing 175 kg and nursing 10 piglets during a 28 day lactation period (based on Everts et al., 1995).

Litter weight gain (g/d)	Lysine	Methionine	Cystine	Threonine	Tryptophan	Isoleucine
2000	41.9	10.9	10.2	26.1	7.4	23.0
2200	45.6	11.9	11.0	28.2	8.0	25.0
2500	51.1	13.3	12.2	31.5	8.9	28.1

The ileal digestible lysine requirements range from 41.9 to 51.1 g/d. Coupled with the information given in Table 12.4, the ileal digestible lysine requirement can be calculated to range from 6.8 to 7.2 g/kg for a diet containing 12.9 MJ ME per kg. The estimated requirement for ileal digestible lysine is somewhat higher than that based on the results of Stahly *et al.* (1990) and Johnston *et al.* (1991). They estimated a total lysine requirement of 46.7 and 53.5 g/d (about 37 and 43 g ileal digestible lysine per day), respectively.

12.3 Effects of undernutrition on reproduction

Many lactating sows do not meet their nutritional requirements (as discussed in section 12.2.4) due to a restricted feed intake capacity. Consequently, mobilisation of body reserves is inevitable. Several studies have demonstrated that sows losing excessive amounts of body weight have a prolonged weaning to oestrus interval and a decreased subsequent litter size.

12.3.1 Mobilisation of body reserves

Based on Everts *et al.* (1995), Kemp *et al.* (1996) calculated the consequences of a restricted feed intake on the mobilisation of body reserves (Figure 12.1) for a sow of 175 kg. They assumed that there are no changes in milk production due to the reduced feed intake.

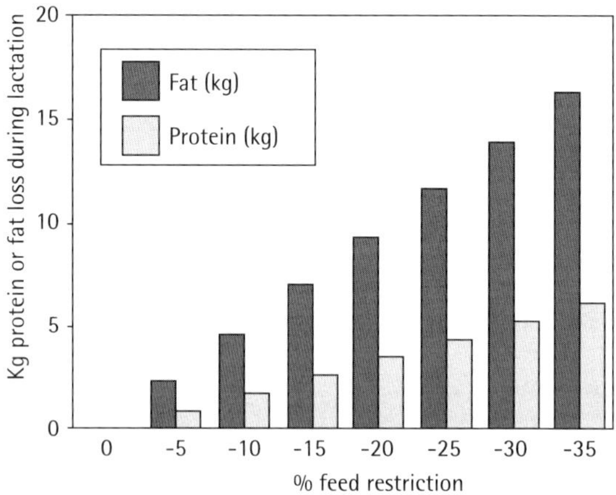

Figure 12.1. Estimated loss of protein (kg) and fat (kg) during a 28 day lactation period in sows fed at various percentages below the energy and protein levels required for no mobilisation of body reserves (based on Everts et al., 1995)

Sows which have a 25% lower energy and protein intake than their requirement, will mobilize about 4.4 kg of protein and 11.6 kg of fat during a 28 day lactation period. A sow weighing 175 kg just after farrowing has about 26 kg of protein and 40 kg of fat (see Table 12.1). This means that body protein and fat are depleted by 17 and 29% respectively, during lactation. In terms of weight loss, the sow will lose about 11.6 + 4.4 * 4.4 (water : protein ratio = 3.4 : 1; Everts and Dekker, 1991) = 31 kg of weight during a 28 day lactation period.

12.3.2 Weaning to oestrus interval

In general, undernutrition and thus catabolism during lactation will lead to an increase in the weaning to oestrus interval. Hughes (1989) reviewed data on the effect of low feeding levels, low energy levels and low protein levels during lactation on the weaning to remating interval (Table 12.6).

Table 12.6. The effects of nutrition during lactation on the length of the weaning to remating interval (days) (from Hughes, 1989)

Number of experiments	Number of animals	Sows/ gilts	Feed intake		Energy intake		Protein intake	
			high*	low	high+	low	high#	low
4[1]	248	gilts	10.5	19.3	-	-	-	-
8[2]	784	gilts	-	-	12.7	14.6	-	-
4[3]	190	gilts	-	-	-	-	10.3	16.6
5[4]	384	sows	5.6	7.1	-	-	-	-
2[5]	658	sows	-	-	4.4	4.3	-	-

* Mean daily DE intake (MJ), gilts 53, sows 81; + mean daily DE intake (MJ), gilts 64, sows 69.
\# Mean daily CP intake (g), gilts 766.
[1] King *et al.* (1984); King and Williams (1984a); Armstrong *et al.* (1986); King and Dunkin (1986a).
[2] Reese *et al.* (1982) - 2 studies; King and Williams (1984b); Reese *et al.* (1984); Johnston *et al.* (1986); Brendemuhl *et al.* (1987); Kirkwood *et al.* (1987a).
[3] King and Williams (1984b); King and Dunkin (1986b); Brendemuhl *et al.* (1987); King and Martin (1989).
[4] Henry *et al.* (1984); Hughes *et al.* (1984); Kirkwood *et al.* (1987a,b); Yang *et al.* (1989).
[5] Reese et al. (1982); Kirkwood *et al.* (1988).

It can be concluded from the information presented in Table 12.6 that low feed, low energy as well as low protein levels during lactation cause a prolonged weaning to remating interval especially in primiparous sows. Vesseur *et al.* (1994a) investigated the effect of body weight loss during lactation on the weaning to oestrus interval (Table 12.7).

Table 12.7. Effect of body weight loss during lactation (as percentage of the body weight after farrowing) on the weaning to oestrus interval (days)

Parity	Body weight loss during lactation %			
	0.0 - 5.0	5.1 - 7.5	7.6 - 12.5	> 12.5
1	9.5	10.0	11.7	14.7
2	6.7	6.7	8.0	8.5
3-5	6.0	6.3	6.5	6.5
≥ 6	6.1	6.0	6.5	6.0

Primiparous sows with a weight loss of more than 7.5% and more than 12.5% during lactation showed a prolonged weaning to oestrus interval. In second parity sows, the effect was less pronounced. The weaning to oestrus interval of third and higher parity sows was not influenced by weight loss during lactation. A delay in oestrus after weaning may result in poor reproductive performance later. Sows inseminated on day 5 after weaning had more piglets born alive and a higher farrowing rate after first insemination than sows inseminated between days 9 and 12 (Vesseur *et al.*, 1994b).
It may be stated that sows losing significant amounts of body reserves as a result of low food intake during lactation have a delayed return to oestrus after weaning. Yang *et al.* (1989), however, concluded that mobilisation of body reserves during lactation was not only influenced by lactation feeding but also by fatness at parturition. It appears that body condition at parturition may partly serve as a metabolic buffer to reproductive problems in first parity sows (Kemp *et al.*, 1996). The degree of weight loss and/or loss of backfat below which a prolonged weaning to oestrus interval occurs, as well as the level of dietary energy intake required to prevent this prolonged interval, is still unknown.

12.3.3 Embryo survival

Catabolism of body tissues during lactation will result in a decrease in subsequent litter size, due to effects on embryonic survival rather than on ovulation rate (Foxcroft *et al.*, 1996). Hughes (1989) reviewed data on the effect of low feeding levels during lactation on embryonic survival and on subsequent litter size (Table 12.8).

Low feeding levels during lactation may have a negative effect on embryonic survival and subsequent litter size. The voluntary food intake of first lactation sows is often too low to meet their metabolic requirements. Zak *et al.* (1997) tested the hypothesis that the pattern of feed restriction and hence weight loss

Table 12.8. The effects of feeding level during lactation on subsequent early embryo survival and litter size in sows and gilts (from Hughes, 1989)

Authors	Number of animals	Sows/ gilts	Early embryo survival (%)		Subsequent litter size	
			high level	low level	high level	low level
Reese *et al.* (1982)	44	gilts	-	-	9.4	9.9
Henry *et al.* (1984)	40	sows	-	-	9.9	8.7
Hughes *et al.* (1984)	26	sows	70	58	-	-
King and Williams (1984a)	80	gilts	71	72	9.7	9.7
Kirkwood *et al.* (1987a)	24	gilts	80	67	-	-
	48	sows				
Kirkwood *et al.* (1987b)	78	sows	83	68	-	-
Kirkwood *et al.* (1988)	201	sows	-	-	10.6	9.6
Prime *et al.* (1988)	80	sows	-	-	11.4	11.6

during lactation has important effects on fertility after weaning. To test their hypothesis, sows were fed to appetite from day 1 to 28 of lactation (group AA) or restricted to 50% from day 22 to 28 (group AR) or from day 1 to 21 (group RA). Feed restriction in the first three weeks or during the fourth week only marginally increased the weaning to oestrus interval (88.7, 122.3 and 134.7 hours for the AA, AR and RA sows, respectively) and reduced the ovulation rate (19.9, 15.4 and 15.4) compared with the *ad libitum* fed sows. This is in contrast to most literature sources. Embryo survival did not differ between *ad libitum* fed sows and sows restricted in feed intake during the first three weeks but was lower in sows restricted in feed intake during the fourth week (87.5% and 86.5% vs 64.4%). These results demonstrate that the pattern of metabolic change in the primiparous lactating sow exerts differential effects on fertility after weaning.

12.4 A physiological concept

In Section 12.3, a relationship was outlined between nutrition during lactation and reproductive performance. The physiological mechanisms by which nutrition affects reproductive performance of sows have not been clearly determined. A physiological concept that explains the impact of nutrition during lactation on the oestrus to weaning interval and on embryonic survival will be presented briefly.

12.4.1 Weaning to oestrus interval

In the relationship between nutrition during lactation and the weaning to oestrus interval, the release of Luteinizing Hormone (LH) seems to be a key factor. The effect of inadequate nutrient intake during lactation on weaning to oestrus interval is mediated through a reduced LH pulsatility before weaning (King and Martin, 1989). Shaw and Foxcroft (1985) demonstrated that LH-levels before and just after weaning were inversely related to weaning to oestrus interval. In normal reproductive sows, LH production is characterised by a high frequency/low amplitude pulse frequency directly after weaning, which induces recruitment of the then existing large follicle population (Kemp *et al.*, 1996). Sows without this pattern of LH production will show a prolonged weaning to oestrus interval. To assess the relationship between LH-secretion during lactation and weaning to oestrus interval, Tokach *et al.* (1992) characterized LH-secretion in the primiparous sow throughout a 28-day lactation period. Sows with prolonged weaning to oestrus intervals had fewer LH peaks per 6 hours and lower LH-concentrations on day 14, 21 and 28 of lactation. The mean LH-concentration and pulsatility increased steadily as lactation progressed. These results demonstrate that alterations in LH profile as early as day 14 of lactation are associated with a delayed weaning to oestrus interval and that insufficient restoration of LH production during lactation will cause a prolonged weaning to oestrus interval.
Restoration of LH production during lactation is influenced by the energy and the protein intake during lactation (King and Martin, 1989; Tokach *et al.*, 1992). Tokach *et al.* (1992) showed that the average daily lysine and ME intake before day 21 affected the mean LH concentration on day 21 in an interactive manner. At low ME intake, increasing lysine intake had little influence on mean LH. The influence of lysine intake on LH secretion increased as energy intake increased. These results reveal that mean LH is reduced by restriction of either lysine or energy intake. King and Martin (1989) also found that sows experiencing restricted protein intake during lactation have a reduced mean LH concentration and fail to develop a high LH pulse frequency during lactation.
Sows with prolonged intervals not only had lower LH concentrations but also lower serum insulin concentrations (Tokach *et al.*, 1992). The insulin concentration on day 7 was correlated with the number of LH peaks on day 14, 21 and 28. Therefore, Tokach *et al.* (1992) suggest that insulin may play a role in the influence of diet on reproductive function. A review by Britt *et al.* (1988) presented evidence that insulin infusions or injections into gilts increased the frequency of LH pulses, oestrogen content in follicular fluid and ovulation rate, whereas atresia of medium-sized follicles decreased. Insulin production can be stimulated by a high feeding level and a low number of suckling piglets (Close *et al.*, 1991) but also by changes in the dietary composition (Kemp *et al.*, 1993 and 1995).

12.4.2 Embryo mortality

The plasma progesterone concentration in early pregnancy seems to be a key factor in the relationship between nutrition and embryo mortality. High feed intakes in the gilt, directly after mating result in a significant decrease in embryonic survival. This effect of nutrition may be progesterone-dependent (Ashworth *et al.*, 1995; Foxcroft *et al.*, 1996; Jindal *et al.*, 1996). Increased embryonic loss is associated with lower concentrations of plasma progesterone in the early pregnancy. The mechanism explaining the reduction in plasma progesterone with increased feed intake after mating is still unknown. Hughes and Pearce (1989) suggested that a high feed intake during early gestation may result in a suboptimal uterine specific protein secretion. This has a negative effect on embryonic survival. Symonds and Prime (1989) reported an increase in hepatic blood flow and in the metabolic clearance of progesterone from plasma when the feed intake was increased.

In sows losing excessive amounts of their body reserves it is also possible that an increased hepatic blood flow after weaning increases the metabolic clearance rate of plasma progesterone and thereby reduces the plasma progesterone (Aherne and Kirkwood, 1985). Einarsson and Rojkittikhun (1993), however, suggested that the effect of low feeding in lactation on embryo survival is the result of suboptimal LH release during the first oestrus after weaning, resulting in inadequate luteinization of the corpora lutea, with concommitant low plasma progesterone in early pregnancy. This hypothesis is supported by a study of Kirkwood *et al.* (1987a). They demonstrated that injection of GnRH at the first oestrus after weaning improved embryo survival and increased progesterone concentrations in early gestation in sows fed low levels during lactation.

Foxcroft *et al.* (1996) suggest that, as the whole process of follicular development occurs over several weeks, the catabolic state of the sow during lactation could already affect the status of the follicles that will eventually enter the final stage of maturation after weaning. The metabolic effects on emerging follicles during lactation could have two important consequences (Foxcroft *et al.*, 1996). Firstly, differences in follicular maturity could affect oocyte maturation and the quality of oocytes available for fertilization and in this way affect embryonic mortality. Secondly, differences in follicular maturation could affect the early steroidogenic activity of the developing corpora lutea, and hence affect embryonic survival indirectly by influencing the secretory activity of the uterus.

It can be concluded, that the reproductive performance of sows will probably depend on an interaction between the effects of metabolic factors on the status of the ovary before and after weaning and effects on the central control of gonadotrophin secretion that will determine the time after weaning when ovulation will occur (Foxcroft et al., 1996). The exact mechanism, however, explaining the effect of nutrition during lactation on embryo survival is still unclear.

12.5 Factors affecting food intake

Due to a restricted food intake capacity, many lactating sows do not meet their nutrient requirements. The food intake during lactation is affected by many factors and there are several possibilities to stimulate food intake during lactation.

12.5.1 Food intake during pregnancy

Several studies have demonstrated that increasing food intake during pregnancy decreases the voluntary food intake during lactation (Mullan and Williams, 1989; Yang *et al.*, 1989; Dourmad, 1991; Xue *et al.*, 1997). Impaired glucose tolerance and decreased insulin sensitivity seems to be responsible for the lower lactational feed intake (Weldon *et al.*, 1994; Xue *et al.*, 1997). Conversely, insufficient food intake during pregnancy cannot always be compensated for by ad libitum food intake during lactation, especially in gilts or high-producing sows (Dourmad, 1991). Yang *et al.* (1989) showed that in primiparous sows, the interval from weaning to conception was longer for sows which were thin at parturition than for fat sows. From this it can be concluded that it is important to feed pregnant sows to their requirements for maintenance, reproduction and maternal gain but not to overfeed the sows. Everts *et al.* (1994) advise an energy intake for primiparous sows of 24.8 and 36.1 MJ ME/d at the beginning and end of pregnancy, respectively. With regard to reproductive performance Yang *et al.* (1989) advise a target backfat thickness (P2) at first parturition of 20 mm.

12.5.2 Ambient temperature

The temperature requirement of a lactating sow is considerably lower than the temperature requirement of her piglets. This difference in the optimum temperature requirements and the fact that the temperature requirements of the piglets are catered for in commercial practice, often leads to heat stress in the sow. Heat stress will decrease the voluntary food intake of sows (Messias de Bragança *et al.*,1997). Results from 9 experiments indicated that for each degree Celsius above 16°C, the daily voluntary food energy intake of lactating sows decreased by 2.4 MJ DE (Black *et al.*, 1993). The milk production is also decreased in heat-exposed sows, more so than can be explained by a reduced nutrient intake (Black *et al.*, 1993). This suggests that there is a direct effect of high ambient temperature on the milk production of sows. An increase in blood flow to the skin to assist heat loss, and a decrease in blood flow to the mammary gland and other organs may explain this phenomenon (Black *et al.*,1993).
The influence of heat stress on sow productivity can be minimized by reducing the heat production or increasing the heat loss to the environment. The sow's heat production can be reduced by decreasing the fibre and increasing the fat content of the diet. Sows fed a lactation diet with a high level of fat have a lower daily heat production, a higher fat content in the milk and a higher energetic

efficiency of milk production compared to sows fed an isocaloric lactation diet with a low level of fat (Babinszky, 1992). Babinsky (1992) suggested that the lower heat production can have a beneficial effect on total energy intake in sows, especially at high ambient temperatures. The heat loss of sows to the environment can be increased by using floors with a low insulatory capacity or by using drip cooling. McGlone *et al.* (1988) concluded that water drip is an effective cooling technique for heat-stressed sows and that snout coolers provide only minor benefits.
Generally, an ambient temperature of 18 to 22°C is advised for a farrowing barn (Everts *et al.*, 1995). The recommended temperature depends, among another things, on floor type and stage of lactation.

12.5.3 Water consumption

The water requirement of lactating sows is high. In the Netherlands it is advised to provide lactating sows water *ad libitum* (Centraal Veevoederbureau, 1997). The ARC (1981) recommendations are in the range of 15 to 20 litres of water per day. Some sows are lethargic in the first days after farrowing and fail to consume adequate amounts of water. This causes low milk production in early lactation and low average bodyweight gains by the piglets (Fraser and Philips, 1989). Choice of drinker type and the flow rate of the drinking nipple may affect the total water consumption. Advisory literature often suggests a flow rate of 2 litres of water per minute for lactating sows to stimulate the water consumption, but a water flow rate of 0.6 litre per minute may be adequate if spillage and management of waste water is a problem (Fraser *et al.*, 1990). In the Netherlands a water flow rate of 1.0 to 1.5 litres per minute is advised (Centraal Veevoederbureau, 1997). Sometimes it is suggested to give sows with a low water intake in the first days after farrowing, some extra water in the trough for a few days. This may increase the overall water consumption.

12.5.4 Feed intake pattern

Lactating sows display diverse feed intake patterns during lactation (Koketsu *et al.*, 1994; Koketsu *et al.*, 1996a). Koketsu *et al.* (1996 a,b) characterized the total feed intake and feed intake patterns of more than 20,000 lactating sows on 30 commercial farms. Each lactation feed record was categorized into one of six feed intake patterns: I rapid increase in feed intake after farrowing with no drop; II a major decrease of > 1.8 kg/d was observed relative to the previous peak feeding level; III a minor decrease of < 1.8 kg/d was observed relative to the previous peak feeding level; IV feed intake was low throughout lactation and did not exceed 4.5 kg/d; V low intake during the first week then an increase in feed intake for the remainder of lactation; VI gradual increase throughout lactation with no drop. The average daily feed intakes during lactation for the patterns II, III, IV and V were lower than those for the patterns I and VI. There were no dif-

ferences in average daily feed intake between patterns I and VI. The pattern of feed intake is also influenced by the reproductive performance and the occurrence of reproductive failure. Sows with patterns IV and V had a longer weaning to first service interval than those exhibiting the other patterns. The group having pattern II also had a higher proportion of sows culled for anoestrus compared to sows with pattern I. Koketsu *et al.* (1996a,b) suggest therefore that both the amount and pattern of feed intake influence subsequent reproduction and that producers should manage their sows to optimize the proportion of sows eating according to either pattern I or VI.
Everts *et al.* (1995) advise a feed intake pattern during lactation which is comparable with pattern I: 1) parity 1, 2 and 3: day 1 after parturition 2.0 kg and then every day 0.5 kg extra until the recommended level of energy intake; 2) parity > 3: day 1 after parturition 2.5 kg and then every day 0.5 kg extra till the recommended level of energy intake.

12.6 Feeding strategy

Energy restriction, regardless of the week when it is imposed, decreases the pulsatile secretion of LH and prolongs the weaning to oestrus interval (Koketsu *et al.*, 1996c). These results suggest that suboptimal feed intake at any stage during lactation can have a negative impact on subsequent reproductive performance. Therefore, it is important to optimize the feed intake of lactating sows during every week of the lactation period. Everts et al. (1995) developed ideal feeding strategies for lactating sows, dependent on litter size, litter weight gain and lactation number of the sows (Tables 12.9 and 12.10). The daily ME-requirement, without mobilisation of body reserves, is presented for every week of the lactation period. Everts *et al.* (1995) assumed that the weekly litter weight gain during a 28-day lactation period was 80, 105, 110 and 105%, respectively. This assumption was based on piglet data from three experimental farms.

Table 12.9. Feed requirement (MJ ME per day) for every week of a 28 day lactation period for sows nursing 10 piglets and a litter weight gain of 2200 g/d (based on Everts et al., 1995)

Lactation number	1	2	3	4	5
week 1	66.8	68.8	70.2	70.9	71.8
week 2	84.2	86.2	87.5	88.4	89.2
week 3	92.4	94.4	95.6	96.5	97.4
week 4	95.1	97.1	98.4	99.3	100.1

For a first parity sow, the energy requirement during lactation increases from 66.8 to 95.1 MJ ME per day or 5.2 to 7.4 kg per day of a diet containing 12.9 MJ per day. For a fifth parity sow the energy requirement during lactation increases from 71.8 to 100.1 MJ ME per day, that is from 5.6 to 7.8 kg per day.

Table 12.10. Feed requirement (MJ ME per day) for every week of a 28 day lactation period for a first parity sow nursing 10 piglets (based on Everts et al., 1995)

Litter weight gain (g/d)	1500	2000	2500
week 1	54.5	63.1	72.3
week 2	65.9	78.9	92.4
week 3	71.5	86.3	101.5
week 4	73.8	89.0	104.4

Litter weight gain has a major influence on the energy requirement of the sow. The higher the litter weight gain the higher the energy requirement of the sow or, stated another way, the higher the energy intake of the sow the higher the litter weight gain.
It can be concluded that the energy requirement of lactating sows, without mobilisation of body reserves, is high. When some mobilisation of body reserves is allowed, the energy requirement will be lower.

12.7 Conclusion

The nutrional needs of lactating sows are very high. When the feed intake of lactating sows is too low to meet the requirements for maintenance and milk production, body reserves will be mobilised. Sows, losing excessive amounts of body weight, have a prolonged weaning to oestrus interval and a decreased subsequent litter size. The level of weight loss and/or backfat loss, below which reproductive failure occurs, is still unknown.
During lactation the feed intake is negatively influenced by a high feed intake during pregnancy, a high ambient temperature in the farrowing stable and a low water intake of the sow during lactation. Suboptimal feed intake at any time during lactation can have a negative impact on subsequent reproductive performance. Therefore it is important to optimize the feed intake of lactating sows during every week of the lactation period.

12.8 References

Agricultural Research Council, 1981. The Nutrient Requirements of Pigs. Commonwealth Agricultural Bureaux, Slough, 307 pp.

Aherne, F.X. & R.N. Kirkwood, 1985. Nutrition and sow prolificacy. Journal of Reproduction and Fertility Supplement, 33, 169-183.

Armstrong, J.D., J.H. Britt & R.R. Krealing, 1986. Effect of restriction of energy during lactation on body condition, energy metabolism, endocrine changes and reproductive performance in primiparous sow. Journal of Animal Science, 63, 1915-1925.

Ashworth, C.J., C. Antipatis & L. Beattie, 1995. Effect of pre- and post-mating nutritional status on embryonic survival and uterine function in the pig. Journal of Reproduction and Fertility, Abstract Series, 16:27.

Babinszky, L., 1992. Energy metabolism and lactation performance of primiparous sows as affected by dietary fat and vitamin E. PhD Thesis, Agricultural University, Wageningen.

Beyer, M., L. Hoffman, R. Schiemann, W. Jentsch, G. Burlacu, M. Iliescu, E.C. Machajew, L. Babinsky, H. Gundel, L. Lassota, M. Walach-Janiak & L. Zeman, 1988. Biological basics for the factorial derivation of the energy and protein requirements for pregnant and lactating sows and suckling piglets. Fifth International Symposium on Protein Metabolism and Nutrition EAAP Publication 35. Wissenschaftliche Zeitschrift der Wilhelm-Pieck-Universität Rostock, 37, 92-93.

Beyer, M., 1986. Untersuchungen zum Energie- und Stickstoffumsatz von graviden und laktierenden Sauen sowie Saugferkeln - ein Beitrag zur Präzisierung des Energie- und Proteinbedarfs. Dissertation Rostock.

Black , J.L., B.P. Mullan, M.L. Lorschy & L.R. Giles, 1993. Lactation in the sow during heat stress. Livestock Production Science, 35, 153-170.

Brendemuhl, J.H., A.J. Lewis & E.R. Peo, 1987. Effect of protein intake and energy intake by primiparous sows during lactation on sow and litter performance and sow thyroxine and urea concentrations. Journal of Animal Science, 64, 1060-1069.

Britt, J.H., J.D. Armstrong & N.M. Cox, 1988. Metabolic interfaces between nutrition and reproduction. Proceedings of the 11th International Congress on Animal Reproduction and Artificial Insemination, 117-125. Dublin, Ireland.

Burlacu, G., M. Iliescu & P. Caramida, 1985. Efficiency of food utilization by pregnant and lactating sows. 2. The influence of isocaloric diets with different protein levels on pregnancy and lactation. In: Energy metabolism of farm animals. Ed. P.W. Moe, H.F. Tyrrell & P.J. Reynolds, EAAP Publication 32, 330-332.

Burlacu, G., M. Iliescu & P. Caramida, 1993. Efficiency of food utilization by pregnant and lactating sows. Archiv Tierernährung, 33, 23.

Carr, J.R., K.N. Boorman & D.J.A. Cole, 1977. Nitrogen retention in the pig. British Journal of Nutrition, 37, 143-155.

Centraal Veevoederbureau, 1997. Voedernormen landbouwhuisdieren en voederwaarde veevoeders. CVB-reeks nr. 22.

Close, W.H., J. Noblet & R.P. Heavens, 1985. Studies on the energy metabolism of the pregnant sow. 2. The partition and utilization of metabolizable energy intake in pregnant and non-pregnant animals. British Journal of Nutrition, 53, 267-279.

Close, W.H., B.P. Mullan, C.E. Sharpe & H.L. Buttle, 1991. Metabolic and endocrine changes in the sow during lactation. British Society of Animal Production: Winter meeting 1991.

Den Hartog, L.A., H. Boer, M.W. Bosch. G.J. Klaassen & H.A.M. van der Steen, 1987. The effect of feeding level, stage of lactation and method of milk sampling on the composition of milk(fat) in sows. Journal of Animal Physiology and Animal Nutrition, 58, 253-261.

Dourmad, J.Y., 1991. Effect of feeding level in the gilt during pregnancy on voluntary feed intake during lactation and changes in body composition during gestation and lactation. Livestock Production Science, 27, 309-319.

Dourmad, J.Y., M. Etienne & J. Noblet, 1991. A contribution to the study of amino acid requirement for lactation in sows. Journées de Recherches Porcines en France, 23, 61-68.

Duee, P.H. & J. Jung, 1973. Amino acid composition of sow's milk. Annales Zootechnie, 22, 243-247.

Einarsson, S. & T. Rojkittikhun, 1993. Effects of nutrition on pregnant and lactating sows. Journal of Reproduction and Fertility Supplement, 48, 229-239.

Elliot, R.F., G.W. van der Noot, R.L. Gillbreath & H. Fisher, 1971. Effect of dietary protein level on composition changes in sow colostrum and milk. Journal of Animal Science, 32, 1128-1137.

Everts, H.& R.A. Dekker, 1991. Reduction of nitrogen and phosphorus excretion by breeding sows using two different feeds for pregnancy and lactation: results of balance trials and comparative slaughtering. Report IVVO-DLO no. 230, Lelystad, The Netherlands.

Everts, H., M.C. Blok, B. Kemp, C.M.C. van der Peet-Schwering & C.H.M. Smits, 1994. Normen voor dragende zeugen (Requirements for pregnant sows). CVB-Documentation Report no. 9. Centraal Veevoederbureau, Lelystad, The Netherlands, 51 pp.

Everts, H., M.C. Blok, B. Kemp, C.M.C. van der Peet-Schwering & C.H.M. Smits, 1995. Normen voor lacterende zeugen (Requirements for lactating sows). CVB-Documentation Report no. 13. Centraal Veevoederbureau, Lelystad, The Netherlands, 45 pp.

Foxcroft, G.R., J.R. Cosgrove & F.X. Aherne, 1996. Relationship between metabolism and reproduction. Proceedings of the 14th IPVS Congress, Bologna, Italy, 6-9.

Fraser, D. & P.A. Philips, 1989. Lethargy and low water intake by sows during early lactation: a cause of low piglet weight gains and survival? Applied Animal Behaviour Science, 24, 13-22.

Fraser, D., J.F. Patience, P.A. Phillips & J.M. Mcleese, 1990. Water for piglets and lactating sows: quantity, quality and quandaries. In: Recent advances in animal nutrition (ed. W. Haresign & D.J.A. Cole), 137- 160.

Goerke, R., 1979. Zur Verwertung der umsetzbaren Energie für die Milchbildung bei unterschiedlicher Proteinversorgung des laktierenden Schweines. Thesis, Göttingen.

Helms, W., 1978. Zur Verwertung von Futterproteinen definierter Zusammensetzung und Ergänzung beim laktierenden Schwein. Thesis, Göttingen.

Henry, R.W., D.W. Pickard & P.E. Hughes, 1984. The effects of lactation length and food level on subsequent reproductive performance in the sow. Animal Production, 38, 527.

Hughes, P.E., 1989. A symposium-Nutrition-Reproduction interactions in the breeding sow. In: Manipulating Pig Production II (ed. J.L. Barnett & D.P. Hennessy), 277-280.

Hughes, P.E & G.P. Pearce, 1989. The endocrine basis of nutrition-reproduction interactions. In: Manipulating Pig Production II (ed. J.L. Barnett & D.P. Hennessy), 290-295.

Hughes, P.E., R.W. Henry & D.W. Pickard, 1984. The effects of lactation food level on subsequent ovulation rate and early embryonic survival in the sow. Animal Production, 38, 527.

Jindal,R., J.R. Cosgrove, F.X. Aherne & G.R. Foxcroft, 1996. Effect of nutrition on embryonal mortality in gilts: association with progesterone. Journal of Animal Science, 74, 620-624.

Johnston, L.J., J.E. Pettigrew & J.W. Rust, 1991. Response of maternal-line sows to dietary protein concentration during lactation. Journal of Animal Science 69 (Supplement): 118.

Johnston, L.R., D.E. Orr, L.F. Tribble & J.R. Clark, 1986. Effect of lactation and rebreeding phase energy intake on primiparous and multiparous sow performance. Journal of Animal Science, 63, 804-814.

Kemp, B., M.W. Bosch, T. Zandstra & N.M. Soede, 1993. The effect of energy source in the diet on plasma glucose and insulin concentrations and ovulationrate of meishan gilts. Proceedings of the 4th international conference on pig reproduction, Columbia, MO, USA, 88.

Kemp, B., N.M. Soede, F.A. Helmond & M.W. Bosch, 1995. Effects of energy source in the diet on reproductive hormones and insulin during lactation and subsequent oestrus in multiparous sows. Journal of Animal Science, 73, 3022-3029.

Kemp, B., H. Everts & L.A. den Hartog, 1996. Nutritional aspects of the lactating sow. EAAP Annual Meeting, Lillehammer, paper 367.

King, R.H. & A.C. Dunkin, 1986a. The effect of nutrition on reproductive performance of first-litter sows. 3. The response to graded increases in food intake during lactation. Animal Production, 42, 119-125.

King, R.H. & A.C. Dunkin, 1986b. The effect of nutrition on reproductive performance of first-litter sows. 4. The relative effects of energy and protein intakes during lactation on performance of sows and their piglets. Animal Production, 43, 319-325.

King, R.H. & G.B. Martin, 1989. Relationships between protein intake during lactation, LH levels and oestrus activity in first litter sows. Animal Reproduction Science, 19, 283-292.

King, R.H. & I.H. Williams, 1984a. The effect of nutrition on the reproductive performance of first litter sows. 1. Feeding levels during lactation and between weaning and mating. Animal Production, 38, 241-247.

King, R.H. & I.H. Williams, 1984b. The effect of nutrition on the reproductive performance of first litter sows. 2. Protein and energy intakes during lactation. Animal Production, 38, 249-256.

King, R.H., I.H. Williams & I. Barker, 1984. The effect of diet during lactation on reproductive performance of first litter sows. Proc. Austr. Society of Animal Production, 15, 412-415.

King, R.H., C.J. Rayner & M. Kerr, 1993. A note on the amino acid composition of sow's milk. Animal Production, 57, 500-502.

Kirkwood, R.N., E.S. Lythgoe & F.X. Aherne, 1987a. Effect of lactational feed intake and gonadotrophin-releasing hormone on reproductive performance of sows. Canadian Journal of Animal Science, 67, 715-719.

Kirkwood, R.N., S.K. Baidoo, F.X. Aherne & A.P. Sather, 1987b. The influence of feeding level during lactation on the occurence and endocrinology of post-weaning estrous sows. Canadian Journal of Animal Science, 67, 405-415.

Kirkwood, R.N., B.N. Mitaru, A.D. Gooneratne, R. Blair & P.A. Thacker, 1988. The influence of dietary energy intake during successive lactations on sow prolifacy. Canadian Journal of Animal Science, 68, 283-290.

Klobassa, F., E. Werhahn & J.E. Butler, 1987. Composition of sow milk during lactation. Journal of Animal Science, 64, 1458-1466.

Koketsu, Y., G.D. Dial, W.E. Marsh, J.E. Pettigrew & V.L. King, 1994. Feed intake patterns in lactation sows. Proceedings of the 13th IPVS Congress, 302.

Koketsu, Y., G.D. Dial, J.E. Pettigrew, W.E. Marsh & V.L. King, 1996a. Characterization of feed intake patterns during lactation in commercial swine herds. Journal of Animal Science, 74, 1202-1210.

Koketsu, Y., G.D. Dial, J.E. Pettigrew & V.L. King, 1996b. Feed intake pattern during lactation and subsequent reproductive performance of sows. Journal of Animal Science, 74, 2875-2884.

Koketsu, Y., G.D. Dial, J.E. Pettigrew, W.E. Marsh & V.L. King, 1996c. Influence of imposed feed intake patterns during lactation on reproductive performance and on circulating levels of glucose, insulin and luteinizing hormone in primiparous sows. Journal of Animal Science, 74, 1036-1046.

McGlone, J.J., W.F. Stansbury & L.F. Tribble, 1988. Management of lactating sows during heat stress: effects of water drip, snout coolers, floor type and a high energy-density diet. Journal of Animal Science, 66, 885-891.

Messias de Bragança, M., A.M. Mounier, J.C. Hulin & A. Prunier, 1997. Could undernutrition explain the effects of high ambient temperatures on performance of sows? Journées de la Recherche Porcine en France, 29, 81-88.

Mullan, B.P. & I.H. Williams, 1989. The effect of body reserves at farrowing on the reproductive performance of first-litter sows. Animal Production, 48, 449-457.

Mullan, B.P., W.H. Close & D.J.A. Cole, 1993. Predicting nutrient responses of the lactating sow. In: Recent developments in pig nutrition 2 (eds. D.J.A. Cole, W. Haresign & P.C. Garnsworthy) Nottingham University Press, 332-346.

Noblet, J. & M. Etienne, 1986. Effect of energy level in lactating sows on yield and composition of milk and nutrient balance of piglets. Journal of Animal Science, 63, 1888-1896.

Noblet, J. & M. Etienne, 1987a. Metabolic utilization of energy and maintenance requirements in pregnant sows. Livestock Production Science, 16, 243-257.

Noblet, J. & M. Etienne, 1987b. Metabolic utilization of energy and maintenance requirements in lactating sows. Journal of Animal Science, 64, 774-781.

Noblet, J. & M. Etienne, 1987c. Body composition, metabolic rate and utilization of milk nutrients in suckling piglets. Réproduction Nutrition Dévelopment, 27, 829-839.

Noblet, J., J.Y. Dourmad & M. Etienne, 1990. Energy utilization in pregnant and lactating sows: modelling of energy requirements. Journal of Animal Science, 68, 562-572.

Pettigrew, J.E., 1993. Amino acid nutrition of gestating and lactating sows. Biokyowa Technical Review 5, 18pp.

Prime, G.R., M.A. Varley & H.W. Symonds, 1988. The effect of food intake during lactation and early pregnancy on plasma progesterone concentrations and prolifacy in multiparous sows. Animal Production, 46, 499.

Reese, D.E., E.R. Peo & A.J. Lewis, 1984. Relationship of lactation energy intake and occurence of post weaning oestrus to body and backfat composition in sows. Journal of Animal Science, 58, 126-144.

Reese, D.E., B.D. Moser, E.R. Peo, A.J. Lewis, D.R. Zimmerman, J.E. Kinder & W.W. Stroup, 1982. Influence of energy intake during lactation on subsequent gestation, lactation and post-weaning performance of sows. Journal of Animal Science, 55, 867-872.

Salmon-Legagneur, E. & A. Aumaitre, 1962. Influence de la quantité de lait et de sa composition sur la croissance du porcelet sous la mère. Annales de Zootechnique, 11, 181-196.

Shaw, H.J. & G.R. Foxcroft, 1985. Relationship between LH, FSH and prolactin secretion and reproductive activity in the weaned sow. Journal of Reproduction and Fertility, 75, 17-28.

Stahly, T.S., G.L. Cromwell & H.J. Monegue, 1990. Lactational responses of sows nursing large litters to dietary lysine levels. Journal of Animal Science 68 (Supplement): 369.

Symonds, H.W. & G.R. Prime, 1989. The influence of volume of food intake by gilts on blood flow in portal vein and clearance of progesterone from plasma. Animal Production, 48, 620-621.

Tokach, M.D., J.E. Pettigrew, G.D. Dial, J.E. Wheaton, B.A. Crooker & L.J. Johnston, 1992. Characterization of luteinizing hormone secretion in the primiparous, lactating sow: relationship to blood metabolites and return-to-oestrous interval.

Verstegen, M.W.A., J. Mesu, G.J.M. van Kempen & G. Geerse, 1985. Energy balances of lactating sows in relation to feeding level and stage of lactation. Journal of Animal Science, 60, 731-740.

Vesseur. P.C., B. Kemp & L.A. den Hartog, 1994. Factors affecting the weaning to oestrus interval in the sow. Journal of Animal Physiology and Animal Nutrition, 72, 225-233.

Weldon, W.C., A.J. Lewis, G.F. Louis, J.L. Kovar and P.S. Miller, 1994. Postpartum hypophagia in primiparous sows: II. Effects of feeding level during gestation and exogenous insulin on lactation feed intake, glucose tolerance and epinephrine-stimulated release of nonesterified fatty acids and glucose. Journal of Animal Science, 72, 395-403.

Whittemore, C.T., A. Aumaitre & I. Williams, 1978. Growth of body components in young weaned pigs. Journal of Agricultural Science, 91, 681-692.

Whittemore, C.T. & C.A. Morgan, 1990. Model components for the determination of energy and protein requirements for breeding sows: a review. Livestock Production Science, 26, 1-37.

Xue, J.L., Y. Koketsu, G.D. Dial, J.E. Pettigrew & A. Sower, 1997. Glucose tolerance, luteinizing hormone release and reproductive performance of first-litter sows fed two levels of energy during gestation. Journal of Animal Science, 75, 1845-1852.

Yang, H., P.R. Eastham, P. Phillips & C.T. Whittemore, 1989. Reproductive body weight and body condition of breeding sows with different body fatness at parturition, differing nutrition during lactation, and differing litter size. Animal Production, 48, 181-201.

Zak, L.J., J.R. Cosgrove, F.X. Aherne & G.R. Foxcroft, 1997. Pattern of feed intake and associated metabolic and endocrine changes differentially affect postweaning fertility in primiparous lactating sows. Journal of Animal Science, 75, 208-216.

13 Lactational effects on the endocrinology of reproduction

B. Kemp

13.1 Introduction

From the lactating sow, we expect a good milk production for the piglets and sound reproduction after lactation. Milk production is given high priority by the sow and in most modern crossbred sows, milk production figures are around 8 to 10 kg per day (Babinszky, 1992; King *et al.*, 1993). Feed intake is often too low to fully account for the demands for milk production and, therefore, the body reserves of fat and protein are depleted. This catabolic state of the animal can result in reproductive failure after lactation typified by a prolonged weaning to oestrus interval (which is especially obvious in the first litter sow), reduced ovulation rate and increased embryonic mortality in the subsequent pregnancy. These effects on reproductive processes give rise to problems in practice including anoestrus after lactation, prolonged intervals between weaning and oestrus and weaning to conception and reduced litter sizes in subsequent pregnancies. The effects of lactation on subsequent reproduction will be discussed in this Chapter, with emphasis placed on the endocrine linkage between milk production and reproduction.

13.2 Consequences of lactation for reproduction

13.2.1 Lactational anoestrus

During lactation the sow generally remains anoestrus. However, lactational oestrus is sometimes seen in sows. Factors increasing the incidence of lactational oestrus seem to be frequent boar contact, group housing systems, low milk production (low number of piglets), high feed intake, litter management factors such as split weaning and interrupted suckling, and advanced parity of the sow. However, oestrus detection during lactation is difficult and successful mating and conception resulting in satisfactorily sized litters has also been shown to be difficult (Varley and Foxcroft, 1990). Therefore, induction of oestrus during lactation is not desirable.

13.2.2 Reproduction after lactation

The majority of the literature describing the effects of lactation on reproduction after lactation covers studies performed with first litter sows (gilts) in which restriction of feed (energy or protein) intake or restriction of suckling intensity (with techniques such as split weaning or interrupted suckling) are applied. This special attention to the first parity sow is probably because, in general, older parity sows have a satisfactory reproductive output and seem less affected by nutritional regimen or litter management as compared to younger sows (Hughes, 1989, Vesseur *et al.*, 1994; Vesseur, 1997). This is most likely caused by the fact that older parity sows have no significant nutrient needs for growth to maturity and have a relatively greater feed intake capacity, higher metabolisable fat and protein stores and a significantly higher rate of ovulation. Higher feed intake capacities make the catabolic state less dramatic and the higher metabolisable stores assist the contribution from maternal stores to milk production. Older parity sows often have ovulation rates of about 24 eggs (Soede *et al.*, 1995) which is well above the uterine capacity for piglets during pregnancy. Therefore such a high ovulation rate may mask possible effects of nutrition or litter management on embryonic mortality.

Reduced feed intake during lactation has been shown to affect the weaning to oestrus interval in first litter sows in many studies. In the literature reviewed by Hughes (1989), first litter sows receiving high amounts of energy or protein during lactation, had mean weaning to oestrus intervals of 10.3 to 12.7 days whereas those receiving low amounts of energy or protein had weaning to oestrus intervals of 14.6 to 19.3 days. In older parity sows, however, the effects of reduced feed intake on weaning to mating interval (which was found to be about 4 to 7 days, Hughes, 1989) are mostly absent or very small (see Hughes, 1989; Whittemore, 1996, for review). Overall, it is clear that underfeeding (energy as well as protein) during lactation causes an extension of the weaning to mating interval, especially in first litter sows.

Hughes (1989) and Whittemore (1996) concluded from their reviews that feed intake during lactation has little effect on ovulation rate. However, Foxcroft *et al.* (1995) demonstrated that the mean ovulation rate of primiparous sows, subjected to a period of reduced feed intake during lactation, was reduced compared to *ad libitum* fed controls (15.4 vs. 19.9 corpora lutea per sow). In this experiment, the effects of undernutrition on weaning to oestrus interval were very small and the weaning to oestrus interval was short (about 4-5 days). It may be that the effects of undernutrition during lactation on ovulation rate are less marked when the weaning to oestrus interval is prolonged.

Hughes (1989) and Whittemore (1996) concluded that low feeding levels during lactation may adversely influence subsequent embryonic survival in gilts and sows. The literature reviewed by Hughes (1989) suggested that low feeding levels, as compared to high feeding levels during lactation, resulted in a 10 % (range 0-15%) lower embryonic survival.

Matte *et al.* (1992) reviewed data on the effects of interrupted suckling (a daily temporary removal of the whole litter) or split weaning (a permanent removal of part of the litter a few days before completing weaning) on subsequent reproduction. In general, such treatments result in a shortened weaning to oestrus interval with no clear effects on subsequent pregnancy rate or litter size. Vesseur (1997) found only a small influence of split weaning on weaning to oestrus interval in first and second parity sows. However, in second parity sows, farrowing rate was increased in sows subjected to split weaning in the previous lactation.

From these data one can conclude that feeding (energy or protein intakes that result in a catabolic state of the animal) or litter management (resulting is variation in suckling stimulation and possible milk production) during lactation may affect weaning to oestrus interval, embryonic survival and possibly ovulation rate.

13.3 Suckling induced milk production and consequences for metabolic state.

Elevated plasma concentrations of prolactin and oxytocin during lactation are dominant lactogenic factors (Varley and Foxcroft, 1990).

Prolactin levels in plasma are elevated during parturition then decrease after parturition but remain much higher than during the oestrus cycle (Bevers *et al.*, 1978; Dusza and Krzymowska, 1981; Stevenson *et al.*, 1981; Edwards and Foxcroft, 1983). During lactation, suckling of piglets results in an elevation of prolactin levels some 10-15 min after initial nuzzling and teat massage, which return to basal levels about 30-40 min after suckling (Kendall *et al.*, 1983; Mattioli *et al.*, 1988; Algers *et al.*, 1991). A gradual decrease in prolactin levels is seen during the course of lactation which appears to be the result of a gradual decrease in suckling frequency (Varley and Foxcroft, 1990). Around parturition, levels of oxytocin are also elevated and during lactation, suckling of the piglets induces a prompt release of oxytocin which induces milk ejection by the sow (Forsling *et al.*, 1979, Kendall *et al.*, 1983).

The suckling stimulated neuro-endocrine response on prolactin and oxytocin promotes utilisation of maternal protein and fat stores for milk synthesis (Einarsson and Rojkittikhun, 1993). In the rat, it has been shown that prolactin increases the number of insulin receptors in the mammary gland and decreases their numbers in maternal fat (Flint *et al.*, 1981; Flint, 1982). Oxytocin seems to stimulate the mobilisation of glucose from maternal stores to the mammary gland (Altzuler and Hampshire, 1981; Stock and Uvnäs-Moberg, 1985). Also, growth hormone levels are elevated during lactation and are increased by suckling behaviour of the piglets (Schams *et al.*, 1994). Growth hormone is important for galactopoiesis and is believed to facilitate the partitioning of glucose and lipids to the mammary gland (Hart, 1983).

Hormones of the thyroid and adrenal gland are also involved in milk production and jointly, these hormones stimulate the production and release of milk.

If the feeding levels are too low to compensate for the energy and protein drain from the body, due to milk production and release, the animal becomes catabolic. This catabolic state of the animal is reflected in changes in the levels of numerous metabolites and metabolic hormones. For instance, increasing levels of urea and free fatty acids are found, indicating protein and fat breakdown from maternal stores. Growth hormone levels are higher and preprandial glucose, insulin and IGF-1 levels are lower in the catabolic sow (Einarsson and Rojkittikhun, 1993; Quesnel and Prunier, 1995).

The concentration pattern of these hormones and metabolites during lactation is dependent on the nutritional balance of the sow during lactation. Milk production normally increases during the first three to four weeks of lactation. Therefore, the effect of the catabolic state of the sow on metabolic hormones and metabolites will be more pronounced as lactation progresses.

In conclusion, the lactation period is characterised by a complex change in hormone and metabolite levels mediated by the suckling induced milk production and depending on the catabolic state of the animal.

13.4 Regulation of reproduction during and after lactation.

13.4.1 The role in reproduction of GnRH/LH release during and after lactation

In the ovary, there is an on-going development from before birth onwards of groups of primordial follicles to antral follicle stages. These follicles will go into atresia (when not recruited), but the on-going development of new groups of primordial follicles results in a more or less constant antral follicle pool (for review see Kemp *et al.*, 1998). This follicle pool is also seen during lactation with maximum follicle diameters of about 6 mm (Palmer *et al.*, 1965; Kunavongkrit *et al.*, 1982). To allow further outgrowth of these follicles to preovulatory follicles (>6mm) (and subsequently oestrus and ovulation), recruitment and selection from this pool is necessary. This recruitment and selection is initiated by a shift in GnRH/LH release by the hypothalamus/pituitary system from a pattern predominated by low frequency/high amplitude pulses to a pattern of high frequency/low amplitude pulses (see Figure 13.1). LH levels and pulsatility are low during lactation and normally such a shift will not be seen during lactation (Cox

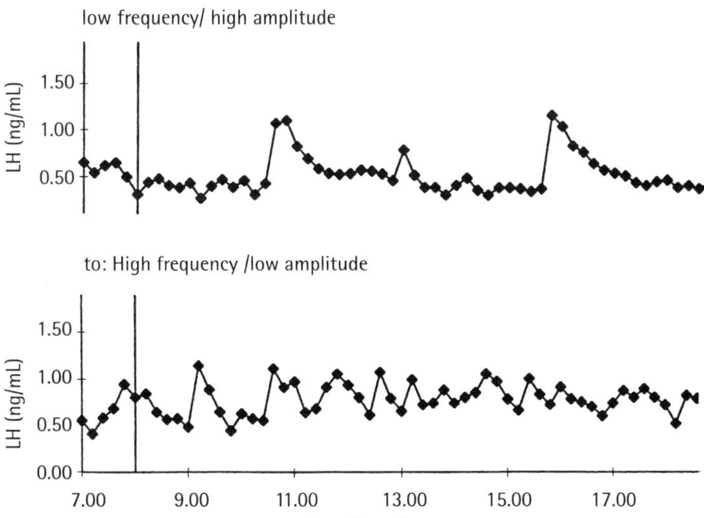

Figure 13.1. Schematic presentation of the change in LH patterns in plasma at initiation of recruitement of follicles resulting in oestrus and ovulation

and Britt, 1982). The suppression of the pulsatile LH release during lactation is an important reason why a sow normally remains anoestrus during lactation.

Directly after weaning, in reproductive sows, LH production shifts from a low frequency/ high amplitude pulse pattern to the high frequency/ low amplitude pulse pattern (see Figure 13.2a) and the sows will ovulate a selected number of follicles from the preovulatory follicle pool at about 4 to 5 days after weaning. However, not all sows will respond to weaning with such a clear change in LH pattern. If the GnRH pulse generator fails to induce this typical high frequency/low amplitude LH release from the pituitary after weaning, sows will have a prolonged interval between weaning and oestrus (Shaw and Foxcroft, 1985) (see Figure 13.2 b, c). Since this study, several studies have shown that LH levels and pulse frequencies at weaning are inversely related to the weaning to oestrus interval (Tokach *et al.*, 1992a; Paterson and Pearce, 1994; Kemp *et al.*, 1995).
The question is, why do some animals fail to show this typical GnRH/LH output after weaning? It has been substantiated that LH levels and pulsatility directly after weaning are related to restoration of LH pulsatility and levels during lactation (Shaw and Foxcroft, 1985; Armstrong *et al.*, 1986; King and Martin, 1989; Barb *et al.*, 1991; Tokach *et al.*, 1992a, Kemp *et al.*, 1995). LH pulsatility and concentrations are reduced during early lactation and the sows in which restoration of LH pulsatility and LH-levels was seen during the course of lactation, showed

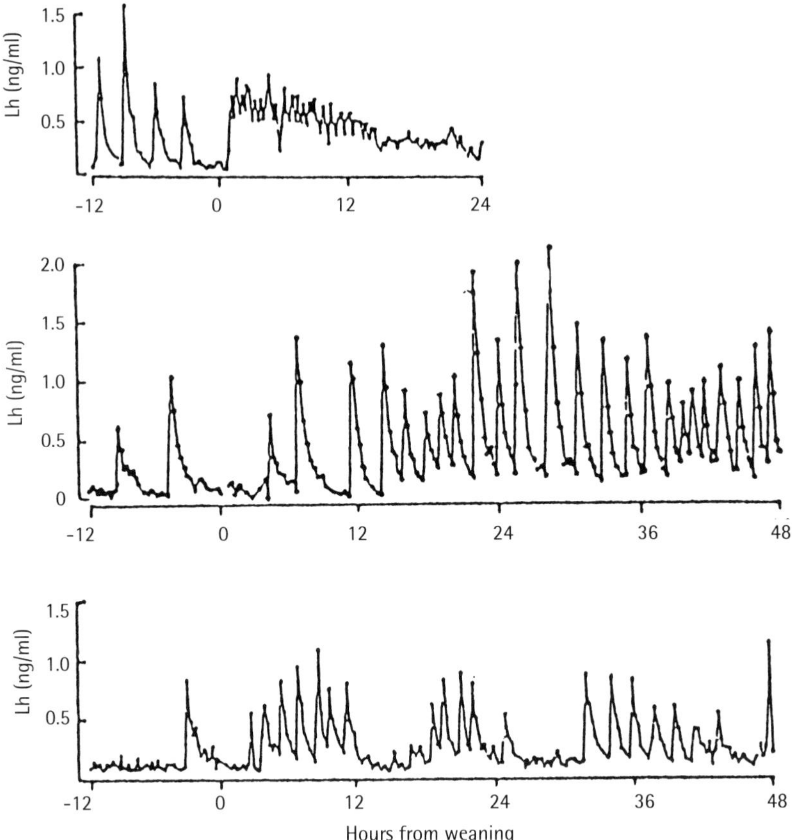

Figure 13.2. Plasma LH in sows weaned at 21 days postpartum and with weaning to oestrus intervals of (a) 4 days, (b) 6 days and (c) > 11 days (from Shaw and Foxcroft, 1985)

high LH levels and pulse frequency directly after weaning, and short intervals from weaning to oestrus. Sows in which LH pulsatility was not restored during lactation showed impaired LH levels and pulse frequencies directly after weaning and a prolonged weaning to oestrus interval (Figure 13.3).

Sesti and Britt (1993) showed that inhibition of LH release during lactation was mainly caused by a blockage of GnRH release and not by depleted pituitary LH pools.

It seems, therefore, that the suppression of GnRH during lactation is an important contributor to anoestrus during and after lactation. Moreover, this was demonstrated in that oestrus and ovulation can be induced during lactation and after lactation in anoestrus sows by mimicking the increased GnRH pulsatility by administration of GnRH at 1-2 h intervals (Armstrong and Britt, 1985; Britt *et al.*, 1985).

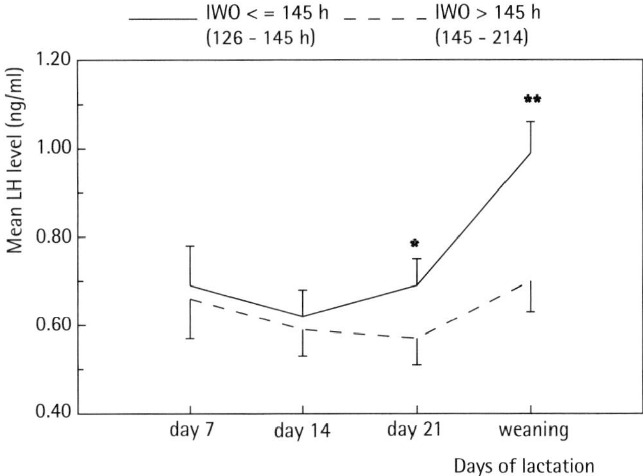

Figure 13.3. Mean plasma LH concentrations over a 12 h period at day 7, 14 and 21 of lactation and after weaning (day 22) for multiparous sows divided into long and short weaning to oestrus intervals (IWO is interval weaning to oestrus, Kemp et al. 1995)

13.4.2 The role of follicular development on reproduction during and after lactation.

Suppressed GnRH release during and after lactation seems to play an important role in re- establishment of oestrus and ovulation during and after lactation. However in the above mentioned studies of Armstrong and Britt (1985) and Britt *et al.* (1985), replacement therapy with GnRH during or after lactation did not result in oestrus and ovulation in all animals (especially early in lactation). Also, effects of lactation on subsequent ovulation rate and embryonic mortality cannot be explained satisfactorily by the GnRH pulse frequency theory.
Moreover, data of Cosgrove and Foxcroft (1996) show that in feed restricted primiparous sows with a normal LH pattern before weaning, negative effects of low feeding levels during lactation on ovulation rate and embryonic survival can still be found.
Baidoo *et al.* (1992) showed that low feeding levels during lactation can result in a depressed preovulatory LH surge. This may adversely influence luteinization of the corpora lutea and result in decreased plasma progesterone levels in early pregnancy which have been shown to be negatively related with embryo survival (Einarsson and Rojkittikhun, 1993). Kirkwood *et al.* (1987) showed that the detrimental effects of low feeding levels during lactation on embryonic survival could be prevented by GnRH injection at the onset of oestrus. They also found higher progesterone levels in early pregnancy in sows treated with GnRH as compared to their low-fed controls.

Such data suggest that a depressed preovulatory LH surge may explain nutritionally induced problems in reproduction. However, the development of the follicle pool during lactation might also play a role in this respect.
During early lactation the follicle pool on the ovaries is characterised by a large number of small sized follicles, a small number of medium sized follicles and the absence of large sized follicles. During lactation there is a gradual shift in numbers of follicles into medium and large size categories and this percentage of atretic follicles decreases (Kunavongkrit *et al.*, 1982).
Miller *et al.* (1996) showed that low feeding levels during the first 14 days of lactation resulted in an impaired follicular development at day 15 of lactation. Quesnel *et al.* (1997) have also shown that follicular development after weaning at 28 days is depressed if low feeding levels are applied during lactation. Therefore, sows can sometimes ovulate after weaning due to a well developed LH pulsatility directly after weaning, while the follicle pool is not yet fully developed. This might result in ovulation of a suboptimal population of eggs and in suboptimal functioning of corpora lutea. This could have consequences for ovulation rate (Foxcroft *et al.*, 1995) and embryonic mortality. This hypothesis is now being tested by Canadian research in which sows with various feed restriction protocols during lactation are slaughtered at the expected time of post weaning oestrus and eggs from the ovaries are studied in an *in vitro* maturation system (G. Foxcroft, personal communication). Moreover, that in first and second parity sows, postponement of ovulation by altrenogest treatment (Johnston *et al.*, 1992; Forgerit *et al.*, 1995) or skipping a heat (Morrow *et al.*, 1989; Clowes *et al.*, 1994; Vesseur, 1997) improves farrowing rates and litter sizes substantially indicates that ovulation after weaning will sometimes take place before an optimal follicle population is established.

Normally a low feeding level during lactation results in both impairment of pulsatile LH release and follicular development. Depression of follicular growth might, therefore, be firstly a result of depressed LH release. Cosgrove *et al.* (1992) studied this possible gonadotrophin independent effect of low feeding levels on follicle development in the gilt. After a period of low feeding levels they refed them but blocked the LH response by treatment with the synthetic progestagen, allyl trenbolone. Despite the lack of LH response to refeeding, significant follicular development was seen, indicating that changes at the ovarian level may be an important component of the reproductive response to changes in metabolic state.

Studies of Guthrie *et al.* (1990) and Bolomba *et al.* (1996), in gilts, have shown that increased LH pulsatility is necessary for outgrowth of follicles from antral stages to preovulatory follicles (recruitment) but follicle development in the antral follicle pool seems more dependent on FSH. There are not many data on FSH secretion during lactation. From the second week of lactation onwards some authors find a continuous increase in plasma FSH and others do not. At weaning, some authors find a rise in FSH and others do not (see Quesnel and Prunier, 1995 for review). Variation between individual animals is remarkable. An explanation for this degree of variation between animals and experiments might be that FSH production is under negative control of inhibin produced by larger follicles. If the follicle pool consists of only small follicles, inhibition of FSH will not occur and a steady increase of FSH levels during lactation and an extra increase after lactation will be seen. If the follicle pool contains larger antral follicles producing inhibin, however, FSH might be blocked and no clear increases in FSH release can be seen. Thus, FSH is more or less inhibited depending on the developmental stage of the follicle pool. This phenomenon might also explain why effects of nutrition on FSH release during and after lactation are variable.

Cosgrove and Foxcroft (1996) suggested that an inadequate nutritional status during lactation influences the development of the follicular pool by metabolites or metabolic hormones influencing the ovaries directly and not only via gonadotropic stimulation as outlined above.

13.5 Regulation of GnRH/LH release and follicle growth by suckling stimulus and catabolic state of the sow

The inhibition of GnRH/LH release and the inhibition of follicle growth during lactation seem to be major contributors to the effects of lactation on subsequent reproduction. As outlined above, suckling stimulus and catabolic state during lactation affect reproduction. Therefore, in the next paragraph, the endocrine links between suckling and catabolic state and GnRH/LH and follicle growth will be discussed.

13.5.1 Causes of inhibition of GnRH/LH release during lactation

LH release during lactation is affected by suckling induced neuroendocrine reflexes, which inhibit GnRH release and by endocrine mechanisms influenced by the metabolic state of the animal. Quesnel and Prunier (1995) hypothesised that at the beginning of lactation (3-14 d post partum), when udder stimulation due to high suckling stimuli is maximal, LH inhibition related to the suckling-induced neuroendocrine reflexes is dominant. During the 3rd and 4th weeks post partum when milk production is maximal (the catabolic state might become more pronounced) and suckling stimuli are lower, the influence of the nutrient deficiency on LH secretion may be increasing.

Inhibition of LH release due to suckling frequency.
Separation of the sow and piglets for periods of 4 h or more per day has been shown to increase basal LH concentrations (Booman and van der Wiel, 1980; Newton *et al.*, 1987; Armstrong *et al.*, 1988a).

There is now accumulating evidence that the suckling induced suppression of LH release may be mediated by opioid peptides. During suckling, endogenous opioids are released from the brain (Varley and Foxcroft, 1990). Experiments in which lactating sows were given naloxone (an opioid antagonist) showed an increase in LH release and pulsatility (Barb *et al.*, 1986; Mattioli *et al.*, 1986; Armstrong *et al.*, 1988a; De Rensis *et al.*, 1993). Moreover, Armstrong *et al.* (1988b) showed that morphine (an endogenous opioid agonist) prevented the normal rise in LH after removal of the litter.

Experiments studying the possible inhibitory role of prolactin on LH release during lactation have been reviewed by Van der Wiel *et al.* (1985) and Dusza and Tilton (1990). These reviews suggest that prolactin or regulators of prolactin release may partly inhibit LH release during lactation. To study the possible role of prolactin, Dusza *et al.* (1984) and Booman *et al.* (1982) studied the effects of post weaning administration of prolactin on plasma LH and oestrus occurrence. After weaning, the suckling mediated (possible opioid regulated) inhibition is absent and administration of prolactin allows the effects of prolactin on LH inhibition to be studied. Dusza *et al.* (1984) found no effects of prolactin administration on mean LH and oestrus post weaning. Booman *et al.* (1982) found a lower LH pulsatility after weaning. In some cases therefore, prolactin might have an inhibitory effect on LH release during lactation although literature is inconclusive. After weaning, prolactin returns to low levels within 4-6 h and delayed oestrus after weaning is not due to a hyperprolactinaemic state (Van der Wiel *et al.*, 1985; Quesnel and Prunier, 1995).

Inhibition of LH release due to catabolic state of the animal.
In primiparous sows given different energy and protein intakes during a 28 day lactation period, Tokach *et al.* (1992a) demonstrated that average daily dietary protein and energy intakes affected mean LH concentration on d 21 of lactation in an interactive manner (see Figure 13.4). At a low dietary Metabolisable Energy (ME) intake, increasing dietary lysine intake had little effect on mean LH concentration. The influence of lysine intake on LH secretion increased as energy intake increased. These results reveal that mean LH at day 21 of lactation is reduced by restrictions of either dietary lysine or energy intake. Similar effects on LH pulse frequency and LH concentration have also been reported by King and Martin (1989) who used protein restriction during lactation. Many studies have shown that inducing a more catabolic state in the animal by feed restriction results in a direct suppression of LH release by the pituitary wich is probably caused by a lower GnRH release in the gilt and the lactating sow (Cosgrove *et al.*, 1993 a, b; Booth *et al.*, 1994; Cosgrove and Foxcroft, 1996).

Tokach *et al.* (1992a) and Pettigrew and Tokach (1993) calculated correlations between LH pulsatility during lactation and the plasma metabolites (glucose, triglycerids, NEFA, lysine, branch-chain amino acids and urea nitrogen) and the

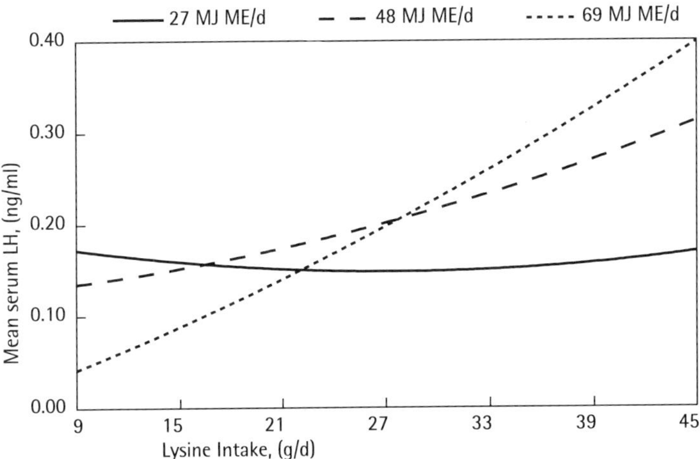

Figure 13.4. Predicted influence of dietary lysine and energy intakes before day 21 on mean LH on day 21 of lactation (redrawn from Tokach et al. 1992a)

metabolic hormones, insulin and IGF-1. LH pulse frequency was sporadically (depending on sample time) found to be weakly positively correlated with plasma glucose concentration and negatively correlated with NEFA concentration. Stronger positive correlations were found with IGF-1 and the strongest correlations were found with insulin. Such data suggest a role for insulin as a linkage between LH production and nutrition.

Pettigrew and Tokach (1993) show in their review that insulin receptors are found in the brain and pituitary and that insulin enhances LH and FSH release *in vitro*. Cox *et al.* (1989) demonstrated that an insulin injection in the cerebroventricular area of the brain had a direct positive effect on LH production, indicating a direct effect of insulin on the hypothalamic/pituitary axis.

Realimentation of feed-restricted gilts by glucose infusions seems to result in a direct restoration of LH pulsatility (Booth, 1990; Cosgrove *et al.*, 1993a) suggesting that glucose or sequelae of the increased glucose levels (insulin or IGF-1) induce restoration of LH release.

Administration of glucose during lactation (Tokach *et al.*, 1992b) increased plasma glucose and insulin levels but failed to restore LH levels. Perhaps inappropriate timing or inadequate duration of infusion might explain this lack of effect. The response may also have been masked by the strong suckling inhibition of LH release in the lactating sow. Insulin administration around and after weaning to shorten the weaning to oestrus interval in primiparous sows (Rojkittikhun *et al.*, 1993) and mixed parity sows (Kirkwood and Thacker, 1991) also failed to result in adequate responses. However, in both experiments the weaning to oestrus interval was very short in the controls and, therefore, no effects would be anticipated.

13.5.2 Possible factors involved in follicle growth

Since follicle growth during lactation and the effects of nutrition and suckling on follicle growth have not been extensively studied only a brief overview can be given.
There is extensive *in vitro* evidence for important effects of glucose, insulin and various growth factors (like IGFs, TGFs) on follicular development (see Cosgrove and Foxcroft, 1996, for review).
A lot of information is available on the role of insulin in follicular development. Cox *et al.* (1987) showed that insulin injections during the follicular phase in gilts increases ovulation rate in the absence of clear effects on gonadotrophins. Matamoros *et al.* (1990, 1991) showed that insulin injections stimulated follicular steroid synthesis and/or decreased follicular atresia in cycling gilts and PMSG treated gilts. Meurer *et al.* (1991) postulated, based on research with diabetic sows, that the positive effect of insulin on ovulation rate could be explained by less follicular atresia in the follicular phase. On the ovarian level, insulin seems to stimulate granulosa cells to form LH receptors and produce oestrogen (Poretsky and Kalin, 1987). Insulin might directly affect granulosa cell glucose utilisation since changes in follicular fluid glucose concentrations did not parallel those in the periphery (Britt *et al.*, 1988). Also realimentation induced increases in follicular aromatase activity and/or follicular development have been associated with a marked increase in insulin status (Cosgrove *et al.*, 1992). These data suggest a direct role for insulin in ovarian follicular development. Many more metabolic factors and growth factors are involved in regulation of follicular development but the possible effects of catabolic state on these factors and/or their role on follicular development are still under study.

13.6 Conclusions

Lactation generally results in anoestrus during the lactation period due to the combined effects of suckling and the catabolic state of the sow. The catabolic state of the sow during lactation can have especially profound negative effects on the weaning to oestrus interval, ovulation rate and embryonic mortality. Anoestrus or a prolonged interval from weaning to oestrus are mainly caused by insufficient restoration of LH release and pulsatility during and after lactation. Insufficient follicular development during lactation might affect ovulation rate and embryonic mortality and could also be an explicatory factor in prolonged anoestrus after weaning. Suckling induced release of endogenous opioids and prolactin are involved and metabolic hormones like insulin and IGF-1 might be involved in the restoration process of LH release during lactation. Insufficient follicular development during lactation may be a result of the inhibited gonadotrophin release during lactation but also direct effects on the ovary of a number of metabolites and metabolic hormones like insulin, IGF-1 and its binding proteins are expected.

However, to increase our understanding of these mechanisms, substantial work is required on follicular dynamics during lactation and the regulation of follicular development during lactation as affected by metabolic state.

13.7 References

Algers, B., A. Madji, S. Rojanasthien & K. Uvnas-Moberg, 1991. Quantitative relationship between suckling-induced teat stimulation and the release of prolactin, gastrin, somatostatin, insulin, glucagon and vaso-active intestinal polypeptide in sows. Vet. Res. Comm.15, 395-407.

Altzuler, N.& J. Hampshire, 1981. Oxytocin infusion increases insulin and glucagon levels and glucose production and uptake in the normal dog. Diabetes 30, 112-114.

Armstrong, J.D.& J.H. Britt, 1985. Pulsatile administration of gonadotropin-releasing hormone to anestrous sows: endocrine changes associated with GnRH-induced and spontaneous estrus. Biol. Reprod. 33, 375-380.

Armstrong, J.D., J.H. Britt & R.R. Krealing, 1986. Effect of restrition of energy during lactation on body condition, energy metabolism, endocrine changes and reproductive performance in primiparous sows. J. Anim. Sci. 63,1915-1925.

Armstrong, J.D., R.R. Kraeling & J.H. Britt, 1988a. Effects of naloxone or transient weaning on secretion of LH and prolactin in lactating sows. J Reprod. Fert. 83, 301-308.

Armstrong, J.D., R.R. Kraeling & J.H. Britt, 1988b. Morphine suppresses luteinizing hormone concentrations in transiently weaned sows and delayed onset of estrus after weaning. J. Anim. Sci. 66, 2216-2223.

Babinszky, L., 1992. Energy metabolism and lactation performance of primiparous sows as affected by dietary fat and vitamin E. PhD Thesis Agricultural University Department of Animal Nutrition, pp 159.

Baidoo, S.K., F.X. Aherne, R.N. Kirkwood & G.R. Foxcroft, 1992. Effects of feed intake during and after lactation on sow reproduction. Can. J. Anim. Sci. 72, 911-917.

Barb, C.R., R.R. Kraeling, G.B. Rampacek & C.S. Whisnant, 1986. Opioid inhibition of luteinizing hormone secretion in the postpartum lactation sow. Biol. Reprod. 35, 368-371.

Barb, C.R., M.J. Estienne & R.R. Kraeling, 1991. Endocrine changes in sows exposed to elevated ambient temperature during lactation. Domest. Anim. Endocrinol. 8, 117-127.

Bevers, M.M., A.H. Willemse & T.A.M. Kruip, 1978. Plasma prolactin levels in the sow during lactation and the post weaning period as measured by radio-immunoassay. Biol. Reprod. 19, 628-634.

Bolomba, D., A. Dunuc, J.J. Dufour & M.A. Sirard, 1996. Effects of gonadotropin treatment on ovarian follicle growth, oocyte quality and in vitro fertilization of oocytes in prepubertal gilts. Theriogenology 46, 717-726.

Booman, P.& D.F.M. van der Wiel, 1980. Lactatie anoestrus bij het varken: mogelijke relatie met hyperprolactineamie. Lactational anoestrus in the pig: Possible relationship with hyper-prolactinaemia. Report B-157. Instituut voor veeteeltkundig onderzoek 'Schoonoord' Zeist, the Netherlands. pp 96.

Booman, P., D.F.M. van der Wiel & A.A.M. Jansen, 1982. Effect of exogenous prolactin on preipheral luteinizing hormone levels in the sow after weaning of piglets. Rapport B-200 Instituut voor veeteeltkundig onderzoek Schoonoord. Zeist, The Netherlands, pp 58.

Booth, P.J., 1990. Metabolic influences on hypothalamic-pituitary-ovarian function in the pig. Contr. of Pig Reproduction III. J. Reprod. Fertil. Suppl. 40, 89-100.

Booth, P.J., J. Craigon & G.R. Foxcroft, 1994. Nutritional manipulation of growth and metabolic and reproductive status in prepubertal gilts. J. Anim. Sci. 72, 2415-2424.

Britt, J.H., J.D. Armstrong, N.M. Cox & K.L. Esbenshade, 1985. Control of follicular development during and after lactation in sows. J. Reprod. Fert. Suppl. 33, 37-45.
Britt, A.H., J.D. Armstong & N.M. Cox, 1988. Metabolic interfaces between nutrition and reproduction in pigs. Proc. 11th ICAR Dublin Ireland 5, 117-125.
Clowes, E.J., F.X. Aherne & G.R. Foxcroft, 1994. Effect of delayed breeding in the endocrinology and fecundity of sows. J. Anim. Sci. 72, 283-291.
Cosgrove, J.R., J.E. Tilton, M.G. Hunter & G.R. Foxcroft, 1992. Gonadotrophin-independent mechanisms participate in ovarian responses to realimentation in feed-restricted prepubertal gilts. Biol. Reprod. 47, 736-745.
Cosgrove, J.R, H.F. Urbanski G.R. & Foxcroft, 1993a. Maturational changes in gonadotrophin secretion: the LH response to realimentation and a nocturnal increment in LH secretion of feed-restricted prepubertal gilts. J. Reprod. Fertil. 98, 293-300.
Cosgrove, J.R., S.G. Cosgrove, G.R. Foxcroft & B.A. Young, 1993b. Modulation of LH, testosterone and cortisol in boars by fasting and re-feeding. 7th World Conf. On Anim. Prod. 28 June-2 July 1993, Edmonton, Alta,Canada.Vol. 2, p 230.
Cosgrove J.R. & G.R. Foxcroft, 1996. Nutrition and reproduction in the pig: Ovarian aetiology. Anim. Reprod. Sci. 42, 131-141.
Cox, N.M. & J.H. Britt, 1982. Relationship between endogenous gonadotropin-releasing hormone, gonadotropins, and follicular development after weaning in sows. Biol. Reprod. 27, 70-78.
Cox, N.M., M.J. Stuart, T.G. Althen, W.A. Bennett & H.W. Miller, 1987. Enhancement of ovulation rate in gilts by increasing dietary energy and administering insulin during follicular growth. J. Anim. Sci. 64, 507-516.
Cox, N.M., C.R. Barb, J.R. Kesner, R.R. Kraeling, I.A. Matamoros & G.B. Rampacek, 1989. Effects of intracerebroventricular (ICV) administration of insulin on luteinizing hormone (LH) in gilts. Proceedings of the 3th international conference on pig reproduction, Nottingham, UK, Abstract No. 7.
De Rensis, F., J.R. Cosgrove & G.R. Foxcroft, 1993. Luteinizing hormone and prolactin responses to naloxone vary with stage of lactation in the sow. Biol. Reprod. 48, 970-976.
Dusza, L. & H. Krzymowska, 1981. Plasma prolactin levels in sows during pregnancy, parturation and early lactation. J. Reprod. Fert. 61, 131-134.
Dusza, L., G. Kotwica, B. Szafranska, R. Ciereszko, A. Milosz, J. Kotwica, A. Ziecik & H. Krzymowska, 1984. Influence of exogenous PRL on hormonal regulation in sows after weaning. Zesz. Probl. Post. Naulk. Rol. 309, 95-104. [In Polish]
Dusza, L. & J.E. Tilton, 1990. Role of prolactin in the regulation of ovarian function in pigs. J. Reprod. Fert., Suppl. 40, 33-45.
Edwards, S. & G.R. Foxcroft, 1983. Endocrine changes in sows weaned at two stages of lactation. J. Reprod. Fert. 67., 161-172.
Einarsson, S. & T. Rojkittikhun, 1993. Effects of nutrition on pregnant and lactating sows. J. Reprod. Fert. Suppl. 48, 229-239.
Flint, D.J., 1982. Regulation of insulin receptors by prolactine in lacating rat mammary gland. J. Endocinoloy 93, 279-285.
Flint, D.J., R.A. Clegg & R.G. Vernon, 1981. Prolactin and the regulation of adipose-tissue metabolism during lactation in rats. J. Mol. Endocr. 22, 265-275.
Forgerit, Y., F. Martina-Botté, F. Bariteau, H. Corbé, C. Macar, P. Poirier, P. Nolibois & M. Terqui, 1995. Utilisation d'un progestagène (Regumate) au moment du tarissement de la primipare. Journée Porc. Rech. en France 27, 45-50.
Forsling, M.L., M.A.M. Taverne, N. Parvizi, F. Elseasser, D. Smidt & F. Ellendorf, 1979. Plasma oxytocin and steroid concentrations during late pregnancy, parturition and lactation in the miniature pig. J. Endocrinol. 82, 61-69.

Foxcroft, G.R., F.X. Aherne, E.J. Clowes, H. Miller & L.J. Zak, 1995. Sow fertility: The role of suckling inhibition and metabolic status. In: Animal Science Research and Development. Centre for Food and Agri-Food Canada Ottawa. (eds.). Ivan. pp. 377-388.
Guthrie, H.D., D.J. Bolt & B.S. Cooper, 1990. Effects of gonadotropin treatment on avarian follicle growth and granulosa aromatase activity in prepubertal gilts. J.Anim. Sci., 68, 3719-3726.
Hart, I.C., 1983. Endocrine control of nutrient partitioning in lactating ruminants. Proc. Nutr. Soc. 42, 181-194.
Hughes, P.E., 1989. A symposium-Nutrition-Reproduction interactions in the breeding sow. In: Manipulating Pig Production II. Barnett, J.L. & D.P. Hennessy (eds.). pp. 277-280, Australian Pig Science Association, Werribee, Victoria, Australia.
Johnston, N.E., M.W. Eastaugh & E.J. Thornton, 1992. The short term use of regumate in first litter sows. Proc. Int. Vet. Soc., The Hague, pp 457.
Kemp, B., N.M. Soede & F.A. Helmond, 1995. Relations between body condition loss, insulin and LH levels during lactation in multiparous sows. Abstracts of the 46th Annual Meeting of the EAAP, Prague. Arendonk, J.A.M. van (ed.). pp333. Wageningen Pers, The Netherlands.
Kemp. B., N.M. Soede & W. Hazeleger, 1997. Control of ovulation. In: Wiseman, J., M.A. Varley & J.P. Chadwick (eds.) Principles in Pig Science. Nottingham press., In press.
Kendall, J.Z., G.E. Richards & L.N. Shih, 1983. Effect of haloperidol, suckling, oxytocin and hand milking on plasma relaxin and prolactin concentration in cyclic and lactating pigs.. J. Reprod. Fert. 69, 271-277.
King, R.H. & G.B. Martin, 1989. Relationships between protein intake during lactation, LH levels and oestrus activity in first litter sows. Anim. Prod. Sci. 19,283-292.
King, R.H., M.S. Toner, H. Dove, C.S. Atwood & W.G. Brown, 1993. The response of first-litter sows to dietary protein level during lactation. J. Anim. Sci. 71, 2457-2463.
Kirkwood, R.N., E.S. Lythgoe & F.X. Aherne, 1987. Effect of lactational feed intake and gonadotrophin-releasing hormone on reproductive performance of sows. Can. J. Anim. Sci. 67, 715-719.
Kirkwood, R.N. & P.A. Thacker, 1991. The influence of premating feeding level and exogeneous insulin on reproductive performance of sows. Can. J. Anim. Sci. 71, 249-251.
Kunavongkrit, A., S. Einarsson & I. Settergren, 1982. Follicular development in primiparous lactating sows. Anim. Reprod. Sci. 5, 47-56.
Matamoros, I.A., N.M. Cox & A.B. Moore, 1990. Exogenous insulin and additional dietary energy effect preovulatory peptides on ovine pituitary gonadotropin secretion in vitro. Peptides, 6, 957-963.
Matamoros, I.A., N.M. Cox & A.B. Moore, 1991. Effects of exogenous insulin and body condition on metabolic hormones and gonadotropin-induced follicular development in prepubertal gilts. J. Anim. Sci. 69, 2081-2091.
Matte, J.J., C. Pomar & W.H. Close, 1992. The effect of interrupted suckling and split-weaning on reproductive performance of sows: a review. Livest. Prod. Sci. 30, 195-212.
Mattioli, M., F. Conte, G. Galeati & E. Seren, 1986. Effects of naloxone on plasma concentrations of prolactin and LH in lactating sows. J. Reprod. Fert. 76, 167-173.
Mattioli, M., G. Galeati & E. Seren, 1988. Control of LH and prolactin secretion during lactational anestrus in the pig. 11th Congress Anim. Reprod. Artificial Insemination, Dublin, Ireland, 1988, 44.
Meurer, K.A., N.M. Cox, I.A. Matamoros & R.C. Tubbs, 1991. Decreaed follicular steroids and insuline-like growth factor-I and increased atresia in diabetic gilts during follicular growth stimulated with PMSG. J. Reprod. Fertil., 91, 187-196.
Miller, H.A., G.R. Foxcroft & F.X. Aherne, 1996. Restricting feed intake suppresses ovarian follicular development and LH pulsatility at Day 14 of lactation in sows. In: Arendonk, J.A.M. van (ed.). Book of abstracts of the 47th Ann. Meeting of the European Assoc. for Anim. Prod. Wageningen Pers, Wageningen , The Netherlands. pp 265.

Morrow, W.E.M., A.D. Leman, N.B. Williamson, R. Moder & C. Pijoan, 1989. Improving parity two litter size in swine. J. Anim. Sci. 67, 1707-1713.
Newton, E.A., J.S. Stevenson & D.L. Davis, 1987. Influence of duration of litter seperation and boar exposure on estrus expression of sows during and after lactation. J. Anim. Sci. 65, 1500-1506.
Palmer, W.M., H.S. Teague & W.K. Venzke, 1965. Histological changes in the reproductive tract of the sow during lactation and early postweaning. J. Anim. Sci., 24 1117-1125.
Paterson, A.M. & G.P. Pearce, 1994. Plasma hormone and metabolite concentrations and the interval from weaning to oestrus in primiparous sows. Anim. Reprod. Sci. 36, 261-279
Pettigrew, J.E. & M.D. Tokach, 1993. Metabolic influences on sow reproduction. Pig News and Information 14-2, 69N-72N.
Poretsky, L. & M.F. Kalin, 1987. The gonadotropic function of insulin. Endocrine reviews 8-2, 132-141.
Quesnel, H. & A. Prunier, 1995. Endocrine bases of lacational anoestrus in the sow. Reprod. Nutr. Dev. 35, 395-414.
Quesnel, H., A. Pasquier, A.M. Mounier & A. Prunier, 1997. Restricted feed intake during lactation inhibits LH pulsatility and follicular development around weaning in sows. In: Program and abstract book of the fifth international conference on pig reproduction. Kerkrade, The Netherlands. pp 73.
Rojkittikhun, T., S. Einarsson, H. Zilinskas, L.E. Edqvist, K. Uvnäs-Moberg & N. Lundeheim, 1993 Effect of insulin administration at weaning on hormonal patterns and reproductive performance in primiparous sows. J. Vet. Med. 40, 161-168
Schams, D., W.D. Kraetzl, G. Brem & F. Graf, 1994. Secretory pattern on metabolic hormones in the lactating sow. Exp. Clin. Endocrinol. 102, 439-447.
Sesti, L.A.C. & J.H. Britt, 1993. Agonist-induced release of gonadotropin-releasing hormone, Luteinizing hormone and follicle-stimulating hormone and their associations with basal secretions of luteinizing hormone and follicle stimulating hormone throughout lactation in sows. Biol. Reprod. 49, 332-339.
Shaw, H.J. & G.R. Foxcroft, 1985. Relationships between LH, FSH and prolactin secretion and reproductive activity in the weaned sow. J. Reprod. Fert. 75, 17-28.
Soede, N.M., C.C.H. Wetzels, W. Zondag, M.A.I. Koning & B. Kemp, 1995, Effects of timing of insemination relative to ovulation, as determined by ultrasonography, on fertilization rate and accessory sperm count in sows. J. Reprod. Fert., 104, 99-106.
Stevenson, J.S., N.M. Cox & J.H. Britt, 1981. Role of the ovary in controlling luteinizing hormone, follicle stimulating hormone and prolactin secretion during and after lactation in pigs. Biol. Reprod. 24, 341-353.
Stock, S. & K. Uvnäs-Moberg, 1985. Oxytocin infusions increase plasma levels of insulin and VIP but not of gastrin in conscious dogs. Act. Physiol. Scan. 125, 205-210.
Tokach, M.D., J.E. Pettigrew, G.D. Dial, J.E. Wheaton, B.A. Crooker & L.J. Johnson, 1992a. Characterization of luteinizing hormone secretion in the primiparous, lactating sow: relationship to blood metabolites and return-to-estrus interval. J.1 Anim.0 Sci. 70, 2195-2201.
Tokach, M.D., J.E. Pettigrew, G.D. Dial, J.E. Wheaton, B.A. Crooker & Y. Koketsu, 1992b. Influence of glucose infusions on luteinizing hormone secretion in the energy restricted, primiparous sow. J. Anim. Sci. 70, 2202-2206.
Van der Wiel, D.F.M., P. Booman, A.H. Willemse & M.M. Bevers, 1985. Relevance of prolactin to lactational and post-weaning anoestus in the pig. In: Ellendorf, F. & F Elsaesser (eds.), Endocrine causes of seasonal and lactational anoestrus in farm animals. M. Nijhoff, Dordrecht, Netherlands, pp. 154-165.
Varley, M.A. & G.R. Foxcroft, 1990. Endocrinology of the lactating and weaned sow. J. Reprod. Fert. Suppl. 40, 47-61.

Vesseur, P.C., B. Kemp, L.A. den Hartog, 1994. The effect of the weaning to oetrus interval on litter size, live born piglets and farrowing rate in sows. J. Anim. Phys. Anim Nutr. 71, 30-38.
Vesseur, P.C., 1997. Causes and consequences of variation in weaning to oestrus interval in the sow. PhD thesis Agricultural University Wageningen, The Netherlands, pp. 165.
Whittemore, C.T., 1996. Nutrition reproduction interactions in primiparous sows. Livest. Prod. Sci. 46, 65-83.

14 Modelling metabolism of the lactating sow

J. E. Pettigrew

14.1 Background

It is important in livestock production to be able to predict the impacts of changes in nutritional programmes or management practices on animal performance. Furthermore, these predictions must be quantitative in order to be of most benefit. The best method of predicting performance of animals systematically and quantitatively under varying conditions is by applying mathematical simulation models.

A recent book edited by Moughan *et al.* (1995) offers a thorough discussion of the relatively advanced application of mathematical modelling to the pig. Most models are directed to the growing pig, but some (e.g. Black *et al.*, 1986; Walker, 1990; Pomar *et al.*, 1991) also predict the lactational and reproductive performance of sows. The growth models operate at the level of lean tissue and fat accretion; whereas the sow models are based more heavily on empirically derived relationships.

Several models of ruminant animals, including lactating dairy cows, have been developed at the metabolic level (e.g. Gill *et al.*, 1984; Baldwin *et al.*, 1987). These models are based on knowledge of tissue metabolism, including quantitative estimates of kinetic parameters, which are aggregated into predictions of nutrient flows and production at the whole-animal level. Most metabolic models have dealt with ruminant animals, not with pigs.

14.2 A metabolic model of the lactating sow

14.2.1 Description

A model of the metabolism of the lactating sow was described in detail by Pettigrew *et al.* (1992a,b) and a modified version has also been described (Pettigrew *et al.*, 1993). The model traces the flow of energy-containing nutrients from absorption through intermediary metabolism, into and out of body stores, and into milk. The diagram of the model (Figure 14.1) shows the principal pools (state variables: metabolites, body stores, and milk components) and transactions (nutrient flows) of the model (Pettigrew *et al.*, 1993).

The model moves through time. At each time step, it estimates the rate of flow along each arrow in Figure 14.1. Then it examines each pool (box in Figure 14.1), and constructs a differential equation describing the amount of material moving

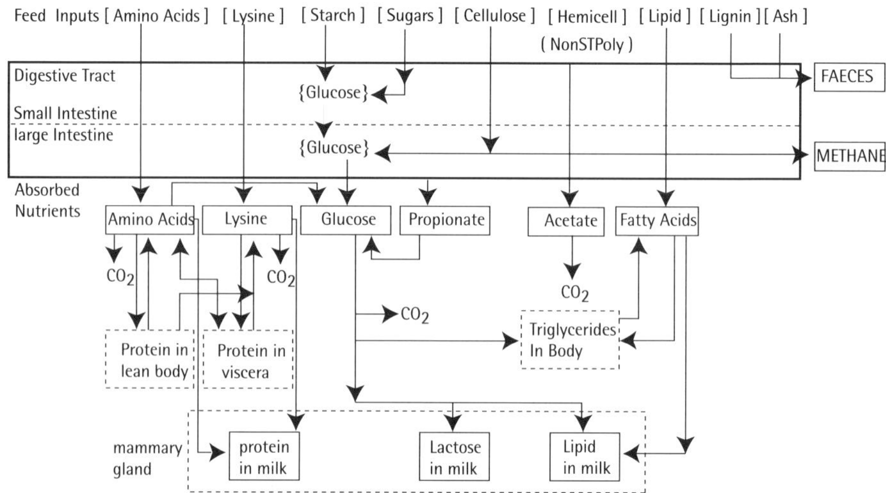

Figure 14.1. Schematic flowchart of a model of metabolism in lactating sows. [ ] indicates feed chemical concentration. Arrows indicate direction of fluxes (uni or bidirectional). Boxes depict inputs or outputs of the metabolism element. The zero pool of glucose in small and large intestines is indicated by brackets: { }. Broken boxes are body pools, which are accumulated or used up, depending on simulated conditions. Feed inputs are in g per day. Absorbed nutrients are in moles per day. Changes in body and milk pools are output as g per day. ATP is produced or utilized stoichiometrically in catabolic and anabolic interconversions, respectively. Reprinted from Livestock Production Science.

into and out of the pool. Finally, it integrates those differential equations, therefore producing new pool sizes, and thus new substrate concentrations, for the next time step. All fluxes are expressed in amounts per day, but the actual integration interval is much shorter (.001 day). This short integration interval is necessary because the turnover time of some pools is very much shorter than a day, resulting in a problem that mathematicians call stiff equations (France and Thornley, 1984).

The following is a description of selected aspects of the model. For more detail, the reader is urged to consult the original publications (Pettigrew *et al.*, 1992a,b, 1993).

Kinetics

The most challenging part of building the model is developing a method for predicting the rate of movement along each of the arrows in Figure 14.1 (the reaction kinetics), under varying circumstances. Four principles guide the reaction kinetics in this model.

1. The kinetics apply to the entire transactions (pathways) shown in Figure 14.1, not to individual reactions within these pathways
2. The rate of a transaction is a function of the state of the animal. Specifically, the rate of each transaction is determined by the concentrations of substrates, and sometimes by concentrations of inhibitors.
3. Most transactions are saturable with substrate, and the kinetics follow established patterns of saturable systems (Mahler and Cordes, 1971). The exceptions to this rule are tissue catabolism transactions.
4. Most rates are expressed per unit of tissue constituting the reaction site, to reflect differences in body size. The only exceptions are the rates of synthesis of milk components.

These principles lead to the following general equation which describes the rate of utilisation of a principal substrate in a transaction:

$$U = V/[1 + (K1/S1)^{\theta 1} + (K2/S2)^{\theta 2} + (I3/J3)^{\theta 3}]$$

where U is the amount of principal substrate utilized, expressed in moles per day, equivalents per day, or kg per day; V is the maximum velocity per unit tissue; K1 and K2 are affinity constants for substrates with concentrations S1 and S2, respectively; $\theta 1$, $\theta 2$ and $\theta 3$ are steepness parameters (described below); and J3 is an inhibition constant for an inhibitor with concentration I3. Each rate equation contains terms for all substrates except oxygen and body stores, but inhibitors are included only if justified on a physiological basis. This mathematical representation is based on accepted principles of biochemical kinetics (Mahler and Cordes, 1971) and has been used in aggregated models of metabolism in other species (Gill *et al.*, 1984; Baldwin *et al.*, 1987). If this equation form seems familiar, it is because it is a modification of the classical Michaelis-Menton equation for the description of enzyme kinetics.

A low affinity constant (K) produces a relatively high rate of the transaction when substrate supply is limiting. Therefore, the priority of one transaction over another for a limiting substrate is produced in the model by assigning a smaller affinity constant to the high-priority transaction. For example, the affinity constant for lysine in protein synthesis is much lower than the affinity constant for lysine in lysine oxidation. This approach is generally consistent with physiological mechanisms for setting priorities.

In some cases, the body's complex control mechanisms produce a different relationship between transaction rate and substrate concentration than is predicted by the simple Michaelis-Menton equation form. For example, the concentration of glucose in the body is under tight homeostatic control so it does not vary much. As part of this homeostatic control, the rate of glycolysis (glucose oxidation) is quite low when glucose concentration is below the target, but quite high when the concentration is above the target. That description is of a sigmoid (S-shaped) function, which can be produced by raising the value of the steepness parameter (θ) above 1. At very high values of θ (e.g. 10) movement of the substrate concentration across the value of K is almost an on-off switch. In the model, steepness parameters are used for low-priority transactions that clear away residual quantities of substrates. Specifically, high steepness parameters are used for lysine in lysine oxidation, for glucose in glycolysis, and for acetate in fatty acid synthesis.

The original version of the model (Pettigrew *et al.*, 1992a) did not explicitly consider metabolic hormones. It was thought that there was inadequate information to estimate quantitatively the rate of hormone release, the rate of hormone degradation, and the tissue sensitivity to each hormone. In fact, the use of steepness parameters is to some extent a substitute for explicit consideration of hormone activity. The revised model (Pettigrew *et al.*, 1993) incorporates a crude approximation of endocrine control in the form of a pool called 'anabolic hormone concentration'. This value, originally used by Baldwin *et al.* (1987) in a metabolic model of the lactating dairy cow, is taken as the ratio of glucose concentration to a reference value (5 mM). This ratio can then alter the values of several kinetic parameters.

Gluconeogenesis

The original version of the model (Pettigrew *et al.*, 1992a) did not consider gluconeogenesis because it was assumed that a nonruminant absorbing most of its energy in the form of glucose would not require extensive glucose synthesis. However, subsequent simulation with the model of experimental data from sows severely restricted in energy intake but still producing a relatively large amount of milk (Tokach *et al.*, 1992) predicted much lower plasma glucose concentrations than were measured in the experiment. Calculations external to the model then revealed that these sows must have been synthesizing large quantities of glucose from amino acids retrieved from body protein stores, in order to support milk production. Therefore, gluconeogenesis was included in the revised model (Pettigrew *et al.*, 1993).

Milk synthesis

Synthesis of milk components (protein, fat and lactose) is driven in the model by a term labeled CHl, perceived as the homeorhetic drive for lactation. The term CHl reflects both the endocrine milieu (Bauman and Currie, 1980) and mammary cell number (Neal and Thornley, 1983). It is primarily a function of the stage of lactation (the lactation curve), but can also be scaled up or down by a milk yield factor that reflects the non-nutritional variation in milk yield caused by such variables as genetics, litter size, and parity, which are not considered within the model. The CHl affects the rates of synthesis of milk protein, fat, and lactose and also the rates of degradation of body protein and fat.

The model does not estimate the amount of water secreted in milk (milk volume), although volume could be estimated from the amount of lactose produced.

14.2.2 Evaluation

Treatments from experiments used in the development of the model were simulated with the complete original model, and simulated outcomes compared to measured outcomes reported in the original papers. The results were encouraging (Pettigrew *et al.*, 1992a). Therefore, treatments from experiments not used in development of the model were similarly simulated (Pettigrew *et al.*, 1992b). Results (Figure 14.2) show close agreement between the simulated and measured values (Pettigrew *et al.*, 1992b). This agreement lends confidence in the structure and parameters of the model.

14.3 Comparison of modelling approaches

As mentioned in the background section (Section 14.1) of this chapter, most models that predict growth of the pig operate at the level of lean tissue and fat accretion, and are often called nutrient-partitioning models. The model described in the previous section operates at the level of metabolic pathways. The two approaches are very different. Each has advantages and disadvantages.

14.3.1 Advantages of metabolic models

Metabolic models can avoid some of the imperfections of traditional energy systems, such as the metabolizable energy system which is often used in nutrient-partitioning level models. They can make appropriate adjustments for the low efficiency of use of metabolizable energy from protein or from non-starch polysaccharides.. Also, they can appropriately reflect the complex variations in energetic efficiency with variation in energy source (starch, non-starch polysaccharides, fats, protein) and with variation in the material produced (protein versus fat in body or milk). For example, a metabolic model can reflect the energetic advantage of the use of dietary fat versus starch for milk fat production, but the lack of that same advantage for synthesis of protein.

One of the difficult tasks in modelling at the nutrient-partitioning level is apportioning a limited supply of energy to competing uses, such as milk production versus body tissue maintenance. The approaches are usually rather empirical, limiting reliability when applied to widely varying feeding levels, genetic lines, etc. This apportionment is conceptually logical and straightforward in a metabolic model, although data to support parameterization are usually inadequate.

Another difficulty in nutrient-partitioning level modelling is describing the

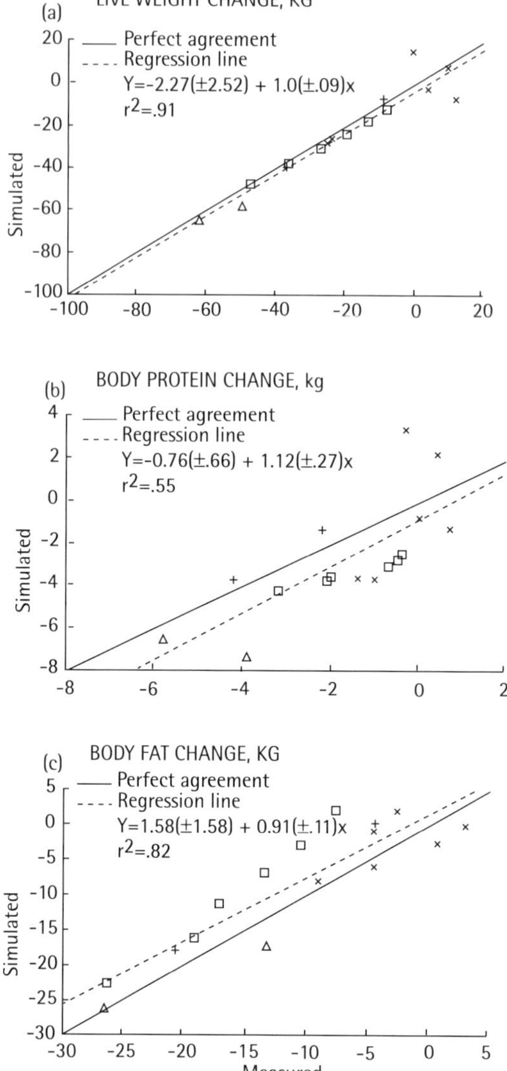

Figure 14.2. Simulated versus determined values for change (gain or loss) of (a) liveweight, (b) body protein, and (c) body fat during lactation. Data points with a common symbol are from the same experiment. Reprinted from the Journal of Animal Science.

marginal efficiency of lysine use for body protein accretion or milk protein production. Some models assume a constant marginal efficiency, while others reflect a reduction in efficiency as the dietary lysine level increases toward the requirement level. The relationships are also built from rather empirical data. Again, a metabolic model offers a more straightforward approach. Incidentally, some nutrient-partitioning level models make no assumptions about the relationship of marginal efficiency to lysine intake, but estimate the various losses of lysine from the body under varying conditions.

There is a predictable increase in milk fat content with supplemental dietary fat (Pettigrew, 1981). This phenomenon can be accommodated easily by a metabolic model, but is more difficult to reflect in a nutrient-partitioning level model.

As discussed in the next section, metabolic models may have specific advantages in modelling nutritional effects on reproduction.

14.3.2 Advantages of nutrient-partitioning level models

To date, nutrient-partitioning level models have been more successful in predicting pig performance than metabolic models, in spite of the greater theoretical accuracy of the metabolic models. Among the important advantages of the nutrient-partitioning level models are:

- More adequate data for parameterization;
- Model inputs are simpler and can be estimated with greater accuracy.

Both types of model can be useful in increasing our knowledge of the quantitative biology of the pig and in improving the efficiency of pork production.

14.4 Special considerations in modelling reproduction

Mathematical models have been applied successfully to livestock production in predicting input-output relationships. For example, pig growth models take quantitative information on nutrient input into the pig in the form of feed, and predict the quantitative output in the form of protein and fat accretion in the pig's body. The metabolic model of lactating sows described above takes quantitative information on nutrient input into the sow and predicts the quantitative output in the form of milk protein, fat and lactose.

However, reproduction presents a different set of challenges. First, in a single animal reproduction is not a continuous variable, but a bivariate variable (it must have one of two values). It either occurs or it does not. In the pig there can be variation in litter size, but each ovarian follicle either produces a liveborn piglet at term or it does not. There is a special challenge in converting quantitative data on a continuous scale (e.g. nutrient intake, metabolite concentration) into outcomes on a bivariate scale.

Second, our knowledge of the mechanisms through which nutrient intake impacts reproduction is inadequate. We have made progress in understanding some aspects of this connection qualitatively (Pettigrew and Tokach, 1993; Foxcroft *et al.*, 1995), but a full and quantitative understanding of the mechanisms involved remains beyond our grasp.

It is clear that nutrient intake of the sow during lactation affects her subsequent reproduction, and that this relationship is enormously important in determining the efficiency of pig production. The pig production industry world-wide and the scientists who support it with research need to be able to predict the impacts of nutrient intake during lactation on subsequent reproductive performance by use of a mathematical model. The following discussion outlines some considerations that need to be addressed in order to produce such a model.

14.4.1 A concept of the connection between nutrient intake and reproduction

An outline of my concept of how nutrient intake during lactation affects subsequent reproduction of the sow is shown in Figure 14.3 (Pettigrew and Tokach, 1993). The basis of this concept is that the metabolic state of the animal affects reproductive function.

The metabolic state, as considered in this concept, is a loosely defined set of conditions that includes:

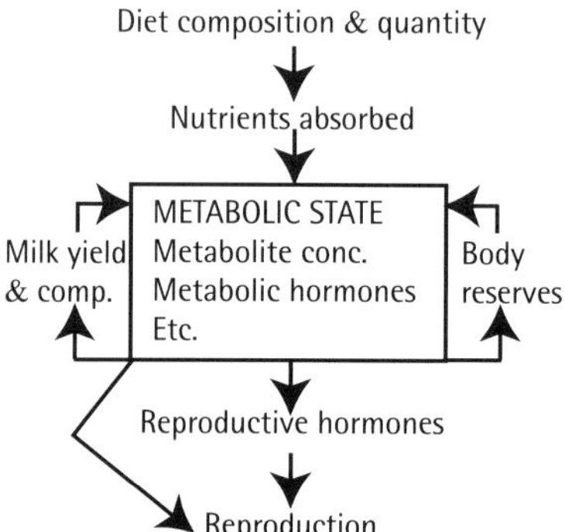

Figure 14.3. Proposed cascade of biological responses connecting nutrition to reproduction in the sow. Reprinted from Pig News & Information.

1. circulating concentrations of metabolites such as glucose, fatty acids, and amino acids;
2. circulating concentrations of metabolic hormones such as insulin, IGF-I, and growth hormone;
3. tissue sensitivity to those metabolic hormones; tissue metabolic capacity and other factors.

This concept holds that the quantity of nutrients absorbed from the intestine largely determines the concentrations of circulating metabolites (nutrients). These metabolite concentrations then affect the release of metabolic hormones. Over time, the metabolic state affects the amount of protein and fat reserves accumulated, and thus the body weight and composition. During lactation, many sows must call upon these reserves of protein and fat to make up for a shortfall in nutrient intake relative to the demands for a high level of milk production. Then the quantities of protein and fat reserves available affect the amounts that can be retrieved, and thus the metabolic state. The metabolic state also influences the quantity and composition of milk produced. Sows that are driven by genetic makeup or large litters to produce a greater amount of milk than others experience a greater nutrient drain, and therefore have a more catabolic metabolic state. The metabolic state of the lactating sow, then, is determined largely by three interacting factors: the quantities of nutrients absorbed, the amounts of body protein and fat reserves, and the amount and composition of milk produced.

The metabolic state is thought to influence the release of reproductive hormones, and also to directly influence the developing ovarian follicle. The mechanisms are not well understood, but are currently under study.

There is a need to identify specific components of the metabolic state that influence reproduction. There is considerable evidence that a high circulating insulin concentration promotes reproductive success (Pettigrew and Tokach, 1993; Foxcroft *et al.*, 1995; Koketsu *et al.*, 1996). Other components, including IGF-I concentrations may also be important.

It appears that good subsequent reproductive performance requires a high level of nutrient intake during every stage of lactation (Koketsu *et al.*, 1996, 1997; Zak *et al.*, 1997). This may be due to effects on the developing ovarian follicles (Foxcroft *et al.*, 1995).

14.4.2 Prospects for development of a model of reproduction

Many aspects of 'normal' reproduction and reproductive endocrinology are well understood. It should be a straightforward matter to develop a mathematical model that would describe these processes. In fact, such a model would not require the quantitative precision of many mathematical models, because most of these processes are described in semi-quantitative terms.

However, development of a mechanistic model that would predict the effects of a change in nutrient intake during lactation on subsequent reproduction would be much more complicated. As described above, our understanding of the connection between the metabolic state and reproduction is far from complete. However, it may be possible to begin the development of such a model. I suggest it be structured as shown in Figure 14.3. Models such as the metabolic model of lactating sows described above cover the upper part of Figure 14.3 (feed intake and composition, nutrients absorbed, body composition, milk production and composition, metabolite concentrations). The model of digestion and absorption described by Bastianelli *et al.* (1996) should be consulted in an effort to strengthen that part of the model.

The main challenge is modelling the connection between the metabolic state and reproduction. I suggest using either insulin concentration or 'anabolic hormone concentration' as the connection. This connection may need to be modelled rather empirically in the first version of the model. Alternatively, a tissue accretion level model could be used as the starting point, and some measure of the rate of tissue loss during lactation could be used as the connection to reproduction.

If such a model were developed, it would highlight areas of inadequate information and clarify the questions that remain to be answered experimentally. I urge the development of such a model.

14.5 Summary

Mathematical simulation models can be powerful tools in managing livestock production systems, because they allow prediction of the effects on production of changes in the diet or other management factors. A model of the metabolism of the lactating sow is described. There is a special need for extending this model or for the development of another model to predict the effects of nutrient intake of the sow during lactation on subsequent reproductive performance. The general structure of such a model is proposed.

14.6 References

Baldwin, R.L., J. France & M. Gill, 1987. Metabolism of the lactating dairy cow. I. Animal elements of a mechanistic model. J. Dairy Res. 54:77.

Bastianelli, D., D. Sauvant & A. Rérat, 1996. Mathematical modeling of digestion and nutrient absorption in pigs. J. Anim. Sci. 74:1873-1887.

Bauman, D.E. & W.B. Currie, 1980. Partitioning of nutrients during pregnancy and lactation: A review of mechanisms involving homeostasis and homeorhesis. J. Dairy Sci. 63:1514.

Black, J.L., R.G. Campbell, I.H. Williams, K.J. James & G.T. Davies, 1986. Simulation of energy and amino acid utilisation in the pig. Res. Dev. Agric. 3:121-145.
Foxcroft, G.R., F.X. Aherne, E.C. Clowes, H. Miller & L. Zak, 1995. Sow fertility: The role of suckling inhibition and metabolic status. In Animal Science Research and Development - Moving Toward a New Century [M. Ivan, editor], pp. 377-393. Ottawa, Ontario, Canada: Centre for Food and Animal Research.
France, J. & J.L. Thornley, 1984. Mathematical Models in Agriculture. Butterworths, London.
Gill, M., J.H.M. Thornley, J.L. Black, J.D. Oldham & D.E. Beever, 1984. Simulation of the metabolism of absorbed energy-yielding nutrients in young sheep. Br. J. Nutr. 52:621.
Koketsu, Y., G.D. Dial, J.E. Pettigrew & V.L. King, 1997. Influence of feed intake during individual weeks of lactation on reproductive performance of sows on commercial farms. Livestock Prod. Sci. 49:217-225.
Koketsu, Y., G.D. Dial, J.E. Pettigrew, W.E. Marsh & V.L. King, 1996. Influence of imposed feed intake patterns during lactation on reproductive performance, circulating levels of glucose, insulin and luteinizing hormone in primiparous sows. J. Anim. Sci. 74:1036-1046.
Mahler, H.R. & E.H. Cordes, 1971. Biological Chemistry (2nd Ed.). Harper and Row, New York.
Moughan, P.J., M.W.A. Verstegen & M.I. Visser-Reyneveld (Editors), 1995. Modelling Growth in the Pig. European Association for Animal Production Publication No. 78. Wageningen Pers, Wageningen. 238 pp.
Neal, H.D.St.C. & J.H.M. Thornley, 1983. The lactation curve in cattle: A mathematical model of the mammary gland. J. Agric. Sci. (Camb.) 101:389.
Pettigrew, J.E., 1981. Supplemental dietary fat for peripartal sows: A review. J. Anim. Sci. 53:107-117.
Pettigrew, J.E., M. Gill, J. France & W.H. Close, 1992a. A mathematical integration of energy and amino acid metabolism of lactating sows. J. Anim. Sci. 70:3742-3761.
Pettigrew, J.E., M. Gill, J. France & W.H. Close, 1992b. Evaluation of a mathematical model of lactating sow metabolism. J. Anim. Sci. 70:3762-3773.
Pettigrew, J.E., J.P. McNamara, M.D. Tokach, R.H. King & B.A. Crooker, 1993. Metabolic connections between nutrient intake and lactational performance in the sow. Lvstk. Prod. Sci. 35:137-152.
Pettigrew, J.E. & M.D. Tokach, 1993. Metabolic influences on sow reproduction. Pig News & Info. 14:69N-72N.
Pomar, C., D.L. Harris & F. Minvielle, 1991. Computer simulation model of swine production systems: II. Modeling body composition and weight of female pigs, fetal development, milk production, and growth of suckling pigs. J. Anim. Sci. 69:1489-1502.
Tokach, M.D., J.E. Pettigrew, B.A. Crooker, G.D. Dial & A.F. Sower, 1992. Quantitative influence of lysine and energy intake on yield of milk components in the primiparous sow. J. Anim. Sci. 70:1864-1872.
Walker, B., 1990. Simulation of Protein and Energy Partitioning in the Reproducing Sow. Ph.D. Dissertation, University of Alberta, Edmonton, Alberta, Canada.
Zak, L.J., J.R. Cosgrove, F..X. Aherne & G.R. Foxcroft, 1997. Pattern of feed intake and associated metabolic and endocrine changes differentially affect postweaning fertility in primiparous lactating sows. J. Anim. Sci. 75:208-216.

15 Thermal requirements of the lactating sow

C.A. Makkink, J.W. Schrama

15.1 Introduction

The thermal environment is an important factor in farm animal husbandry. For growing pigs it is relatively easy to assess and maintain an environmental temperature range in which production (growth, feed conversion) levels are optimal. The situation in the farrowing room is more complicated, since lactating sows and their sucking piglets differ greatly in their temperature requirement.
After a short description of thermoregulation in general, this chapter deals with the climatic requirements of lactating sows and their litters. The effects of ambient temperature as part of the thermal environment on lactating sows and on sucking piglets will be discussed. Practical recommendations are made to deal with the different thermal requirements of the lactating sow and her piglets.

15.2 Theory of thermoregulation.

Pigs are homeothermic animals. Homeothermic animals maintain a constant body temperature under varying environmental conditions by balancing heat loss and heat production (Mount, 1979). The principles of this thermoregulation have been extensively described (e.g. Mount, 1974, 1979; Curtis, 1983). In Figure 1a, the effect of ambient temperature on heat production demonstrates the general concept of thermoregulation. Irrespective of the ambient temperature, animals are able to maintain their body temperature constant within the zone *AC*. Temperatures below temperature *A* and above *C* (Figure 1a) will induce hypothermia and hyperthermia, respectively. The zone *AC* can be divided into two zones, according to the type of body temperature regulation: in zone *BC* by regulation of heat loss; and in zone *AB* by regulation of heat production. In zone *BC*, the thermal neutral zone, heat production is independent of climatic conditions, but is influenced by other factors such as: feeding level, physical activity and physiological status (e.g. lactation). Total heat loss is kept constant by regulation of both sensible heat loss (conduction, convection and radiation) and evaporative heat loss. With increasing temperature in zone *BC*, the sensible heat loss diminishes, because the temperature gradient between the animal and its environment is reduced. Therefore, the animal needs to increase its evaporative heat loss by perspiration and/or panting. In zone *AB*, mechanisms to reduce and control heat loss are depleted. Hence, with decreasing ambient temperature the heat loss increases. To maintain homeothermia, the animal has to increase its heat production.

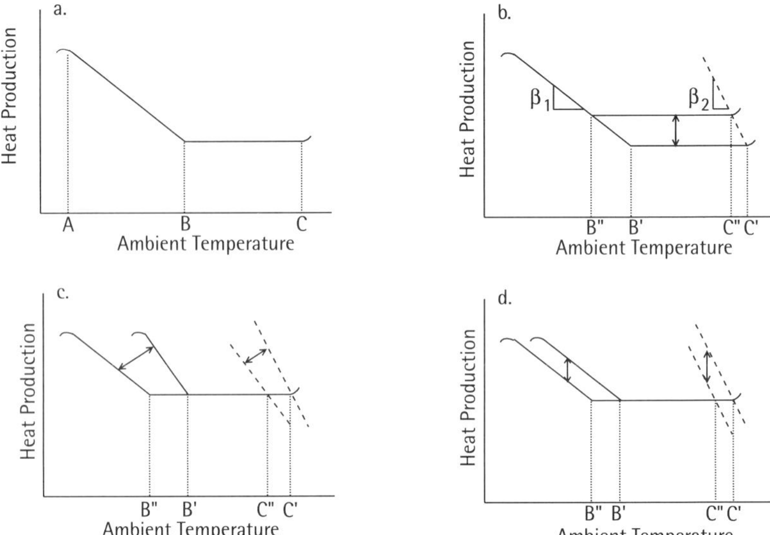

Figure 15.1. The general concept of thermoregulation
a: Relation between ambient temperature and heat production.
b: Consequences of changes in feeding level.
c: Consequences of changes in insulation value.
d: Consequences of changes in evaporative heat loss.

The lower limit of the thermoneutral zone (*B*) is called the lower critical temperature (LCT) and the upper limit (*C*) the upper critical temperature (UCT). The thermoneutral zone (TNZ) can be regarded as a thermal indifferent zone. The climatic conditions in this zone are optimal for the animal. Hence, LCT and UCT are the threshold values (in terms of temperature) regarding cold and heat stress, respectively. It is important to keep animals within their thermoneutral zone, because this will require minimal effort to maintain body temperature. When temperatures are below LCT, animals need to increase their heat production and therefore will need more feed energy for maintenance and less feed energy will be available for production. Above UCT respiration rate and rectal temperature will increase and feed intake will decrease.

LCT and UCT are not fixed values. Both LCT and UCT depend on animal related factors (e.g. age, breed, body condition) and environmental factors (e.g., feeding level, group size, floor type, and climatic factors other than ambient temperature). The effects of these factors are illustrated in Figure 15.1:

Figure 15.1b: The heat production in the TNZ is increased with increasing feeding level. Consequently, LCT and UCT are lower.

Figure 15.1c: The insulation value of the whole animal (slope) is affected by body condition (e.g. backfat thickness). With low insulation, slopes will be steeper and LCT and UCT will be higher.

Figure 15.1d: The evaporative heat loss depends on the body surface area and on wetness of the skin. Wet skin increases evaporative heat loss and therefore LCT and UCT are increased.

15.3 Thermal requirements of sucking piglets and lactating sows

It is generally accepted that the thermal requirements of lactating sows differ from the thermal requirements of sucking piglets. According to Mullan (unpublished, cited by Black *et al.*, 1993) the zone of thermal comfort lies between 12 and 22 °C for the sow and between 30 and 37 °C for the piglets. This discrepancy causes practical problems in housing and climate regulation in the farrowing barn. Usually the environmental temperature is kept at a compromise value which means that the room temperature is too low for the piglets (especially shortly after birth) and too high for the sow. This may cause cold stress and mortality in the piglets and heat stress and depressed feed intake in the sow, leading to reproductive problems.

15.3.1 Sucking piglets

The first week of life seems to be the critical period with regard to thermoregulation. Piglets are born behind the sow, usually on a slatted floor, in a relatively cold environment. Newborn piglets have a liveweight of 0.7 to 1.5 kg and a fat content of only 1 to 1.5 % on a liveweight basis (Mullan *et al.*, 1989). At birth, their skin is wet and the piglets will lose an appreciable amount of evaporative heat (Close, 1989).
Newborn piglets have a LCT of 32-35 °C. At this temperature their heat loss amounts to 5 MJ per m^2 of skin surface per day, while at 20 °C, heat production doubles (Mount, 1979). With increasing age of the piglets the LCT decreases, to 24-27 °C at 4 weeks of age (weaning). According to Rousseau *et al.* (1992), the skin temperature of sucking piglets is 32 to 33 °C, and even at 10 days of age, piglets prefer a floor temperature of 35 °C when no radiant heat (lamps) is provided.

15.3.2 Lactating sows

The animal factors affecting LCT and UCT are difficult to assess in lactating sows. Skin temperature, for example, may vary considerably over the animal's body For lactating sows, the udder is especially important; skin temperature and tissue insulation values differ greatly between udder and, for example, the back of the animal. Udder skin temperature is less susceptible to changes in environmental temperature than back skin temperature in lactating sows (Welch and Baxter, 1986). Udder temperature is 5 to 8 °C higher than back temperature according to Welch and Baxter (1986).

The thermoneutral heat production of lactating sows depends on their feed intake, liveweight and milk production. The desired feed intake depends on the liveweight of the sow (maintenance requirements) and on the milk production (requirements for production). The daily maintenance requirements for a lactating sow amount to 460 kJ per kg $BW^{0.75}$ (see Chapter 6). The energy requirements for milk production (kJ per day) may be estimated by 28.6 x Litter gain (kg/d) - 0.52 x Litter size (see Chapter 6).

Little information on LCT and UCT of lactating sows is available from the literature. It is not possible to make accurate measurements of the heat production of lactating sows in respiration chambers, since their litters must always be present to allow undisturbed milk production.

In Figures 15.2 and 15.3, the effects of milk production and bodyweight on LCT and UCT of lactating sows are illustrated. The LCT of a 140 kg non-lactating sow fed according to maintenance requirements is assumed to be 21 °C (Holmes and Close, 1977). From this starting point we have calculated the decrease in LCT with increasing daily milk production (Figure 15.2a) and the increase in LCT with increasing bodyweight (Figure 15.2b). The changes in UCT with increasing milk production and increasing bodyweight are illustrated in Figures 15.3a and 15.3b, respectively. The starting value for UCT (non-lactating 140 kg sow fed on maintenance) was again derived from Holmes and Close (1977).

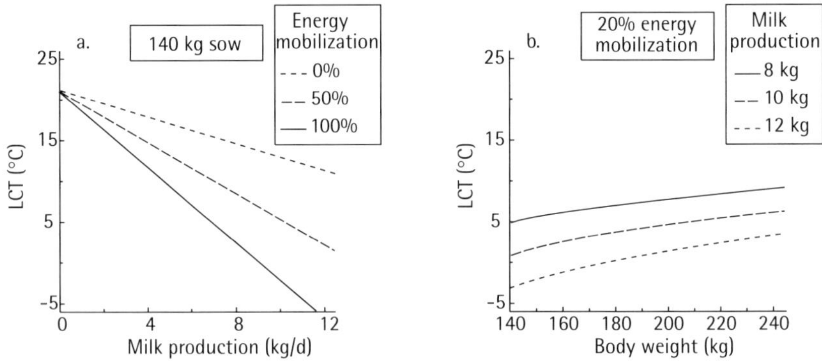

Figure 15.2. Lower critical temperature (LCT) for lactating sows.
a: Effect of milk production on LCT, assuming that milk energy is derived only from feed energy (0% energy mobilisation), or milk energy is derived from feed energy and body energy mobilisation on a fifty-fifty basis (50% energy mobilisation) or milk energy is formed entirely through mobilisation of body energy reserves (100% energy mobilisation).
b: Effect of body weight on LCT at three levels of milk production. It is assumed that 20% of milk energy is derived from body energy mobilisation.

For non-lactating sows, LCT and UCT decrease slightly with increasing bodyweight. This is due to the change in the ratio of surface area to bodyweight. With lactating sows, however, we find an increase in UCT with increasing bodyweight (Figure 15.3b). Figure 15.3a illustrates the options the lactating sow has when the ambient temperature exceeds her UCT; the sow may mobilise more body reserves to maintain milk production at the same level, or she has to lower milk production. In practice, the sow probably has some in-built maximal value for body energy mobilisation. When this value is reached, the sow has no other option than to decrease her milk production and sacrifice litter growth.

With ongoing selection, sows are becoming heavier and producing more milk, which will aggravate the situation when the ambient temperature in the farrowing room is high.

It is clear that the LCT of a lactating sow is much lower than the LCT of sucking piglets. This complicates the situation in the farrowing room; young piglets require much higher temperatures than the lactating sow. The room temperature in a farrowing barn will be too high for the sows and too low for the piglets.

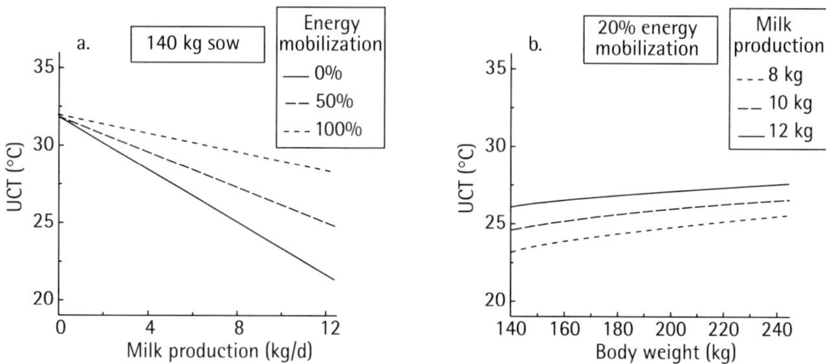

Figure 15.3. Upper critical temperature (UCT) of lactating sows
a: Effect of milk production on UCT, assuming that milk energy is derived only from feed energy (0% energy mobilisation), or milk energy is derived from feed energy and body energy mobilisation on a fifty-fifty basis (50% energy mobilisation) or milk energy is formed entirely through mobilisation of body energy reserves (100% energy mobilisation).
b: Effect of body weight on UCT at three levels of milk production. It is assumed that 20% of milk energy is derived from body energy mobilisation.

15.4 Effects of room temperature on sucking piglets

Figure 15.4 summarizes literature data on the effects of ambient temperature on growth and mortality in sucking piglets.

Low ambient temperatures generally lead to extra thermoregulatory heat produc-

tion (ETH), behavioural adaptation (increased feed intake, huddling, shivering) and increased tidal volume, minute volume and oxygen consumption. This implies that energy requirements for maintenance will be higher and less feed energy will be available for growth. Higher temperatures (within TNZ) are expected to cause higher growth rates. However, Figure 15.4 shows that the growth of sucking piglets decreases with increasing temperature. This indicates that milk intake is probably lower at high temperatures. It seems that milk production by the sow is depressed, which affects the growth rate of her piglets (Barb *et al.*, 1991).
The relationship between ambient temperature and piglet mortality is less clear from the literature (Figure 15.4); some authors report higher mortality with higher temperature (e.g. Lynch, 1977), while others find the opposite (e.g. McGlone *et al.*, 1988b). Most researchers compared only two ambient temperatures. Stansbury *et al.* (1987) compared three ambient temperatures (18, 25 and 30 °C) and they found the lowest mortality at 25 °C, while litter growth was highest at 18 °C. Stansbury *et al.* (1987) explain this by assuming that litters at 18 °C experience higher mortality due to chilling, while at 30 °C milk production by the sow is reduced and therefore reduced energy intake by the piglets is the cause of higher mortality.

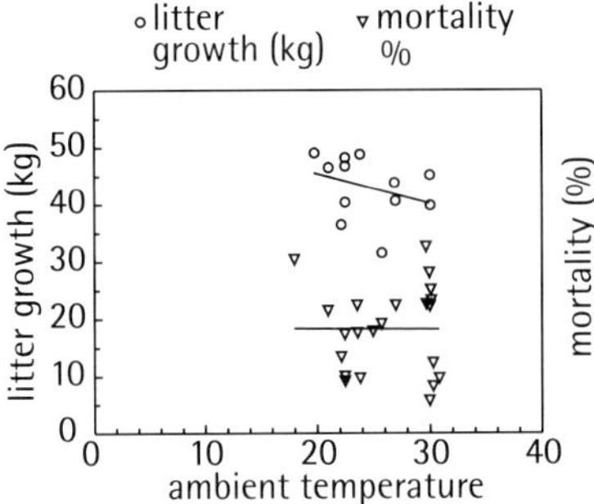

Figure 15.4. Effect of ambient temperature on litter growth and mortality. Literature sources: Lynch, 1977; Stansbury et al., 1987; McGlone et al., 1988a; McGlone et al., 1988b; Murphy et al., 1989; Barb et al., 1991; Johnston et al., 1993; Dove & Haydon, 1994; Prunier et al., 1994; Biensen et al., 1996

15.5 Effects of room temperature on lactating sows

Figure 15.5a summarises the effects of environmental temperature on body temperature and respiration rate in lactating sows. In Figure 15.5b, feed intake and energy intake of lactating sows in relation to room temperature are shown. Figure 15.5c depicts the effects of temperature on the mobilisation of body reserves during lactation.
From Figure 15.5a (body temperature and respiration rate) it is clear that lactating sows are suffering from heat stress when ambient temperatures rise from 20

to 30 °C. The sow will decrease her feed intake and energy intake to reduce her heat production. This is evident from Figure 15.5b. To maintain her milk production, the sow will have to mobilise more body reserves. This strategy leads to higher losses of bodyweight and back fat thickness, as shown in Figure 15.5c.
From the literature data shown in Figure 15.5 it appears that the lactating sow under heat stress is setting a new balance between energy from feed and energy from body reserves. However, it seems that she is not totally succeeding in keeping her milk production at the same level: in the previous section, it was shown that piglet growth is negatively affected at high ambient temperatures. In Chapter 16 (Section 16.5), some recent literature is discussed which indicates that the negative effects of high temperatures on milk production are not solely related to depressed energy intake but also to physiological adaptations to heat stress, such as changes in the direction of blood flow.
The room temperature in the farrowing barn will also influence reproduction. Negative effects of high temperatures on the incidence of anoestrus, oestrus length, conception rate, weaning-conception interval, embryo survival and foetal growth

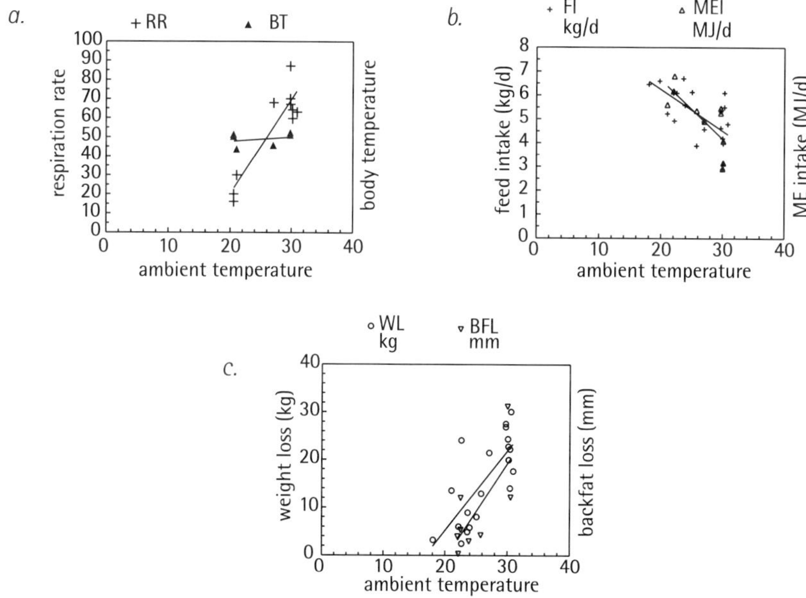

Figure 15.5. Effect of ambient temperature on lactating sows. Literature sources: Lynch, 1977; Kelly & Curtis, 1978; Stansbury et al., 1987; McGlone et al., 1988a; McGlone et al., 1988b; Murphy et al., 1989; Barb et al., 1991; Johnston et al., 1993; Dove & Haydon, 1994; Prunier et al., 1994; Biensen et al., 1996
a: Body temperature and respiration rate.
b: Feed intake and energy intake.
c: Weight loss and backfat loss.

and survival have been reported (Hsia, 1984; Whittemore and Morgan, 1990).
The effects of high environmental temperatures on endocrine changes during lactation were investigated by Barb *et al.* (1991). They found that in sows exposed to 30 °C, LH (luteinizing hormone) pulse frequency was decreased and LH pulse amplitude was increased compared to sows kept at 22 °C. These effects could be mediated by the differences in body reserves mobilisation brought about by the temperature induced differences in energy intake.
Koketsu *et al.* (1996) analyzed feed intake patterns for more than 20,000 sows on 30 commercial farms during lactation and subsequent reproductive performance. They found that low feed intake, either during the entire lactation or during the first week, prolonged the weaning to conception interval and impaired litter weaning weight. The occurrence of a major drop in feed intake (> 1.6 kg decrease for 2 days or more) at any time during lactation also increased the weaning to conception interval and decreased litter weaning weight.

The effects of feed intake patterns during lactation have been studied by Zak *et al.* (1997). They fed primiparous sows either *ad libitum* during the entire four weeks lactation period or restrictedly (50 %) during either the first three weeks or the last week. Observed differences in post-weaning reproduction were due to the extent and timing of catabolic losses during lactation. Feed restriction reduced plasma LH secretion and realimentation for 7 days increased pulsatile LH secretion. These results indicate that targeting some particular feed intake or change in body condition score over the whole of the lactation period may not be very useful for improving reproductive performance if this management leads to increasing catabolism toward the end of lactation.
The effects of high ambient temperatures during lactation on fertility in the sow merit further study. From the literature (e.g. Barb *et al.*, 1991, Zak *et al.*, 1997) it seems that the effects of experimentally imposed energy restriction on endocrine changes are not identical to the effects of depressed energy intake caused by elevated ambient temperatures. Endocrine function is altered in lactating sows exposed to high temperatures and this alteration is at least partly independent of changes in energy intake and/or the mobilisation of body reserves.

15.6 How to solve the dilemma

In practice, the thermal situation in the farrowing barn is a compromise between sow and piglet requirements. This means, that generally the temperature will be too high for the sow and too low for her litter. It is preferred to create two microclimates in a farrowing pen, a warm environment for the piglets and a cool environment for the sow. Local heating devices for the piglets and/or cooling devices for the sow may help to obtain such microclimates.
From literature data it appears that LCT is lower at night than during the day (Verstegen and Schrama, 1992). This implies that nocturnal temperatures may be

kept at a lower level than daytime temperatures in pig housing systems. Optimal diurnal temperature patterns need to be developed and evaluated.
It may be possible in the future to decrease the farrowing barn temperature to comfortable values for the sow (e.g. 15 °C), provided that the piglets are comfortable in their creep area. Near the mammary tissue of the sow, the climate should also be attractive to the piglets, so that they are encouraged to visit the sow regularly for sucking.
Improving the climate control systems in farrowing barns may also substantially reduce the energy costs of heating.

15.6.1 Relief of cold stress for piglets

The room temperature in the farrowing barn is generally too low for the piglets, so provisions have to be made to keep the piglets comfortable and to reduce mortality. Radiating heat lamps create a microclimate for the piglets in a corner of the farrowing pen. Floor heating (electric or hot water) is generally the most energy-efficient means to heat the creep area (Kuhn, 1990). The provision of straw bedding is also helpful to keep sucking piglets warm.
The use of heat lamps may have a general disadvantage, because of the bright light accompanying the heat. Rohde Parfet and Gonyou (1991) determined various sensory preferences in newborn piglets and they found that the animals showed a strong preference for dim or dark areas over bright light.
Floor heating should not be combined with bedding. When no straw or other bedding material is used, hot water floor heating is an economic way of heating creep areas. Covering the creep area is effective in reducing heat losses from the piglets. Improvement of the temperature control units (more refined regulation) will be an important means to save energy in the farrowing house (Geers and Goedseels, 1993).

15.6.2 Relief of heat stress for sows

To enable heat stressed sows to dissipate heat, several methods may be used. Generally, increasing means for evaporative heat loss will be most effective, since at high temperatures, evaporation will account for 44% to 63% of total heat loss (Clark and McQuitty, 1989).
Wetting the animal's skin may help to increase evaporative heat losses and thus alleviate heat stress and improve feed intake, feed conversion and gain (Baccari *et al.*, 1993).
Wallowing in mud is very effective for evaporative thermolysis: it may cause a heat loss of more than 43 MJ per m^2, while sweating (actually passive diffusion through the skin), which is minimal in pigs, releases only 1.7 MJ per m^2 (Curtis, 1983).
Murphy *et al.* (1989) studied drip cooling during the last 19 days of lactation with a room temperature of ± 30 °C. Drip cooling decreased sow respiration rate,

increased litter weaning weight and sow feed intake, and decreased sow lactation weight loss. Using the drip cooling system will decrease ventilation needs and thus save energy.
Stansbury *et al.* (1987) investigated the effect of snout coolers on sow and litter performance at different ambient temperatures. They found that only at the higher temperatures (> 25 °C) did snout coolers increase feed intake for the sow, but there was also an increased piglet mortality, probably due to increased heat loss.
McGlone *et al.* (1988a) compared water drip, snout coolers, floor type (partially slotted concrete vs plastic-coated expanded metal) and an energy-dense diet (14.2 vs 12.8 MJ per kg) to evaluate heat stress relief in lactating sows. They concluded from their results (sow feed intake, weight loss, and respiratory rate) that drip cooling was the most effective way to reduce heat stress. However, wetting the pen floor, causing cold stress to the piglets, must be avoided.
Feeding high energy lactation diets (with higher fat levels and lower fibre and crude protein levels) to sows kept at high environmental temperatures may improve energy intake and reduce the interval from weaning to oestrus (Reese *et al.*, 1982; Cox *et al.*, 1983; Reese *et al.*, 1984; Britt, 1986; Shurson *et al.*, 1986; Schoenherr *et al.*, 1989c). However, extending the possibilities for heat loss generally has a more beneficial effect than reducing the rate of heat production through nutritional measures (Black *et al.*, 1993).
Floor material may affect conductive heat loss, as was shown by Johnston *et al.* (1987), who found higher lactation feed intake and shorter rebreeding interval with sows housed on concrete than with sows housed on plastic-coated expanded metal. Cold floors may, however, predispose the mammary gland to mastitis, as was suggested for cows by Ewbank (1968).
Heat loss also occurs through the heating of ingested feed and water to body temperature. Therefore, it may be useful to provide cold water or liquid feeding to pigs in warm environments (Holmes, 1970). However, during early lactation sows may be lethargic and fail to consume sufficient amounts of feed and water (Fraser and Phillips, 1989).

15.7 Conclusions

It is clear that the climate in the farrowing room is still a point of concern. Until now only compromise solutions have been possible to maintain the room temperature at a desirable level for both sows and piglets.
The effects of low temperatures on piglets (survival rate, growth) are most severe during the first few days after birth, while the negative effects of high temperatures on sow milk production are predominant during mid and late lactation. Therefore, it might be beneficial to adjust the environmental temperature in the farrowing room towards the requirements of the piglets during early lactation and to shift the room temperature to lower levels (sow requirements) towards the end of the lactation period. More knowledge should be obtained concerning the

changes of the thermal requirements of sow and piglets during the lactation period. Optimal patterns of room temperature in farrowing houses may be developed when this knowledge becomes available.
Possibilities for solving the dilemma of contrary requirements for sows and piglets include methods to cool the sow locally and methods to warm the piglets locally. The creation of microclimates in the farrowing room is the only way to keep both the sow and her piglets content and productive.

15.8 References

Baccari, F., A.L.B.A. Gayão & J.R.V. Nunes, 1993. Effect of water cooling on growth rate of Large White-Landrace gilts during thermal stress. In: E. Collins & C. Boon (Editors), Livestock Environment IV. Fourth Intern. Symp., Univ. of Warwick, Coventry, England. 6-9 July 1993. Publ. by ASAE, St Joseph, Michigan, USA. p. 889-894.
Barb, C.R., M.J. Estienne, R.R. Kraeling, D.N. Marple, G.B. Rampacek, C.H. Rahe & J.L. Sartin, 1991. Endocrine changes in sows exposed to elevated ambient temperature during lactation. Dom. Anim. Endocrinol. 8(1):117-127.
Biensen, N.J., E.H. von Borell & S.P. Ford, 1996. Effects of space allocation and temperature on periparturient maternal behaviours, steroid concentrations, and piglet growth rates. J. Anim. Sci. 74:2641-2648.
Black, J.L., B.P. Mullan, M.L. Lorschy & L.R. Giles, 1993. Lactation in the sow during heat stress. Livest. Prod. Sci. 35:153-170.
Britt, J.H., 1986. Improving sow productivity through management during gestation, lactation and after weaning. J. Anim. Sci. 63:1288-1296.
Clark, P.C. & J.B. McQuitty, 1989. Heat and moisture loads in farrowing rooms. Can. Agric. Engineering 31:55-59.
Close, W.H., 1989. The influence of the thermal environment on the voluntary food intake of pigs. In: J.M. Forbes, M.A. Varley & T.L.J. Lawrence (Editors), The Voluntary Food Intake of Pigs. Occasional Publication No 13, British Society of Animal Production 1989. p. 87-96.
Cox, N.M., J.H. Britt, W.D. Armstrong & H.D. Alhusen, 1983. Effect of feeding fat and altering weaning schedule on rebreeding in primiparous sows. J. Anim. Sci. 56:21-29.
Curtis, S.E., 1983. Environmental Management in Animal Agriculture. Part II The Animal and its Thermal Environment. p. 23-133.
Dove, C.R. & K.D. Haydon, 1994. The effect of various diet nutrient densities and electrolyte balances on sow and litter performance during two seasons of the year. J. Anim. Sci. 72:1101-1106.
Ewbank, R., 1968. An experimental demonstration of the effect of surface cooling upon the health of the bovine mammary gland. Vet. Rec. 83:685-686.
Fraser, D. & P.A. Phillips, 1989. Lethargy and low water intake by sows during early lactation: a cause of low piglet weight gain and survival? Appl. Anim. Behav. Sci. 24:13-22.
Geers, R. & V. Goedseels, 1993. An improved system of temperature control in commercial pig houses: some effects on performance. Pig News and Inform. 14(2):73N-75N.
Holmes, C.W., 1970. Some thermal effects on the pig of the ingestion of liquid feed at various temperatures. Anim. Prod. 12:485-492.
Hsia, L.C., 1984. High environmental temperatures and pig production. In: L.C. Hsia (Editor), Environment and Housing for Livestock. Proceedings of the 1st International Conference on Environment and Housing for Livestock. May 22-23, 1984. Pig Research Institute, Taiwan, Republic of China.

Johnston, L.J., L.D. Jacobson & K.A. Janni, 1993. Effect of hovers for baby pigs on energy usage and animal performance during lactation. Minnesota Agric. Exp. Stat. Paper No 20,414 of the scientific journal article series.
Johnston, L.J., D.E. Orr, L.F. Tribble & J.R. Clark, 1987. Effect of body condition and floor material on sow performance. J. Anim. Sci. 64:36-42.
Kelley, K.W. & S.E. Curtis, 1978. Effects of heat stress on rectal temperature, respiratory rate and activity rates in peripartal sows and gilts. J. Anim. Sci. 46:356-361.
Koketsu, Y, G.D. Dial, J.E. Pettigrew & V.L. King, 1996. Feed intake pattern during lactation and subsequent reproductive performance of sows. J. Anim. Sci. 74:2875-2884.
Kuhn, J., 1990. Klimatisierung von Abferkelställen. Deutsche Geflügelwirtschaft und Schweineproduktion 28:830-835.
Lynch, P.B., 1977. Effect of environmental temperature on lactating sows and their litters. Irish J. Agric. Res. 16(2):123-130.
McGlone, J.J., W.F. Stansbury & L.F. Tribble, 1988a. Management of lactating sows during heat-stress: effects of water drip, snout coolers, floor type and a high energy-density diet. J. Anim. Sci. 66:885-891.
McGlone, J.J., W.F. Stansbury, L.F. Tribble & J.L. Morrow, 1988b. Photoperiod and heat stress influence on lactating sow performance and photoperiod effects on nursery pig performance. J. Anim. Sci. 66:1915-1919.
Mount, L.E., 1974. The concept of thermoneutrality. In: J.L. Monteith & L.E. Mount (Editors), Heat Loss from Animals and Man. Butterworths, London, UK. pp 425-439.
Mount, L.E., 1979. Adaptation to Thermal Environment. Man and his productive animals. Edward Arnold (Publishers) Ltd., London, UK. 333 pp.
Mullan, B.P., W.H. Close & D.J.A. Cole, 1989. Predicting nutrient responses of the lactating sow. In: W. Haresign & D.J.A. Cole (Editors), Recent Advances in Animal Nutrition 1989. Butterworths, Londen, UK. pp 229-243.
Murphy, J.P., D.A. Nichols & F.V. Robbins, 1989. Drip cooling of lactating sows. Pigs (May/June 1989) 5(3):8-9.
Prunier, A., J.Y. Dourmad & M. Etienne, 1994. Effect of light regimen under various ambient temperatures on sow and litter performance. J. Anim. Sci. 72:1461-1466.
Reese, D.E., B.D. Moser, E.R. Peo, A.J. Lewis, D.R. Zimmerman, J.E. Kinder & W.W. Stroup, 1982. Influence of energy intake during lactation on the interval from weaning to first estrus in sows. J. Anim. Sci. 55:590-598.
Reese, D.E., E.R. Peo & A.J. Lewis, 1984. Relationship of lactation energy intake and occurrence of postweaning estrus to body and backfat composition in sows. J. Anim. Sci. 58:1236-1244.
Rohde Parfet, K.A. & H.W. Gonyou, 1991. Attraction of newborn piglets to auditory, visual, olfactory and tactile stimuli. J. Anim. Sci. 69:125-133.
Rousseau, P., I. Hamon & J. Le Dividich, 1992. Des dalles chauffantes pour les porcelets: Mesures des températures superficielles et du gradient thermique sans animaux. Comportement du porcelet sur deux dalles soumises à des températures différentes. Journ. Rech. Porc. en France 24:287-294.
Schoenherr, W.O., T.S. Stahly & G.L. Cromwell, 1989. Influence of dietary fiber and fat additions on the lactation performance of sows housed in a warm or hot environment. Swine Res. Rep., Univ. of Kentucky, Agric. Exp. Stat., Lexington, USA, 1989. p. 46-51.
Shurson, G.C., M.G. Hogberg, N. DeFever, S.V. Radecki & E.R. Miller, 1986. Effects of adding fat to the sow lactation diet on lactation and rebreeding performance. J. Anim. Sci. 62:672-680.
Stansbury, W.F., J.J. McGlone & L.F. Tribble, 1987. Effects of season, floor type, air temperature and snout coolers on sow and litter performance. J. Anim. Sci. 65:1507-1513.
Verstegen, M.W.A. & J.W. Schrama, 1992. Climatic conditions, metabolic rate and health. Proc. 8th Internat. Conf. on Production Diseases in Farm Animals. 24-27 August 1992. Bern, Switzerland.

Welch, A.R. & M.R. Baxter, 1986. Responses of newborn piglets to thermal and tactile properties of their environment. Appl. Anim. Behav. Sci. 15:203-215.
Whittemore, C.T. & C.A. Morgan, 1990. Model components for the determination of energy and protein requirements for breeding sows: a review. Livest. Prod. Sci. 26:1-37.
Young, B.A., B. Walker, A.E. Dixon & V.A. Walker, 1989. Physiological adaptation to the environment. J. Anim. Sci. 67: 2426-2432.
Zak, L.J., J.R. Cosgrove, F.X. Aherne & G.R. Foxcroft, 1997. Pattern of feed intake and associated metabolic and endocrine changes differentially affect postweaning fertility in primiparous lactating sows. J. Anim. Sci. 75:208-216.

16 The influence of some sow and piglet characteristics and of environmental conditions on milk production

M. Etienne, J.-Y Dourmad, J. Noblet

Age at weaning of piglets has considerably decreased during the last 30 years. In order to improve sow productivity through a reduction of the interval between farrowings, duration of lactation has been shortened from 2 months to 3-4 weeks in practical conditions, and weaning at 10 days has even been considered. The duration of lactation is now stabilised at about 4 weeks (26.9 days as a mean in France in 1996, according to the Technical sow herd management). Milk production has retained all its importance since piglets ingest only very small amounts of dry food until weaning. Survival and growth depend almost completely on colostrum and milk intake. Quantity and quality of milk produced are thus determining criteria of the maternal qualities of sows. The genetic and nutritional influences on milk production and composition are discussed in previous chapters. The present chapter deals with the effects of certain characteristics of sows and piglets and of environmental conditions on milk production.

16.1 Determination of milk production

Direct determination of milk production is not possible in the sow since oxytocin release, in response to stimulation of the teats by the nuzzling and sucking of piglets, is necessary for milk ejection. Many indirect methods have been proposed. The milking of sows by machine after an oxytocin injection was proposed by Hartman and Pond (1960) and Hartman *et al.* (1962). This procedure, however, requires docile sows or the use of a tranquillizer, and massage of the glands increases the amount of milk obtained by about 10%. Moreover, the results of Hartman *et al.* (1962) after single measurements showed low correlations between the amounts of milk obtained by machine and the weight of the pigs during the three first weeks of lactation. This method therefore seems more appropriate for determining milk composition than milk production. Estimation of milk production by determining sow weight loss during sucklings was used by Clausen (1952, cited by Salmon-Legagneur, 1956). But the small weight variation (200-600 g) compared to the sow's weight limits the precision of this method, especially if the sow is not completely still.

16.1.1 The weigh-suckle-weigh method

The weigh-suckle-weigh technique is the most commonly used method for estimating milk intake by piglets. Piglets are separated from the sow on the days of measurement and are allowed to suckle at regular intervals. Litter weight is determined before and after each suckling, the difference between the two weights corresponding to the milk produced during that suckling. This procedure is repeated many times on the day of measurement, and the total quantity of milk produced during the period of measurement is extrapolated to a 24-h duration. Many factors can affect the precision of this technique. The intervals between sucklings and the number of determinations on the same day are of importance. In the first experiments involving this technique, variable intervals of 2 to 5 hours between sucklings were used. But these intervals affect milk production over the whole day, and a frequency of sucklings close to the natural one (1/60 to 75 min: Salmon-Legagneur, 1956) is recommended. Variable numbers of measurements per day are performed. Speer and Cox (1984) showed that the yields in the first and probably the second hour underestimate yields obtained in subsequent hours. Mahan *et al.* (1971) concluded that an 8-hour estimate would provide an adequate measure of milk production, although a 10% gain in precision may be obtained by going to a 12-hour or longer period. Hourly determinations for 6 to 10 hours/day are more often used.
Other difficulties are linked to the piglets. The scales must be accurate to allow the measurement of a small weight variation of a litter weighing between 10 and 100 kg. Moreover, piglets are often active during weighing. This can be solved now by using electronic weighing machines equipped with an integration device. All the piglets' weight variations which are not due to milk intake must also be evaluated. Piglet weight losses due to metabolism, evaporation, activity and salivation during suckling must be taken into consideration. Estimations of these losses based on the age of the piglets were obtained by Klaver *et al.* (1981) and Noblet et Etienne (1986). Moreover, weight losses due to urination and defecation of the piglets between the weighings preceding and following sucklings must be accounted for. Corrections based on piglet weight were also proposed by Klaver *et al.* (1981). But Etienne and Noblet (unpublished data) found important variations within and between piglets in the quantity of urine voided. This shows that it is important to evaluate the true weight of excreta. The weigh-suckle-weigh technique is time consuming and requires a lot of care to be reliable. Even when used cautiously, it usually leads to an underestimation of milk production in comparison with other methods (Pettigrew *et al.*, 1985; Noblet and Etienne, 1989).

16.1.2 The isotope dilution method

A more recent method based on the dilution of an isotope in body water has been developed in pigs (tritium-labelled water: Yang *et al.*, 1980; deuterium oxide: Rudolph, 1984, cited by Schoenherr *et al.*, 1989; Pettigrew *et al.*, 1985, 1987;

Prawirodigdo *et al.*, 1987). Labelled water is injected i.v., i.m. or intraperitoneally into the piglets. After a 2-h rest period for equilibration with body water, a first blood sample is taken to measure the initial isotope concentration in the water component of the blood. Piglets are then returned to the sow. Assuming that milk water is the only water consumed by the young, water intake from the milk can be estimated through the decrease of isotope concentration in blood water. A correction must be made for water derived from metabolism of milk solids. Milk intake is then estimated through the measurement of milk composition. The quantity of labelled water injected needs to be determined with precision, generally by weighing the syringe and needle before and after injection. The injection must be done carefully: Pettigrew *et al.* (1987) obtained only 45 usable observations out of 71 measurements attempted, mainly because of D_2O loss from the injection site. Alternatively, a venous catheter may be used. This technique has been validated with piglets trained to drink an artificial milk replacer. A good level of accuracy was found over measurement periods of 1 to 7 days by Pettigrew *et al.* (1987) and Prawidodigdo *et al.* (1987). The longer measurement periods, however, gave slightly less precise values and required corrections for changes in water pool size. According to Pettigrew *et al.* (1985), the isotope dilution technique and the weigh-suckle-weigh method give similar results when used simultaneously. The latter technique, however, decreases the milk consumption of the piglets, due to the disruption of piglets and sows and suppression of udder massage by the piglets after suckling (Algers and Jensen, 1991). More recently, it has been shown that the determination of D_2O directly in pig serum instead of blood water obtained after vacuum sublimation gives sufficiently precise values (Pluske *et al.*, 1997).

16.1.3 Estimation through piglet growth rate

Since piglets do not ingest significative amounts of dry food before three weeks of age, their growth during that period originates almost solely from sucked milk. Many attempts have been made to estimate milk ingestion through litter growth rate during a 3-week lactation period. However, most of the relationships provided a limited estimate of sow milk production, and the part in the variance of milk output explained by piglet weight gain differs greatly between the published estimations: 54% (Salmon-Legagneur, 1958), 34% (Allen and Lasley, 1960), 76% (Salmon-Legagneur and Aumaître, 1962), 18% (Hemsworth *et al.*, 1976), 34% (Lewis *et al.*, 1978) ; 68% (King *et al.*, 1989). Milk composition, and especially lipid and energy content, varies between sows and between diets. More accurate figures are obtained when milk nutrient output is estimated instead of milk production (Beyer, 1985; Noblet and Etienne, 1989). Noblet and Etienne (1989) estimated dry matter, energy and protein output in milk using the weigh-suckle-weigh technique, but the values obtained were corrected by coupling gas exchange measurement between sucklings to the determination of body composition of piglets at weaning. In these conditions, Noblet and Etienne (1989) obtained determination coefficients of 96%, 97% and 93% for the regressions between piglet growth rate (ADG) combined to their gain composition and dry matter (DM), energy (E) and nitrogen (N) output in milk during a 20 to 25 day lactation, respectively:

$DM = 0.60 \times ADG + 31.7\ E_G - 62$

$E = 4.09 \times ADG + 230\ E_G - 485$

$N = 0.0270 \times ADG + 1.12\ N_G - 2.59$

where DM and N are in $g.piglet^{-1}.d^{-1}$, E in $kcal.piglet^{-1}.d^{-1}$, ADG in $g.piglet^{-1}$, E_G is energy in piglet weight gain in $kcal.g^{-1}$ and N_G is nitrogen in piglet weight gain in %.

From a practical point of view, determination of milk production based on litter growth rate is sufficiently accurate to be used for estimating nutrient requirements of lactating sows in pig herds.

16.2 Influence of sow characteristics on milk yield

16.2.1 Effect of litter size

According to most studies, litter size is the major factor influencing milk production. In a review of literature, Elsley (1971) reported that milk yield of sows increases by more than 100% if litter size increases from four up to twelve pigs. This is mainly due to the greater number of functional mammary glands.

More recently, linear relationships between litter size and daily milk production were also found by King *et al.* (1989) and Auldist *et al.* (1994). All of these data are presented in Figure 16.1. They show that the slope of the relationship is quite similar in the different publications, but for a given litter size, milk production is higher by about 2 kg/day in the more recent than in the older estimations. Differences in lactation duration and differences in the methods of estimation used may explain part of this difference. However, a real increase in milk output over the last two decades has surely resulted from genetic improvement through selection for growth rate and for weaning weight of the piglet. Better energy and amino acid feeding of sows during the reproductive cycle is certainly also involved. Consequently, the sows from the hyperprolific lines which are now present in herds produce more than 10-12 kg milk daily, which is almost twice the amount sows yielded thirty years ago. This figure corresponds to the milk production peak of the sow with the greater milk yield measured by Salmon-Legagneur (1958). This emphasises the importance of nutrition during lactation and of body reserves for modern day sows.

Milk production, however, does not increase proportionally to litter size (Salmon-Legagneur, 1965). As a consequence, milk intake per piglet nursed decreases in a linear manner when litter size increases. Milk intake/piglet for example decreased from 1.0 to 0.7 kg/day when litter size increased from 4 to 12 according to Elsley (1971), or from 1.3 to 0.9 kg/day between 6 and 14 piglets/litter according to Auldist *et al.* (1994). This effect may be explained through many factors: an increased solicitation of the glands in the case of small litters due to greater piglet vigour, less fighting between litter mates and fewer unsuccessful nursings (Fraser and Thompson, 1986), the opportunity for piglets to suckle more than one gland and, finally, the only small increase in sow voluntary feed intake when litter size increases (see Chapter 6).

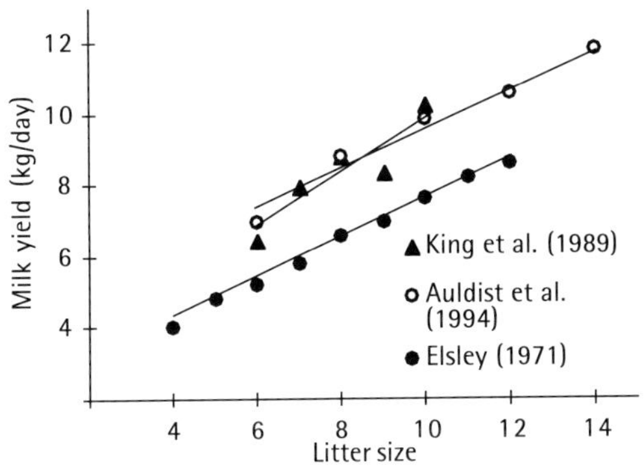

Figure 16.1. Effect of litter size on milk yield in sows (Auldist and King, 1995)

16.2.2 Effect of parity

Differences in milk yield have been found between parities in sows. However, experiments in which valid conclusions are found are scarce, since estimates must be made during successive cycles. Salmon-Legagneur (1958) found that milk production was significantly lower during the first lactation, remained constant from the second to the fourth lactation, and decreased thereafter. According to Vanschoubroek and Van Spaendonck (1966), milk production amounted to 85% of the mean in the first and sixth lactation, 115% in the second and third lactation, compared to 100% in the fourth and fifth lactation.

Walkiewicz (1978) and Ferreira *et al.* (1988) found also that primiparous sows produced less milk than multiparous sows, whereas Lima *et al.* (1988) did not find any significant effect of lactation number during the first three parities. No significant correlation was found by Salmon-Legagneur between the weight of sows at mating or at farrowing and their milk production. The evolution of milk yield with parity number which is generally found is partly explained by the variation of litter size over the successive reproductive cycles (Table 16.1).

Table16.1. Influence of parity on milk yield during an 8-week lactation (Salmon-Legagneur, 1958)

Lactation number	1	2	3	4	5	6
Total milk production (kg)	264	337	316	309	251	176
Litter size at weaning	7.8	9.1	8.1	8.0	8.1	7.7

16.2.3 Effect of lactation stage

As in other animal species, milk yield varies with the stage of lactation. Most of the results show that milk production is lowest during the first week, increases until the third week, remains fairly constant up to the sixth week, and decreases thereafter (Salmon-Legagneur, 1958; Allen and Lasley, 1960; Vanschoubroek and Van Spaendonck, 1966; Elsley, 1971). However, important variations occur between sows (Smith, 1959; Allen and Lasley, 1960). Salmon-Legagneur (1958) described different lactation curves depending on the period when the maximum yield is achieved. Such differences were also recorded between sows of different breeds (Allan and Lasley, 1960). More recent results on shorter lactations confirm that maximal milk production mostly occurs during the third week (Klaver *et al.*, 1981; Noblet and Etienne, 1986). This means that under current conditions, weaning occurs when milk production is at its maximum.

Milk production is the main factor contributing to nutrient requirements during lactation (see Chapters 6 and 11). Since milk production increases by about 100% between small and large litters, litter size is the most important source of variation of the nutrient balance in lactating sows.

16.3 Influence of piglets weight on milk yield

An influence of piglet weight at birth on growth rate during lactation has been found in many studies (Winters and Cummings, 1947; Lodge and McDonald, 1959; Fraser and Jones, 1975). Moreover, Hartman *et al.* (1962), Hemsworth *et al.* (1976) and Campbell and Dunkin (1982b) reported that heavier piglets at birth ingested more milk than their lighter litter mates. Conversely, Lodge and Elliot (1979) showed that a lower birth weight inhibited growth in hysterectomy-derived piglets which were artificially reared to a lesser extent than piglets kept sucking the sow. Campbell and Dunkin (1982a) also concluded that in piglets weaned from the sow at 24h of age, subsequent growth and body composition were not affected by birth weight. All these data agree with Hemsworth *et al.* (1976) who concluded that heavier piglets may be more efficient at draining the teats than lighter piglets and, therefore, may stimulate a greater subsequent milk flow or, alternatively, that this may be due to the influence of birth weight on the ability of the piglet to keep a high-yielding teat.

In a more recent experiment, van der Steen and de Groot (1992) evaluated pre-natal and post-natal effects on milk intake and growth of piglets. They formed cross fostering pairs composed of Meishan and Dutch sows, and at 12-24 h of life exchanged half of each litter between the sows within each pair. At an average birth weight (1.38 and 0.89 kg at birth for the Dutch and Meishan pigs, respectively), growth rate to weaning at 35 days was 27% higher and milk intake 37% higher in the Dutch than in the Meishan piglets, whereas differences between the sows of the two genotypes were small (Table 16.2). Heavy Meishan which had the same birth weight than light Dutch newborn piglets had also the same growth rate. The lower growth rate of Meishan piglets is not caused then by the competition with the heavier Dutch piglets but is related to birth weight itself. King *et al.* (1997) compared piglets fostered at different ages to sows at different lactation stages. Sows which received after farrowing piglets between 17 and 29 days of age produced 26% more milk between 4 and 8 days of lactation than control sows which received newborn piglets. But there was no more difference thereafter. Conversely, sows which received newborn piglets at 17 days of lactation produced 22% less milk than the control sows between 18 and 22 days of lactation, but again there was no more difference thereafter. In agreement with earlier results, this experiment confirms that, together with litter size, piglet's milk intake is affected by their body weight and, therefore, is an important factor contributing to milk production of sows.

Differences in milk production according to teat position have been proposed as an explanation. In fact, some studies on a low number of sows where milk production was determined for each teat concluded that the anterior teats yield more milk than the posterior ones (Donald, 1937 ; Barber *et al.*, 1955). Based on 63 pairs

Table 16.2. Effect of piglet's birth weight on growth rate and milk intake (adapted from van der Steen and de Groot, 1992)

Breed of the nursing sow	Dutch		Meishan	
Breed of the nursed piglet	Dutch	Meishan	Dutch	Meishan
Piglets birth weight, kg	1.38	0.89	1.38	0.89
Piglets ADG, 0 to 35 days (g/day)	221	164	208	173
Milk intake at day 13 (g.hour^{-1}.piglet^{-1})	36	23	36	29
Milk intake at day 30 (g.hour^{-1}.piglet^{-1})	41	28	35	28

of measurements, Salmon-Legagneur (1958) found that after an oxytocin injection, the two anterior pairs of teats produced 34.2 g milk instead of 19.0 g for the three posterior pairs. It is usually considered that the piglets compete for anterior teats at birth, and these teats are generally suckled by heavier piglets which then have a greater growth rate. Most of these assumptions are based on correlations between birth weight and teat number. However, these correlations are very low, -.09 to -.24 (Fraser, 1983). According to the same author, piglets clearly prefer the anterior teats, but there is only a slight tendency for heavier pigs to obtain them. The reasons are unclear: sow's grunts are more audible from the anterior teat position, or these teats have a better milk flow during the first hours of lactation, or the piglets avoid smaller teats which are common at the posterior end. Another possible explanation for the higher milk intake in heavy pigs was given by Algers and Jensen (1991) who showed that at least during the first two days of lactation, the duration of the teat massage performed by the piglets after letdown influenced the amount of milk produced by the teat. They suggested that the heavier piglets will stimulate their teat more vigorously resulting in a higher milk production rate. The final massage could modulate the blood flow through the particular teat, and consequently the subsequent milk production (Algers and Jensen, 1985). Whatever the reason, the heavy piglets seem to be more efficient for obtaining milk during suckling than their lighter litter mates, which contributes to maintenance of or even an increase in intra-litter variation of weight.

16.4 Influence of suckling interval on milk yield

The influence of suckling interval on milk yield was investigated by Auldist *et al.* (1995). First-litter sows nursing litters of 6 or 12 piglets and a crossed-suckle treatment involving two litters of 6 piglets for each sow were compared. Teats in excess were taped to ensure that piglets did not suck more than one teat. The two litters of 6 were alternated every 30 min to be with the sow from day 6 to 27 of lactation. The six functional glands of the cross-suckled sows allowed almost similar piglet growth as the 12 glands of the sows with litters of 12, whereas litter growth rate was lower in the sows with litters of 6 (Table 16.3). Milk production

Table 16.3. Effect of increased suckling frequency on milk yield of sows (Auldist et al., 1995)

Litter treatment	6	12	6+6
Litter growth rate (g/day)	1762	2571	2195
Mean gland weight (g DM)	110.5	64.9	124.0
Suckling interval (min)	46.3	47.4	38.6

per functional gland was about two times greater, which suggests a greater rate of milk synthesis when the suckling interval was reduced.

Spinka *et al.* (1997) obtained similar conclusions in an experiment in which sows were forced to nurse every 35 or every 70 min during 24 hours at 7 to 8 days postpartum. The piglets suckling every 35 min, despite missing more sucklings and receiving 23% less milk per nursing than the other group, consumed 27% more milk and gained 44% more weight during the experimental day. As in the preceding work, this demonstrates that changing nursing frequency strongly affects milk output. According to Spinka *et al.* (1997), the sow can adjust the demand for milk by changing intervals between nursings, and the pigs can try to get more milk by initiating nursings sooner after the previous one. In another experiment, Spinka *et al.* (1997) showed that when nursing intervals were enforced every 35, 70 or 100 min at 8-12 days postpartum, milk output per nursing did not differ from that performed at 50 min intervals (Figure 16.2). This indicates that there is an almost full ration of milk ready in the glands by 35 min after the last milk release. Piglets suckling more frequently will receive this dose more frequently, and hence have a higher total milk intake and induce a higher milk yield. Thus, any condition which affects suckling interval would consequently change milk yield.

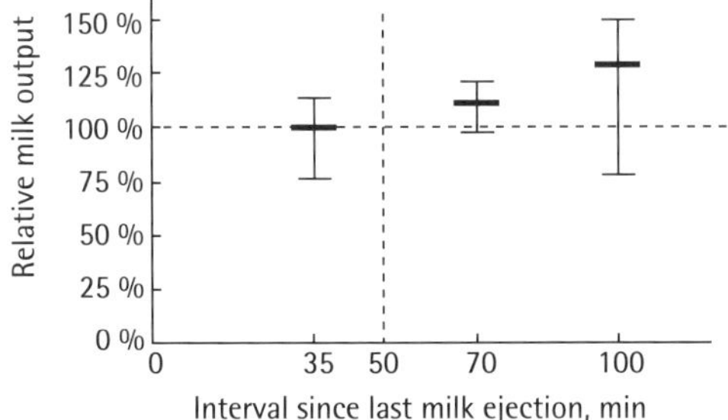

Figure 16.2. Influence of interval between nursings on milk output (Spinka et al., 1997) (milk outputs are expressed in percent of the output after 50 min ; median and lower and upper quartiles are depicted)

16.5 Influence of environmental conditions on milk yield

An increased milk production was reported by Mabry *et al.* (1982) when sows were submitted to a 16-hour light/day instead of 8 hours from 103 days of pregnancy to weaning at 21 days (7.17 vs. 5.76 kg at day 15 of lactation, respectively). Litter weight and individual piglet weight at weaning were increased, and piglet survival was improved. Under the same photoperiod conditions, Mabry *et al.* (1983)

observed that sows exposed to 16 hour light/day suckled significantly more often than those exposed to only 8 hour light/day (Figure 16.3). They concluded that this pattern of more frequent suckling could be a possible explanation for the increased milk yield, survival rate and weaning weight reported previously.

Stone *et al.* (1974) found that auditory stimuli such as the cyclic playback of recorded feeding sounds can shorten the interval between nursings and increase milk production. Conversely, when sows with litters were exposed to high levels of continuous noise such as that of a 85 dB(A) fan, normal nursing-suckling pattern was disrupted and fighting frequency amongst piglets increased (Algers and Jensen, 1985). The piglets exposed to noise massaged the teats for shorter periods, and mean consumption of milk at each suckling together with overall milk intake measured on days 1 and 2 of lactation were lower than in the controls exposed to noise below 45 dB(A) (Algers and Jensen, 1991). Algers and Jensen (1985) suggested that noise would make the piglets unable to perceive the grunt pattern during lactation and, therefore, affect the suckling behaviour of the litter.

Ambient temperature also affects milk production. Smith (1959) reported that in New Zealand, the cool environment in spring was more favourable for milk production than the hotter conditions of summer. Lynch (1977) showed that when sows were maintained at 27 vs. 21°C from 110 days of gestation until weaning, mean piglet weight at 4 weeks and at weaning was lower. Stansbury *et al.* (1987) found that litters were lighter at weaning when sows were kept at 30°C instead of 18 or 25°C, and that individual pig weaning weight was higher in the 18°C environment. These data suggest that piglet milk intake is lower in hot condi-

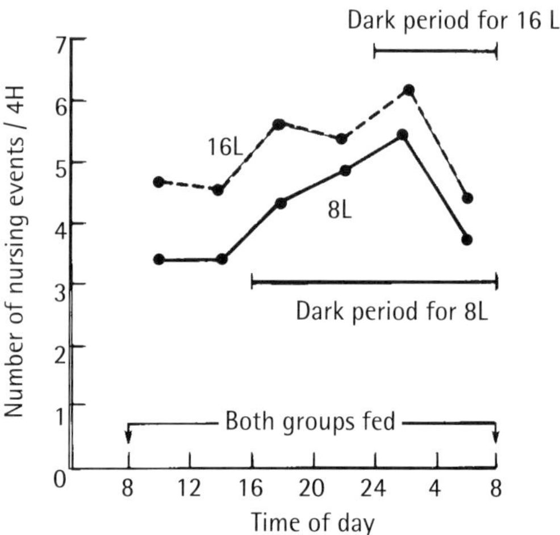

Figure 16.3. Influence of photoperiod conditions on suckling frequency (Mabry et al., 1983). 16L group: 16 h light/24 h; 8L group: 8 h light/24 h

tions. Indeed, a decreased milk production was found by Stansbury *et al.* (1987) in sows maintained at a high temperature during lactation (30 vs. 22°C), and by Vidal *et al.* (1991) at 30 vs. 20°C. Schoenherr *et al.* (1989) reported that heat exposure (32°C vs. 20°C) decreased milk energy yield, whereas effects on milk yield were less clear. In these experiments, hot conditions also depressed voluntary feed intake and increased weight loss of the sows.

In a recent experiment, Messias de Bragança *et al.* (1997) compared lactating sows fed *ad libitum* and maintained at 20 or 30°C and sows at 20°C pair fed with the sows at 30°C. Piglet growth rate was depressed by 20% at 30°C, but not in the restricted sows maintained at 20°C (Table 16.4). The liveweight and backfat losses were highest in the restricted sows at 20°C and lowest in those fed *ad libitum* and kept at 20°C. The decreased milk yield in sows maintained in hot conditions seems to be not only related to their lower feed intake. Deep body temperature of sows submitted to high environmental temperatures is increased (Lynch, 1977; Messias de Bragança *et al.*,1997). Black *et al.* (1993) suggested that blood flow is redirected to the skin to increase heat losses, at the expense of blood flow to the mammary gland and other organs. Nutrients would then be diverted from the mammary gland, resulting in a decreased milk synthesis. Lower levels of T3, T4 and cortisol were found by Messias de Bragança *et al.* (1997) in plasma of sows in hot conditions. These physiological adaptations would allow a reduction in heat production, but are also unfavourable to milk production. Altered endocrine function at 30°C (decreased frequency of LH pulses, modification of the response of prolactin, growth hormone and T4 after TRH injection, suppression of cortisol concentration) was found by Barb *et al.* (1991) who suggested that the responsiveness of the hypothalamic-pituitary-adrenal axis is suppressed by chronic exposure to elevated ambient temperature. The decreased milk yield due to heat stress appears to be due not to an alteration of piglet behaviour, but to deep physiological and metabolic changes in the sows.

Table 16.4. Effects of temperature and feeding level on lactation performance of sows (adapted from Messias de Bragança et al., 1997)

Temperature °C	20	20	30
Feeding level	*Ad libitum*	Restricted	*Ad libitum*
Mean food intake (kg/day)	4.9	3.1	2.8
Sow body weight loss (kg)	8.3	31.5	21.7
Backfat depth loss (mm)	0.9	3.5	2.8
Litter size at weaning	8.5	8.3	8.2
Piglet mean weight at weaning (kg)	6.44	6.29	5.80
Litter growth rate (kg/day)	2.05	1.97	1.62

These results clearly show that milk production in sows can be affected by environmental conditions. A shorter light duration or noise decrease milk output. A high ambient temperature, as usually found in some countries or during summer in more temperate regions, also reduces milk output.

16.6 Conclusion

Milk yield of sows appears to be highly variable and to depend on many factors. The most important is litter size: milk production of a given sow can double only because of differences in the number of piglets nursed. Differences in litter size between parities also explain the lower milk yield in first-litter sows and the decrease in milk yield after the fourth lactation. As well as litter size, the duration of the interval between sucklings can greatly affect milk production. It seems that the milk suckled during a nursing needs a limited period, about half an hour, to be replaced. If the piglets suckle more frequently, they will obtain more milk, and milk production will increase. However, the question remains as to what extent the piglets are able to change their suckling behaviour and adapt their milk intake to their requirements. Piglet weight at birth also affects milk production. The heavier piglets stimulate teats to a greater extent than the lighter ones, maybe because of a more efficient massaging, and thus obtain higher amounts of milk at each suckling. Milk production can also be affected by environmental conditions. It is depressed in hot and noisy conditions and under short day lengths. The mechanisms have still not been studied, but the interval between nursings seems to be involved in the effects of photoperiod and noise, whereas physiological disturbances are more likely responsible for the decreased milk yield of sows kept under high temperatures. Finally, it is important to stress the considerable increase of milk yield in sows during the last decades, mainly due to selection for greater litter sizes and higher weaning weights of the piglets. Added to the fact that sows are now weaned when their milk yield is maximal, this may contribute to the increased frequency of reproductive problems after weaning. Contrary to what was thought thirty years ago, milk production remains a major component, possibly the most important one, to take into account in the management of sows.

16.7 References

Algers, B. & P. Jensen, 1985. Communication during suckling in the domestic pig. Effects of continuous noise. Appl. Anim. Behav. Sci., 14, 49-61.
Algers, B. & P. Jensen, 1991. Teat stimulation and milk production during early lactation in sows: effects of continuous noise. Can. J. Anim. Sci., 71, 51-60.
Allen, A.D. & J.F. Lasley, 1960. Milk production of sows. J. Anim. Sci., 19, 150-155.

Auldist, D.E., L. Morrish, C. Wakeford & R.H. King, 1995. Effect of increased suckling frequency on mammary development and milk yield of sows. In Hennessy D.P. & P.D. Cranwell Ed., Manipulating Pig Production V, 137. Australasian Pig Science Association, Werribee, Australia.
Auldist, D.E. & R.H. King, 1995. Piglet's role in determining milk production in the sow. In 'Hennessy D.P. & P.D. Cranwell Ed., Manipulating Pig Production V', 114-118. Australasian Pig Science Association, Werribee, Australia.
Auldist, D.E., L. Morrish, M. Thompson & R.H. King, 1994. Response of sows to varying litter size. Proc. Nutr. Soc. Aust., 18, 175.
Barb, C.R., M.J. Estienne, R.R. Kraeling, D.N. Marple, G.B. Rampacek, C.H. Rahe & J.L. Sartin, 1991. Endocrine changes in sows exposed to elevated ambient temperature during lactation. Domest. Anim. Endocrinol., 8, 117-127.
Barber, R.S, R. Braude and K.G. Mitchell, 1955. Studies on milk production of Large White sows. J. Agric. Sci., Cambridge, 46, 97-118.
Beyer, M., 1986. Untersuchungen zum Energie- und Stoffumsatz von gravieden und laktierenden Sauen sowie Saugferkeln - Ein Beitrag zur Präzisierung des Energie- und Proteinbedarfes. Promotionsarbeit aus dem Forschungszentrum für Tierproduktion Dummerstorf-Rostock.
Black, J.L., B.P. Mullan, M.L. Lorschy & L.R. Giles, 1993. Lactation in the sow during heat stress. Livest. Prod. Sci., 35, 153-170.
Campbell, R.G. & A.C. Dunkin, 1982a. The effects of birth weight and level of feeding in early life on growth and development of muscle and adipose tissue in the young pig. Anim. Prod., 35, 185-192.
Campbell, R.G. & A.C. Dunkin, 1982b. The effect of birth weight on the estimated milk intake, growth and body composition of sow-reared piglets. Anim. Prod., 35, 193-197.
Donald, H.P., 1937. The milk production and growth of suckling pigs. Emp. J. Exp. Agric., 5, 349-360.
Elsley, F.W.H., 1971. Nutrition and lactation in the sow. In I.R. Falconer Ed., Lactation, 393-411. Butterworths, London.
Ferreira, A.S., P.M. de Costa, J.A.A. Pereira & J.C. Gomes, 1988. Estimation of milk yield of sows. Rev. Soc. Brasil. Zootec., 17, 203-211.
Fraser, D., 1984. The role of behaviour in swine production: a review of research. Appl. Anim. Ethol., 11, 317-339.
Fraser, D. & R. M. Jones, 1975. The 'teat order' of suckling pigs. I. Relation to birth weight and subsequent growth. J. Agric. Sci., 84, 387-391.
Fraser, D. & B.K. Thompson, 1986. Variation in piglet weights: relationship to suckling behavior, parity number and farrowing crate design. Can. J. Anim. Sci., 66, 31-46.
Hartman, D.A. & W.G. Pond, 1960. Design and use of a milking machine for sows. J. Anim. Sci. 19, 780-785.
Hartman, D.A., T.M. Ludwick & R.F. Wilson, 1962. Certain aspects of lactation performance in sows. J. Anim. Sci. 21, 883-886.
Hemsworth, P.H., C.G. Winfield & P.D. Mullaney, 1976. Within-litter variation in the performance of piglets to three weeks of age. Anim. Prod., 22, 351-357.
King, R.H., B.P. Mullan, F.R. Dunshea & H. Dove, 1997. The influence of piglet body weight on milk production of sows. Livest. Prod. Sci., 47, 169-174.
King, R.H., M.S. Toner & H. Dove, 1989. Pattern of milk production in sows. In Barnett J.L. & D.P. Hennessy Ed., Manipulating Pig Production II, 98. Australasian Pig Science Association, Werribee, Australia.
Klaver, J., G.J.M. van Kempen, P.G.B. de Lange, M.W.A. Verstegen & H Boer, 1981. Milk composition and daily yield of different milk components as affected by sow condition and lactation/feeding regimen. J. Anim. Sci., 52, 1091-1097.
Lewis, A.J., V.C. Speer & D.G. Haught, 1978. Relationship between yield and composition of sows' milk and weight gains of nursing pigs. J. Anim. Sci., 47, 634-638.

Lima, G.J.M.M., R.G. Elkin & T.R. Cline, 1988. Effects of energy nutrition and parity of the sow on milk yield and composition. Proc. 10th Congress I.P.V.S., 359.
Lodge, G.A. & J.I. Elliot, 1979. The influence of birth weight on the subsequent growth of hysterectomy-derived pigs. Can. J. Anim. Sci., 59, 215-216.
Lodge, GA & I. McDonald, 1959. The relative influence of birth weight, milk consumption and supplementary food consumption upon the growth rates of suckling piglets. Anim. Prod., 1, 139-144.
Lynch, P.B., 1977. Effect of environmental temperature on lactating sows and their litters. Irish J. Agric. Res., 16, 123-130.
Mabry, J.W., M.T. Coffey & R.W. Seerley, 1983. A comparison of an 8- versus 16-hour photoperiod during lactation on suckling frequency of the baby pig and maternal performance of the sow. J. Anim. Sci., 57, 292-295.
Mabry, J.W., F.L. Cunningham, R.R. Kraeling & G.B. Rampacek, 1982. The effect of artificially extended photoperiod during lactation on maternal performance of the sow. J. Anim. Sci., 54, 918-921.
Mahan, D.C., D.E. Becker, H.W. Norton & A.H. Jensen, 1971. Milk production in lactating sows and time lengths used in evaluating milk production estimates. J. Anim. Sci., 33, 35-37.
Messias de Bragança, M., A.M. Mounier , J.C. Hulin & A. Prunier, 1997. La sous-nutrition explique-t-elle les effets d'une température ambiante élevée sur les performances des truies? Journ. Rech. Porcine en France, 29, 81-88.
Noblet, J. & M. Etienne, 1986. Effect of energy level in lactating sows on yield and composition of milk and nutrient balance of piglets. J. Anim. Sci., 63, 1888-1896.
Noblet, J. & M. Etienne, 1989. Estimation of sow milk nutrient output. J. Anim. Sci., 67, 3352-3359.
Pettigrew, J.E., A.F. Sower, S.G. Cornelius & R.L. Moser, 1985. A comparison of isotope dilution and weigh-suckle-weigh methods for estimating milk intake by pigs. Can. J. Anim. Sci., 65, 989-992.
Pettigrew, J.E., S.G. Cornelius, R.L. Moser & A.F. Sower, 1987. A refinement and evaluation of the isotope dilution method for estimating milk intake by piglets. Livest. Prod. Sci., 16, 163-174.
Pluske, J.R., T.W. Fenton, M.L. Lorschy, J.E. Pettigrew, A.F. Sower & F.X. Aherne, 1997. A modification of the isotope-dilution technique for estimating milk intake of pigs using pig serum. J. Anim. Sci., 75, 1279-1283.
Prawirodigdo S., R.H. King, A.C. Dunkin & H. Dove, 1987. Estimation of milk intake by pigs using deuterium oxide dilution. In Barnett J.L., E.S. Batterham, G.M. Cronin, C. Hansen, P.H. Hemsworth, D.P. Hennessy, P.E. Hughes, N.E. Johnston & R.H. King Ed., Manipulating Pig Production I, 135. Australasian Pig Science Association, Werribee, Australia.
Salmon- Legagneur, E., 1956. La mesure de la production laitière chez la truie. Ann. Zootech. 5, 95-110.
Salmon- Legagneur, E., 1958. Observations sur la production laitière des truies. Ann. Zootech. 7, 95-143-162.
Salmon- Legagneur E. & A. Aumaître, 1962. Influence de la quantité de lait et de sa composition sur la croissance du porcelet sous la mère. Ann. Zootech. 11, 181-196.
Schoenherr W.D., T.S. Stahly & G.L. Cromwell, 1989. The effects of dietary fat or fiber addition on yield and composition of milk from sows housed in a warm or hot environment. J. Anim. Sci., 67, 482-495.
Smith, D.M., 1959. The yield and composition of milk from sows fed varying proportions of separated milk and concentrates. New Zeal. J. Agric. Res., 2, 1057-1070.
Speer, V.C & D.F. Cox, 1984. Estimating milk yield of sows. J. Anim. Sci., 59, 1281-1285.
Spinka, M., G. Illmann, B. Algers & Z. Stetkova, 1997. The role of nursing frequency in milk production in domestic pigs. J. Anim. Sci., 75, 1223-1228.

Stansbury, W.F., J.J. McGlone & L.F. Tribble, 1987. Effects of season, floor type, air temperature and snout coolers on sow and litter performance. J. Anim. Sci., 65, 1507-1513.
Stone, C.C., M.S. Brown & G.H. Waring, 1974. An ethological means to improve swine production. J. Anim. Sci., 39, 137 (Abstr.).
Van der Steen, H.A.M. & P.N. de Groot, 1992. Direct and maternal breed effects on growth and milk intake of piglets: Meishan versus Dutch breeds. Livest. Prod. Sci., 30, 363-373.
Vanschoubroek, F. & R. Van Spaendonck, 1966. Nutrition des truies en lactation en fonction de leurs besoins énergétique et protidique. In L'alimentation de la truie, 31-55. Journée d'étude organisée par l'Association professionnelle des fabricants d'aliments composés pour animaux, Bruxelles.
Vidal, J.M., S.A. Edwards, O. MacPherson, P.R. English & A.G. Taylor, 1991. Effect of environmental temperature on dietary selection in lactating sows. Anim. Prod., 52, 597 (Abstr).
Walkiewicz, A., 1978. Milk production and composition of Pulawy sows. Roczniki Nauk Rolniczych, B, 99, 115-117.
Winters, L.M., J.N. Cummings & H.A. Stewart, 1947. A study of factors affecting survival from birth to weaning and total weaning weight of the litter in swine. J. Anim. Sci., 6, 288-296.
Yang, T.S., B. Howard & W.V. Macfarlane, 1980. A note on milk intake of piglets measured by tritium dilution. Anim. Prod., 31, 201-203.

17 Behaviour of sows and piglets during lactation

P.H. Brooks and J. Burke

17.1 Introduction

Domestic sows have one function, namely to give birth to piglets and rear them until they have achieved sufficient physiological maturity that they can function successfully, as individuals, independent of their mothers. During the period from late pregnancy through to weaning, the sow exhibits a rich and varied repertoire of behaviours. The way in which the sow interacts with her piglets and responds to her environment has a significant influence on her success in rearing her piglets and on their subsequent growth and development. Lactation behaviour is multidimensional, comprising a complex series of interactions between component behaviours which cumulatively determine the sow's success in nurturing her piglets. The component behaviours and their interactions (summarized in Figure 17.1) are considered in this chapter.

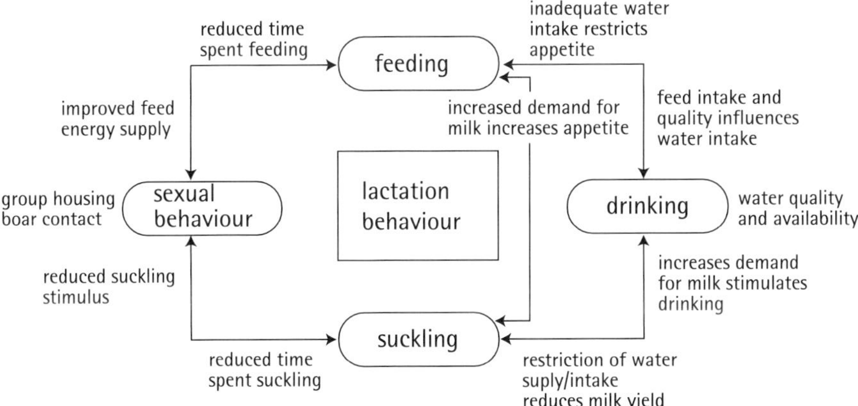

Figure 17.1. The interrelationship of different behaviours during lactation

17.2 Suckling behaviour of sow and piglets

17.2.1 Birth of the piglets

During the 24 hours prior to farrowing sows become increasingly restless. Wild boar sows and domestic sows in semi-natural environments spend much of this time seeking a suitable nest site, collecting vegetation and building an elaborate farrowing nest. In the confinement of a farrowing crate this activity is largely prevented and sows may become increasingly agitated. Attempts to perform nest building movements even when no nesting substrate is provided, frequently result in stereotyped behaviours such as bar biting and pawing (Baxter, 1980; Hansen and Curtis, 1981; Lammers and De Lange, 1986).

As a rule, piglets are born while the sow is in lateral recumbency. This is true of wild boar (Gundlach, 1968), domestic sows in semi-natural conditions (Jensen, 1986a) and sows farrowing in conventional farrowing crate systems (Fraser, 1984). Unlike other ungulates, the sow does not lick the newly born piglets and offers them no assistance in finding the udder (Petersen, Recen and Vestergaard, 1990; Rohde Parfet and Gonyou, 1991). However, wild boar sows and domestic sows in semi-natural conditions are reported to stand and sniff their piglets during farrowing, before turning to lie on the other side (Gundlach, 1968; Jensen, 1986a; Petersen *et al.*, 1990). Randall (1972) noted that sows in farrowing crates and pens got up on several occasions during farrowing.

17.2.2 Suckling development of the neonatal piglet

Location of udder

The development of a regular suckling routine by a litter of piglets follows a distinct pattern (Figure 17.2). Immediately following birth piglets struggle to free their head from birth membranes and upper respiratory tract of fluids (Randall, 1972; Welch and Baxter, 1986). Within minutes of birth young piglets are mobile and begin to make their way towards the udder of the sow. If not already severed during birth, the umbilical cord is broken at this stage, easing progress as piglets nose and nuzzle along the body of the sow. Occasionally piglets travel around the back of the sow, but more usually climb over or push between the hind legs to reach the udder (Welch *et al.*, 1986; Petersen *et al.*, 1990).

Teat seeking

Having reached the vicinity of the udder, the teat seeking phase of suckling development begins (Hartstock *et al.*, 1976). It appears that although piglets are born with their eyes open, they do not search visually for a teat. They will often pass very close to a teat without appreciating its presence (Randall, 1972; Hartstock *et al.*, 1976). Nosing and nuzzling intensify as developing suckling movements are directed towards the surface of the udder. Barber (1955) noted that during this exploratory phase piglets had some nose contacts with the sow. In the majority of cases, the first nose to nose contact between piglet and sow occurred before any suckling began (Petersen *et al.*, 1990).

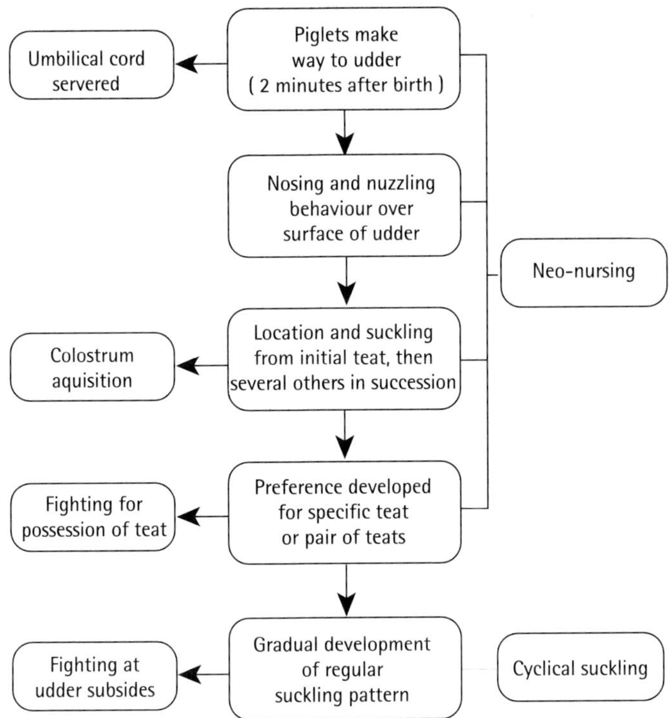

Figure 17.2. The development of nursing behaviour in piglets

Teat sampling

Once piglets establish contact and suckle from a teat they move along the udder, suckling from several teats in succession (Randall, 1972; Petersen *et al.*, 1990). Hartstock (1976) classified this behaviour, occurring at between 2 and 6 hours after parturition, as the teat sampling phase of suckling development. It is suggested that during this phase, the first fights at the udder occur as piglets compete with their littermates for possession of teats (Hartstock *et al.*, 1976; Petersen *et al.*, 1990). More recently De Passille (1989b) reported that piglets suckled from 2 to 13 teats during the first 8 hours after birth and that those suckling high numbers of teats had more agonistic interactions with litter mates. In sharp contrast, Rosillon-Warnier (1984) reported that no agonistic behaviour between piglets occurred during teat-order establishment.

Colostrum aquisition

The energy reserves of newborn piglets, in the form of liver glycogen, are rapidly depleted after birth, leaving piglets highly susceptible to chilling, hypoglycaemia, weakness and death from crushing by the sow (Dividich and Noblet, 1981; Moser, 1983). In addition, the neonatal piglet has only low levels of immunoglobulins for protection from disease (De Passille, Rushen & Pellether, 1988). Colostrum is the source of dietary energy which also contains immunoglobulins which can be absorbed intestinally by piglets for up to 36 hours after birth, prior to 'gut closure' (Hartstock & Graves, 1976; De Passille et al., 1988). The speedy acquisition of colostrum by the piglet soon after birth is therefore essential to provide the energy and antibody protection necessary for survival. During farrowing and in the first few hours of lactation colostrum may be expressed relatively easily from the sow's teats. However, Fraser (1984) demonstrated that after 15 minutes yield declined sharply, after which colostrum could be collected during discrete ejections lasting 1 to 4 minutes, occurring every 5 to 30 minutes, depending upon the stimulation received by the sow. More recently Castren (1993) demonstrated that discrete milk ejections during parturition and 4 hours post partum, frequently occurred in the absence of oxytocin peaks. However, it was pointed out that at this time basal oxytocin concentrations may be high enough for milk ejection to occur without further secretion of the hormone.

During this time the sow emits rhythmical grunting sounds which increase in rate at intervals during the first 5 hours post partum (Castren *et al.,* 1989b). An investigation conducted by Castren (1993) demonstrated that both oxytocin secretion and milk ejection must occur to induce an increased grunting rate by the sow.

The teat sampling phase of suckling is the first opportunity for piglets to obtain the colostrum, essential for their survival and fitness. As farrowing typically lasts for 3 to 4 hours, earlier born piglets have a greater opportunity to benefit from the energy and immunoglobulins contained in colostrum than their later born littermates (Graves, 1984). According to De Passille et al. (1988) piglets which suckled earlier, suckled from several teats, won more teat disputes and had the highest within litter immunoglobulin levels, whereas later born piglets had much lower antibody protection.

Teat order establishment

According to Lewis (1985) this early period is a distinct phase of 'neo-nursing', during which individual piglet activity gradually polarises towards specific areas of the udder as their teat preferences become better established. Once a definite teat order for suckling has developed, piglets generally suckle from the same teat or pair of teats throughout lactation (McBride, 1963; De Passille *et al.,* 1989b). During this teat defence phase, aggressive encounters become limited to piglets occupying neighbouring teats (Hartstock *et al.,* 1976). It is generally presumed that the anterior teats are claimed by the stronger more vigorous piglets, however there is little evidence to support this. Barber (1955) suggested that the heavier, earlier born piglets fight for possession of the anterior teats. Hartstock (1977) claimed that as these teats are more productive, they were defended by the more successful, heavier fighters which achieved greater early weight gains. However, De Passille *et al.* (1989b) considered there was little evidence that piglets fought specifically for anterior teats or that heavier piglets had greater access to them. In addition, Rosillon-Warnier (1984) found that although there was a tendency for piglets suckling the first four teats to have slightly higher weight gains, birth weight and birth order had no effect on teat-order. Studies conducted by Fraser (1979b) demonstrated that piglet growth was influenced by the relative weight of littermates and not by the position of the teat suckled. There is evidence which suggests that piglet weight gain, dependent on milk intake, is influenced by the power of the piglet to suckle (Fraser & Thompson, 1979a; King *et al.*, 1997).

Transition from neo-nursing to cyclical nursing

As teat ownership becomes established, the incidence of fighting reduces and a regular suckling pattern develops, which Hartstock (1976) classified as the teat maintenance phase. This change in suckling behaviour signals the transition from 'neo-nursing' to more regular, synchronised or 'cyclical' bouts of nursing (Lewis *et al.*, 1985). The same author claims this transition occurs 10.7 ± 4.5 hours after parturition, whilst Castren *et al.* (1989b) and Rosillon-Warnier *et al.* (1984) state that the change begins to occur from 5 and 3 hours after birth, respectively. More recently De Passille *et al.* (1989b) concluded that although the estimate of Lewis *et al.* (1985) might be the more realistic, the change was a gradual one so that no definite point in time when continuous suckling gave way to regular, synchronised bouts of suckling could be identified.

17.2.3 Suckling frequency

Once cyclical suckling has been established, nursings involving all or most of the litter occur at regular intervals throughout lactation (Table 17.1). According to Schouten (1986), piglets spent approximately 30% of their time engaged in suckling behaviour during the first two weeks of lactation. Thereafter suckling activity decreased over time, occupying only 15% of time when piglets were six weeks of age.

Table 17.1. Mean intra-suckling intervals reported in the literature

Interval (minutes)	Day of lactation	Reference
48 to 52	10 to 24	(Auldist & King, 1995)
76	3	(Spinka *et al.*, 1997)
52 (range 42 to 68)	14 to 5	(Wechsler & Brodmann, 1996)
44 (range 21 to 92)	7 to 28	(Ellendorf *et al.*, 1982)
51 and 63 (range 26 to 96)	6 and 51	(Barber *et al.*, 1955)
29 to 78	1 to 42	(Newberry & Wood-Gush ,1984)
40 to 45	1 to 13	(Arey & Sancha 1996)

The milk yield of the sow is influenced by litter size, piglet liveweight and suckling demand (Auldist *et al.*, 1995; King *et al.*, 1997). The more frequent the opportunities for piglets to suckle, the higher their milk intake and subsequent liveweight gain over lactation (Barber *et al.*, 1955; Newberry *et al.*, 1984; Spinka *et al.*, 1997). The results of studies of the effect of nursing frequency on piglet weight gain and sow milk yield are summarised in Table 17.2.

Table 17.2. The effect of nursing frequency on sow milk yield and piglet weight gain

Nursing frequency per 24 hours	Sow milk yield	Piglet weight	Reference
8	241g/24hrs	-	(Barber *et al.*, 1955)
9.6	304g/24hrs	-	"
24	553g/24hrs	-	"
25.25	5.07kg/21days	39 (21 days)	(Mabry *et al.*, 1983)
30.75	6.07kg/21days	44.8 (21 days)	"
20.2	595g/24hrs	135g/24hrs	(Spinka *et al.*, 1997)
33.9	755g/24hrs	198g/24hrs	"

Suckling frequency may be increased by exposure to an extended photoperiod (Mabry *et al.*, 1983) and by auditory stimuli (Auldist *et al*,. 1995). Indeed, studies conducted by Wechsler (1996) revealed that nursing bouts could be stimulated by playback of sounds made by sows and piglets during suckling. Similarly, Newberry (1984) suggested that sows responded to the suckling vocalisations of each other, resulting in synchrony of sucklings within the sow group. An investigation conducted by Algers (1985) indicated that high levels of continuous noise, such as that emanating from ventilation fans, affected communication between sow and piglets. As a result, suckling routines were disrupted, leading to lower milk yields and reduced piglet weight gains.

17.2.4 Sow and piglet behaviour during suckling

The nursing and suckling behaviour of the pig is complex and consists of several distinct phases (Whittemore & Fraser, 1974; Fraser, 1980; Algers *et al.*, 1985) (Figure 17.3). Initial observations distinguished four distinct suckling phases of udder nosing, quiet interval, milk ejection phase and renewal of udder nosing (Barber *et al.*, 1955). Following further studies,Whittemore (1974) described five phases of suckling behaviour, beginning with a phase of jostling for teats, followed by a phase of nosing the udder, then a phase of quiet suckling with slow mouth movements of high amplitude, a phase of sucking with rapid mouth movements of lower amplitude and finally a further phase of slow sucking and nosing of the udder.

Piglet vocalisations and repeated gruntings from the sow accompany these phases of suckling and play an important role in the interaction between sow and litter (Algers *et al.,* 1985). The grunting of the sow follows a distinct pattern related to the suckling behaviour of the piglets, oxytocin release and milk letdown (Whittemore *et al.,* 1974; Fraser, 1980; Ellendorf *et al.,* 1982; Algers *et al.*, 1990b).

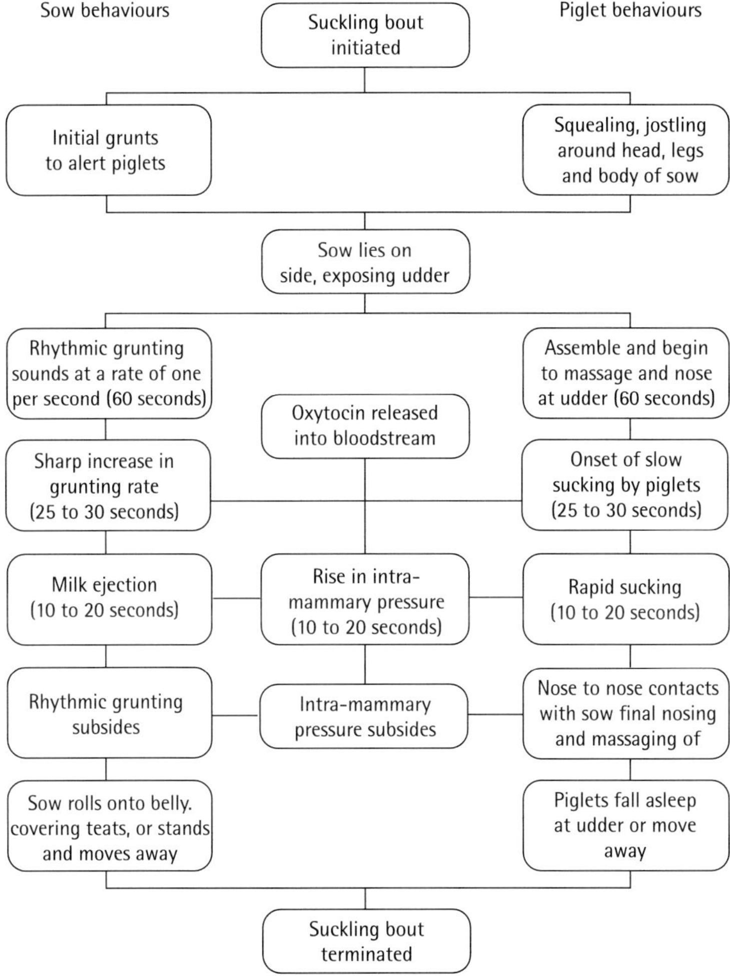

Figure 17.3. The sequence of behaviours of sow and piglet during nursing

lactating sow

Sucklings may be initiated by either the sow grunting to alert her litter and attract them to her udder or by the piglets congregating around the sow, squealing and massaging the udder (Fraser, 1980; Ellendorf *et al.*, 1982; Lewis and Hurnik, 1986; Castren *et al.*, 1989b). At this point the sow will generally lie on one side with both rows of teats exposed as the nursing bout begins. Once piglets assemble at the udder and perform the udder nosing phase of suckling, the sow begins rhythmic grunting, at a rate of about 1 grunt per second. After about one minute a sharp increase in sow grunting rate occurs, which coincides with the onset of slow sucking by the piglets and the release of the hormone, oxytocin into the blood stream (Fraser, 1980; Algers *et al.*, 1990b). According to Ellendorf (1982) a rise in intra-mammary pressure occurs approximately 23 seconds after the onset of fast grunting by the sow. The timing of this rise in intra-mammary pressure corresponds to the 25 second circulation time reported for oxytocin and results in milk ejection (Fraser, 1980; Algers *et al.*, 1990b).

The start of the rapid sucking phase of piglet suckling behaviour, occurring 25 to 30 seconds after the increase in sow grunting rate, also coincides with milk ejection (Whittemore *et al.*, 1974; Fraser, 1980).

Milk is only available to piglets for between 10 and 20 seconds (Barber *et al.*, 1955; Whittemore *et al.*, 1974; Fraser, 1980), corresponding to the duration of the rise in intra-mammary pressure (Ellendorf *et al.*, 1982). Once the pressure subsides, the milk supply ceases as the mammary glands of the sow have no teat cistern for storing milk (De Passille *et al.*, 1989b). Once milk flow ceases, the rapid sucking of piglets immediately stops, to be replaced by the final period of udder massage, whilst sow grunting gradually subsides (Fraser, 1980). The whole sequence of suckling behaviours may last for no more than 2 to 3 minutes (Fraser, 1980).

The nose to nose contacts made between sow and piglet prior to initial sucklings immediately after birth continue during later more established sucklings. However, the number of pre-suckling contacts reduces during days 1 and 2 after birth, to be largely replaced by contacts which increasingly occur after the cessation of milk flow (Whatson and Bertram, 1982; Jensen, Stangel and Algers, 1991). This mainly piglet initiated behaviour is the only reciprocal interaction which occurs between sow and piglets and is considered to play an important part in the establishment and maintenance of close social bonds between sow and piglets (Whatson *et al*,. 1982; Petersen *et al.*, 1990).

17.2.5 Incomplete nursings

Studies conducted by Whittemore (1974) revealed that when the sow grunt rate did not increase, the rapid sucking phase of suckling did not follow and milk ejection did not occur. These incomplete nursings are a relatively common occurrence (Whittemore *et al.*, 1974) and have been reported for domestic sows in semi-natural surroundings (Newberry *et al.*, 1984; Castren, Algers and Jensen, 1989a; Jensen *et al.*, 1991) and in sows in conventional farrowing accommodation (Whatson and Bertram 1980). There was concern that, as the mean interval between two successful sucklings was shorter than that between two successful sucklings separated by one or more unsuccessful suckling, frequent unsuccessful nursings might reduce overall milk intake and decrease piglet growth rates (Newberry *et al.*, 1984; Castren *et al.*, 1989a).

It was postulated that sounds of nursing by other sows might cause premature nursing in others, housed in the same room. However, Whatson (1980) found no difference in frequency of incomplete nursings in groups of sows housed in individual pens with farrowing crates and single sows housed in isolation in individual loose pens. In contrast, Arey *et al.* (1996) reported that sows in the family pen system had fewer false nursings than sows in farrowing crates. Incomplete nursings were most common during week 2 of lactation and accounted for 27% of all suckling bouts (Whatson *et al.*, 1980). Unsuccessful sucklings in sows kept in semi-natural conditions were most frequent during days 1 to 5 post partum, accounting for 30.5% of all sucklings, before decreasing to 23.4% during days 6 to 10 of lactation (Jensen *et al.*, 1991). This is in accordance with findings of Newberry (1984) who reported a mean of 22.6% unsuccessful sucklings over a 10 week period and results of Castren (1989a) who found that milk ejection failed in 31% of sucklings during the first 3 days post partum in sows kept in a semi-natural enclosure.

It was noted that sows which had recently suckled would start a subsequent suckling bout in synchrony with another sow, even though she was unlikely to let down milk (Newberry *et al.*, 1984). The same author suggests that, notwithstanding the number of unsuccessful sucklings and their effect of increasing the interval between successful sucklings, social stimulation in farrowing houses promotes increased milk production and piglet weight gain, by initiating an overall increase in the frequency of suckling bouts. Unsuccessful sucklings are considered to be part of the natural behaviour of pigs and not caused specifically by intensive housing systems (Castren *et al.*, 1989a).

17.2.6 Changes in nursing behaviour over time

Sows in group farrowing systems tended to stay inside the farrowing enclosure with their piglets during the night and spent time away from their litters during the day (Boe ,1993). The same author found that sows spent increasing amounts of time lying sternally, during weeks 2 and 3 of lactation. Sows in farrowing crates were also observed to increase sternal lying time over a 27 day lactation (De Passille and Robert, 1989a). The frequency of sternal lying was greater during the day time than at night, when more time was spent in lateral recumbency (De Passille *et al.*, 1989a).

At first, sucklings were initiated by the sow with the piglets taking a passive role, but as they grew older, more and more sucklings were begun by piglet stimulation (Jensen *et al.*, 1991). During the first week of lactation the number of sucklings terminated by sows in a semi-natural environment gradually rose from less than 5% to 60% of sucklings (Jensen *et al.*, 1991). According to Jensen (1988), the number of suckling terminations by free-ranging sows had increased to 90% by the fourth week of lactation. Suckling terminations by sows in indoor group farrowing systems followed a similar pattern (Boe, 1993; Burke, J. unpublished data). The number of sow and piglet suckling terminations which occurred daily, from day 1 to day 17 of lactation in a group farrowing system are presented in Figure 17.4. The time spent foraging by free-ranging sows increased between weeks 1 and 4, whilst the time spent lying decreased along with the frequency of sucklings (Jensen, 1988). The same author noted that piglets reduced the time spent nosing and massaging the udder, following milk ejection, during weeks 1 to 4 of lactation. The percentage of sucklings with piglets missing increased over time, from 1.8% in week 1 to 7.8% in week 4 (Jensen, 1988).

In the Edinburgh family pen system, pigs are able to carry out more normal patterns of behaviour and form normal social groups (Arey *et al*, 1996). In this system, sows began to suckle their piglets outside the farrowing area, at between 10 and 14 days postpartum.

In contrast, sows in a fully integrated, group farrowing system, in which piglets were confined to the farrowing enclosure, reduced the time spent with their piglets from over 90% during the first week of lactation, to only 58% of each 24 hour period in week 2 (Boe, 1993). By week 3, this had reduced further to a mere 17.1% of the day. Houwers (1992) also found that sows in a free access farrowing

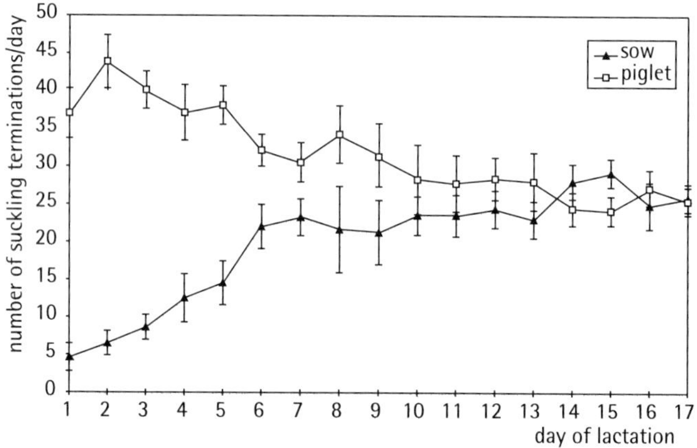

Figure 17.4. Sow and piglet nursing terminations from day 1 to day 17 of lactation in a group farrowing system (error bars denote SEM) (Burke, J. unpublished

system gradually increased the amount of time away from their litters and reduced the number of sucklings, over lactation. In a natural situation the sow and piglets would leave the farrowing site approximately 10 days post-partum and join other sows and litters (Jensen and Redbo, 1987). Sow behaviour in the family system was similar to that of free-ranging sows which abandon the farrowing nest when piglets were about 10 days of age. The reduction in time sows spent with their piglets which were confined to the farrowing enclosure, also coincided with the time when sows and litters would leave the farrowing nest and re-join the herd. As the confined piglets were unable to follow the sow, her interest in them declined, resulting in weaning before 3 weeks of age in some instances (Boe, 1994).

17.2.7 Reasons for suckling behaviour development

Parturition in the sow may take between 1 and 5 hours (Whittemore, 1993). The physiology of the sow ensures that colostrum is freely available from before farrowing onset and for several hours afterwards. All newborn piglets have an opportunity to find their way to the udder and acquire energy and disease protection so essential for survival (Fraser, 1980). It is hypothesised that the period of neo-nursing may allow learned responses to develop in the piglets, preparing them for the more advanced cyclical nursing which follows (Lewis *et al.*, 1985). According to McBride (1963), Fraser (1980) and Whittemore (1993), the formation of a teat order may promote orderly feeding and eliminate competition between piglets when feeding. It is also suggested that as sows in natural conditions farrow in isolation, the establishment of a teat order would ensure that milk is only produced in teats regularly used by that particular litter, thus reducing opportunities for intruder piglets to suckle (Newberry *et al.*, 1984; Jensen, 1986a).

Piglets of up to 14 days of age were found to move towards the sound of sow nursing vocalisations, which are an important cue for milk release, regardless of their level of hunger (Lewis *et al.*, 1986). It was hypothesised that this response maintained contiguity of the litter and was the method by which sucklings were initiated by the sow (Lewis *et al.*, 1986) and piglet behaviour during suckling was synchronised (Castren *et al.*, 1989b).

The prolonged period of udder massage performed by piglets and the grunting sounds emitted by the sow at the start of a suckling bout give every member of the litter a chance to find a place at the udder before the short period of milk ejection occurs (Fraser ,1980; Algers *et al.*, 1990b). However, this does not mean that all piglets need be assembled at the udder for milk ejection to occur, as if this was the case, all piglets would suffer if nursing did not proceed due to the absence of one litter member, which might have died (Newberry *et al.*, 1984).

The slow sucking phase of nursing behaviour may serve to position piglets (Fraser, 1980), following a change in sow grunting rate, in readiness for the short milk ejection which follows (Algers *et al.*, 1985).

The 'restaurant hypothesis' was suggested by Algers (1985) to explain the function of the final udder massage. This means that by spending more or less time massaging their particular teat, the blood flow through that teat and subsequent milk production are stimulated, so that in effect, piglets order the size of their next meal (Algers *et al.*, 1985). This stimulation effect appeared to be greatest during the first few days of lactation, after which the teat order stabilised (Rosillon-Warnier *et al.*, 1984) and milk production adjusted to individual piglet requirements (Jensen *et al.*, 1991). More recently Spinka (1995) concluded that although nursings on day 3, which were preceded by sucklings with longer final massage times, produced more milk, there was still no firm evidence to support the 'restaurant hypothesis'.

It is possible that the synchrony of sucklings among groups of sows and litters, whether in free-ranging conditions or in a conventional farrowing house, might be an adaptation to minimise the incidence of cross suckling (Newberry *et al.*, 1984; Wechsler *et al.*, 1996).

The changes in nursing behaviour of sows and piglets during lactation are linked to a gradual process of weaning which begins around 10 days post partum (Jensen and Recen, 1989). This timing coincides with when sows and piglets in a natural environment vacate the farrowing nest (Jensen, 1988). According to Jensen (1987), the piglets change from being hiders -remaining in the place where they were born, to become followers - keeping in close contact with the mother when she moves. The 'fast food hypothesis' was proposed by Jensen (1989) to explain the process of weaning. They suggest that by terminating more sucklings and shortening the time for final udder massage, which may decrease the amount of milk produced over time, the sow reduces the benefit of suckling. In addition, the cost of obtaining milk was gradually increased by the sow as she initiated fewer sucklings, increased the pre-massage time and made final massage difficult to perform.

As this process continues, piglets' dependence on milk reduces and they increase their intake of solid food until weaning in a natural environment is completed by around 17 weeks of age (Jensen *et al.*, 1989; Petersen, 1994).

17.3 Sow and piglet activities not directly associated with suckling

17.3.1 Exploratory behaviour of piglets

Over the first 8 weeks of piglet life the amount of time spent suckling decreases to be replaced by a rapid increase in exploratory behaviour, including sniffing of objects and substrate, chewing, biting, rooting, walking and standing (Schouten, 1986; Petersen, 1994). Piglets in a semi-natural environment were engaged in these activities for 40% of the time during the nest occupation phase, after which activity increased (Petersen, 1994). The amount of exploration carried out may be influenced by the quality of the environment in which pigs are kept. Pigs in straw bedded pens spent 44% of time exploring compared with only 24.9% of time for pigs reared in a farrowing crate pen with no bedding substrate (Schouten, 1986).

Walking and standing occurred during week 1 and increased from nest leaving time to week 8 in free-ranging piglets (Petersen, 1994), whereas in piglets in straw-bedded pens and crates, locomotion gradually decreased over this time (Schouten, 1986). This difference may have been an effect of reduced interest in surroundings as the novelty value diminished over time in housed pigs, whilst free-ranging animals continued to receive stimulation from a changing environment.

Rooting behaviour began in the first week of life, and increased in frequency over subsequent weeks (Schouten, 1986; Petersen, 1994). Chewing, present from the first week of life, was considered to be an important behaviour, as piglets in straw bedded pens spent up to 20% of their time in the activity by week 4 (Schouten, 1986). Piglets in natural conditions chewed earth and other objects from the first week of life, and gradually increased time spent chewing to week 4, after which grazing behaviour began (Petersen, 1994). According to Petersen (1994), piglets learn to identify food sources, whilst involved in these investigative behaviours, so that they are prepared for the time when nutritional requirements must come from the wider environment.

17.3.2 Social interactions between littermates and sow

Physical interactions

Social behaviour amongst piglets, which included nosing between piglets, considered to be important for individual recognition, decreased with age (Schouten, 1986). Nibbling and massaging of littermates was higher in crate piglets than those in straw bedded pens (Schouten, 1986). These behaviours did not occur in free-ranging piglets (Petersen, 1994). After suckling, the sow in a semi-natural environment, would move off to resume foraging while the piglets foraged, rested or played close by (Newberry *et al.*, 1984; Stangel and Jensen, 1991). Sows housed in farrowing crates and straw bedded pens were the focus of attention by piglets, whose nosing and nibbling resulted in sows standing for many hours (Whatson *et al.*, 1982). According to Schouten (1986) and Arey (1996), nibbling and massaging of the sow continued for longer in farrowing crates than in straw bedded pens, whereas Whatson (1982) concluded that there was no difference in this behaviour between the two types of environment. Observations of De Passille (1989a) demonstrated that sows in farrowing crates use postural changes including increased sitting, standing and sternal lying to limit piglet access to the udder and other vulnerable body parts. It is suggested that the well-being of confined sows may suffer as a result of a reduction in the quality and total duration of resting time (De Passille *et al.*, 1989a; Arey *et al.*, 1996) and that the amount of irritating interactions between sow and piglets might be reduced with the provision of alternative forms of stimulation for the piglets (Whatson *et al.*, 1982).

Piglet vocalisations

Piglets have a well developed auditory discrimination and a substantial repertoire of vocal communication (Rohde Parfet *et al.*, 1991; Horrell and Hodgson, 1992). Jensen (1983/84) identified five different classes of piglet vocalisations related to suckling behaviour. According to Jensen (1983/84), piglets make croaking sounds most frequently at the beginning of nursing. Other vocalisations include the scream and the squeak, both associated with aggressive interactions, and deep and high grunts which were uttered throughout nursing (Jensen *et al.*, 1983/84).

Suckling piglets vocalise a great deal when isolated from the sow and their littermates and the sow vocalises when separated from her litter (Weary *et al.*, 1997). Weary (1995) demonstrated that the extent of calling made by isolated piglets varied according to their level of need as small, slow growing piglets and those which missed a suckling bout called more, using longer, higher pitched sounds than large, faster growing piglets and those which had just suckled. There were similar differences in vocal behaviour between piglets isolated in an enclosure at 14°C and piglets isolated at 30°C (Weary *et al.*, 1997). Sows responded to piglet calls by vocalising and approaching the source of the sounds (Weary *et al.*,1995), showing a stronger response to playback sounds from more needy piglets than from less needy piglets by vocalising more, moving more and spending more time near the playback speaker (Weary, Lawson and Thompson, 1996). As piglet isolation calls provide reliable information about the young animal's needs, they might be used as an indicator of welfare (Weary *et al.*, 1995; Weary *et al.*, 1997). However, Horrell (1992) found no evidence to suggest that sows could discriminate between vocalisations of their own piglets and those of others. In support of these findings, Gundlach (1968) reported that if a wild boar piglet was threatened, its squeals brought other sows with young in the vicinity, to its defence.

There is evidence to suggest an effect of the farrowing environment on maternal behaviour of the sow (Cronin and van Amerongen, 1991; Arey *et al.*, 1996;

Herskin, Jensen and Thodberg, 1997). Sows confined in a farrowing crate covered with hessian cloth and bedded with chopped straw prior to parturition, were more responsive to piglet vocalisations than sows in unmodified crates without bedding (Cronin *et al.*, 1991). Herskin *et al.*, (1997) demonstrated that sows in 'get away' farrowing pens, provided with sand substrate for bedding, were more responsive to piglet distress calls and spent more time in the farrowing enclosure during days 1 to 12 post partum than sows on bare concrete. A greater proportion of sows provided with both straw and sand bedding responded to playback of piglet distress calls by standing, compared with those without environmental stimuli (Herskin *et al.*, 1997). Similarly, Arey (1996) reported that sows in the family pen system stood more frequently in response to the playback of piglet squeals than sows in farrowing crates.

17.3.3 Behaviours affected by the environment

Excretory behaviour
Free-ranging sows leave the farrowing nest to eliminate, whereas sows in farrowing pens are forced to soil the area in which they farrow (Stangel *et al.*, 1991). Stangel (1991) suggested this restriction may be stressful for sows in intensive units. Free-ranging sows have been observed to clean the nest of piglet faeces and afterbirth during the first days after farrowing (Stangel *et al.*, 1991). It was suggested that this behaviour decreased the risk of infections, improved insulation properties of the nest (Stangel *et al.*, 1991) and reduced the chance of attracting predators to the area (Graves, 1984). Sows housed in straw bedded pens were observed to lick up piglet faeces from the floor of the pen, during the first 7 days post partum, whereas sows in farrowing crates were unable to perform these cleaning operations (Whatson *et al.*, 1982).

From about 4 days of age free-ranging domestic piglets and wild boar piglets left the birth place to eliminate, moving further away as they grew older (Buchenauer, Luft and Grauvogl, 1982, 1983; Stangel *et al.*, 1991). Buchenauer (1982, 1983) observed that piglets in farrowing pens began to eliminate in a more specific part of the pen from day 4 onwards, preferring to do so on straw bedding than on bare concrete and frequently close to the walls. Piglets born in farrowing crates, only soiled the creep area during the first 2 days of life, after which they excreted mainly in corners and close to the wall (Petherick, 1982).

Thermo-regulatory behaviour
Domestic breeds of neonatal piglets chill rapidly as they have low energy reserves, sparse pelage and a poorly developed subcutaneous adipose layer which provides only minimal insulation (Dividich *et al.*, 1981). The lower critical temperature of the neo-natal piglet is around 32°C (Whittemore, 1993). Hypothermic piglets become lethargic and may not suckle successfully (Edwards *et al.*, 1994). These piglets are more susceptible to disease and to crushing by the sow. Up to

30% of all piglets alive at parturition do not survive until weaning (Edwards and Furniss, 1988). The majority of these perish within the first three days after birth (Dividich *et al.*, 1981).

Neonatal wild piglets and domestic piglets in semi-natural environments have been observed to huddle together, close to the sow, for warmth, during the initial days of life (Gundlach, 1968; Algers and Jensen, 1990a; Stangel *et al.*, 1991). Whilst huddled together, piglets moved from time to time, so that no individual stayed on the top or outside of the heap for more than a few minutes (Algers *et al.*, 1990a). Welch (1986) demonstrated that newborn piglets were attracted by a combination of warmth and softness, characteristics possessed by the udder of the sow. The same author described how the surface of the udder rose in temperature by 3°C around parturition, resulting in a skin temperature of 36-37°C in the region of the teats. It is believed that as piglets lie close to the sow during the first days post partum, the risk of death by crushing is increased. In most commercial farrowing systems newborn piglet survival is aided by the provision of a protected, heated creep area for the piglets, which often incorporates some form of insulated flooring material. However, attempts to induce piglets to lie in heated creep areas were unsuccessful in attracting the newborn away from the sow before 3 days of age (Rohde Parfet *et al.*, 1991). Arey (1996) suggests that the lower ambient temperature in the family pen system resulted in increased use of the creep area by piglets in the family system, compared with piglets in a farrowing crate system.

In cold conditions newborn piglets were less active than piglets in warm housing and huddled together, shivering and altering posture to reduce the amount of body contact with the floor (Dividich *et al.*, 1981). The intake of colostrum by neonatal piglets exposed to cold, for short periods of time, was markedly reduced (Dividich *et al.*, 1981). As a result these piglets were more susceptible to disease, hypothermia and death. The provision of straw will reduce conductive heat loss to the floor. Using the relationship between O_2 consumption of new born piglets and the ambient temperature, Stephens (1971) demonstrated that a straw covered floor at 10°C was equivalent to a concrete floor at 18°C in terms of thermal demand upon the piglet. This benefit was revealed by placing piglets on top of the straw and could reasonably be expected to be greater if piglets were covered by straw as would occur in a nest constructed by a sow.

Algers (1990a) investigated the thermal microclimate within the nests of free ranging domestic pigs during a Scandinavian winter. The nest structures and lining materials afforded considerable protection for the young piglets against the outside climate. The results of the study revealed that when outside temperatures averaged -1.5°C, temperatures inside the nests, 5 cm from the piglets, averaged 20.3°C. It is suggested that the nest material acts as insulation against the outside cold, retaining the heat generated by the sow and piglets, enabling them to maintain a suitable microclimate within the nest.

17.4 Feeding Behaviour

Although the nutritional requirements of the lactating sow have been extensively researched, feeding and drinking behaviour have received much less attention. As a consequence, at farm level, there are often failures to translate nutritional recommendations into satisfactory production practices.

The voluntary feed intake of the animal is the cumulative expression of the sow's physiological and biochemical requirements, moderated by feeding and drinking behaviour. Subtle changes in the feeding and drinking behaviour of the sow can significantly modify nutrient intake and thus negate advances that have been made in our understanding of the sows nutrient requirements. A number of factors interact to influence individual sow feed intakes and feeding strategies (Figure 17.5).

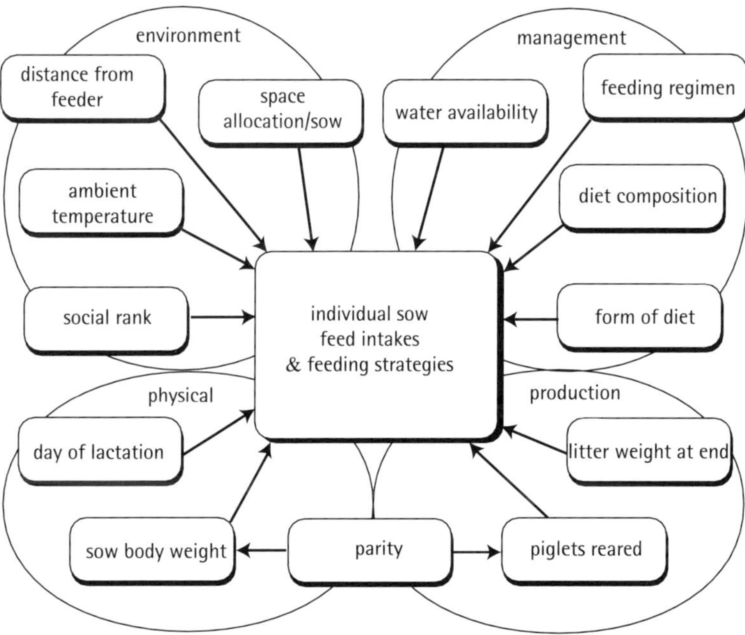

Figure 17.5. Factors influencing individual sow feed intakes and feeding strategies

In this section we consider how the major influences affect voluntary feed intake and where there is information indicate how these operate through the modification of feeding behaviour and feeding strategies.

17.4.1 Feeding strategies

In considering feeding strategies it is necessary to make a distinction between the foraging behaviour (activities associated with finding food) and feeding behaviour (the consumption of readily available food). A study of groups of lactating wild boar sows in a 1 hectare enclosure indicated that they spent between 24.8% and 59.1% of their time foraging and feeding, respectively (Teilland, 1986). Similarly, Mauget (1981) reported that wild boar spend 25.2% of their time foraging and feeding, although the proportion may reduce considerably when food is plentiful. De Passille *et al.* (1989) found that sows spent 5.5% of their time feeding on Day 17 (1.32h) of lactation and 4.0% (0.96h) on Day 27. They spent respectively 8.2% of the light period (15h) and 1.3% of the dark period feeding. In recent studies of group housed lactating sows, fed using a sow operated feed dispenser, sows spent 1.3 to 2.0 hours per day feeding (Burke *et al.*, 1997) (Table 17.3).

Table 17.3. The mean ±SEM daily feed intake, number of visits to the feeder per day and time spent feeding per day by farrowing and lactating sows in two different pen areas (Burke et al., 1997)

Area/sow	13.4m²/sow			8.6m²/sow		
Time period(days)	-5 to -1	1 to 7	8 to 17	5 to -1	1 to 7	8 to 17
intake/day(kg)	6.9 ± 0.42	5.8 ±0.46	9.0 ±0.35	6.8 ±0.54	6.8 ±0.58	8.4 ±0.40
visits/day	8.3[1] ±0.68	7.4[2] ±0.60	9.5[3] ±0.45	5.5[1] ±0.45	5.6[2] ±0.45	8.0[3] ±0.46
time/day(hrs)	2.6[4] ±0.16	1.5 ±0.11	2.0[5] ±0.07	2.1[4] ±0.17	1.3 ±0.11	1.7[5] ±0.05

pairs of means with the same following letter in the same row differ at [1]=P<0.001; [2]=P<0.05; [3]=P<0.05; [4]=P<0.05; [5]=P<0.001

When feed is presented in discrete meals the time spent consuming feed may be quite low. Blackshaw *et al.*, (1994) found that sows given two feeds per day spent 19.0±4.6 minutes eating in the morning and 13.6±1.1 minutes in the afternoon. Martin *et al.* (1994) found that gestating domestic sows fed outdoors took an average of 18.1 minutes to consume their diet when it was spread on the ground. In outdoor sow systems social rank may be important in determining the sow's success in obtaining an adequate feed supply. High ranking sows appropriate areas of high food density and defend the area aggressively against lower ranking individuals (Csermely *et al.*,1990). However, Martin *et al.* (1994) concluded from their studies that when feed distribution is adequate, outdoor feeding of sows imposes relatively little disadvantage on low ranking animals.

Information about feeding strategies adopted by lactating sows is relatively sparse. Nutritional studies generally concentrate on total feed intake and pay little attention to the pattern and temporal variation in feed consumption of individual sows. In many studies, and in much of commercial practice, the sow's preferred pattern of consumption is subjugated to the needs of management with sows being fed in discrete meals rather than being given access to feed *ad libitum*. Lactating sows, fed *ad libitum*, exhibit a marked diurnal pattern of feeding (Dourmad, 1993; J. Burke *unpublished data*, 1997) with most feeding occurring during daytime, peaking in early morning and mid afternoon (Figure 17.6).

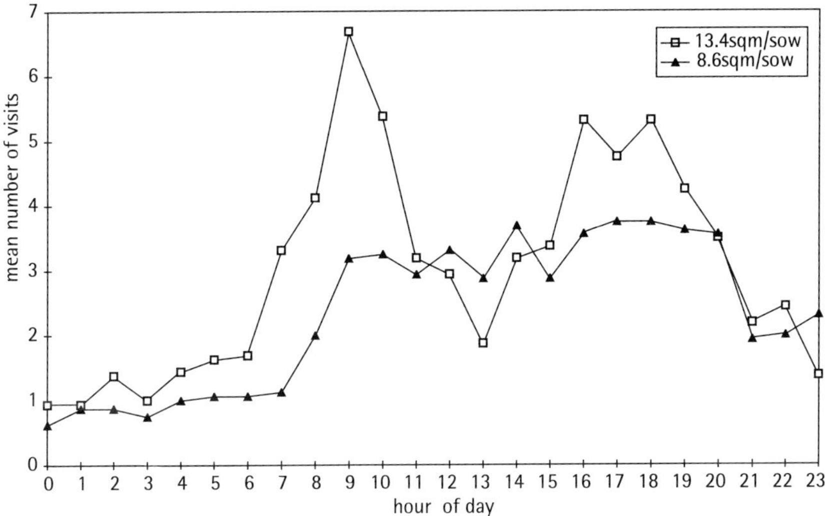

Figure 17.6. Time of day of feeding visits made by group housed sows in two different space allocations, providing 13.4m² and 8.6m² per sow, from day 1 to day 17 of lactation. (Burke et al., 1997)

The pattern of consumption and the number of meals taken is conditioned by the extent to which the dietary regimen creates a feeling of satiety. Thus growing pigs fed *ad libitum* made several visits to the feeder and took their daily feed allowance in a series of meals (de Haer *et al.*,1992; Nielsen, 1995). As the group size and competition for food increased, pigs reduced the meal duration, increased the meal size and reduced the number of meals taken. In contrast gestating sows, ration fed using electronic sow feeders, usually consumed the whole of their daily feed allowance during a single feeder visit. However, all sows made more than one feeder visit per day on some occasions (Eddison *et al.,* 1995).

Lactating sows confined in farrowing crates and fed four times per day to appetite, took a mean of 8.7 meals each day (Dourmad, 1993). Sows that had lower feed intakes took a similar number of meals but reduced the duration of each meal and the amount eaten on each occasion. Burke *et al.*, (1997) found that group housed lactating sows also took a number of meals each day (Table 17.3) and that the number of meals was influenced by the floor area provided per sow in the farrowing enclosure. Sows provided with 8.6 m^2 took fewer meals and spent less time feeding than sows provided with 13.4 m^2 but had similar feed intakes, implying a faster eating rate. This suggests that where the sow perceives competition, both the frequency and rate of feeding are adjusted to maintain intake.

Feeding sows *ad libitum* simplifies management. More importantly it removes the association between the presence / appearance of the stockperson in the farrowing house and anticipation of a feeding event. Sow activity tends to be particularly high during parturition and around the regular feeding periods with the risk of overlying being correspondingly higher at these times (English, 1969). In some situations adoption of *ad libitum* feeding has been shown to reduce the peaks of sow activity and increase piglet survival (English, 1969). However, in studies in which sows were fed once or twice per day or *ad libitum* no significant effects on piglet survival were found (Stahly *et al.,* 1979; Anderson *et al.,* 1990; NCR-89 Committee on Confinement Management of Swine 1990; Rudd *et al.,* 1994). A range of other management strategies and housing provisions probably make a greater contribution to the reduction of overlaying deaths than differences in the feeding pattern of the sow (English *et al.,* 1982a). These include:

- the use of farrowing crates designed to control the way in which the sow moves from the upright to the prostrate position
- the provision of heated safe areas (creeps) to attract the piglets away from the immediate vicinity of the sow
- the provision of floor surfaces which ensure good mobility of piglets and a good foothold for the sow

A discussion of the wide range of management strategies which can be adopted to improve the survival of the neonatal pig are outside the scope of this review but see reviews by Brooks, 1989; English *et al.,* 1982b; England, 1986.

17.4.2 Imposed feeding strategies and their effects on feed consumption and performance

There is a great diversity in the feeding strategies imposed on lactating sows on commercial units. Many producers are concerned that if sows are fed *ad libitum* in the early stages of lactation the udder will become overstocked with milk and that this in turn will lead to mastitis and agalactia. Consequently, many producers restrict the feed intake of the sow during early lactation, feeding the sow a restricted ration in one or more feeds per day.

Restriction of feed intake at any stage of lactation should be avoided unless there are serious health contraindications, as the feed intake of the lactating sow is often insufficient to meet nutrient requirements for maintenance and milk production (Lynch 1989; Mullan *et al.*, 1990; Dourmad, 1993). Nutrient intakes in lactation affect the overall productivity of the herd by influencing piglet growth rates and the post weaning reproductive performance of the sow (Lynch, 1989; Mullan *et al.*, 1990; Koketsu *et al.*, 1996a; Koketsu *et al.*, 1996b).

The feed intake of normal sows fed *ad libitum* on conventional diets may vary between 2 and 8 kg per day (see review by Whittemore, 1990) and the maximum intake of a sow, at a single feed, is generally between 3 and 4kg. Data collected by Handley *et al.* (1996) (Table 17.4) demonstrate the variation in intake achieved by sows of the same genotype on five different farms.

On *ad libitum* feeding, feed intake normally falls on the day of parturition and then increases progressively after weaning reaching a peak after approximately 7 days (for example see Figure 17.7). However, the pattern can become disrupted with adverse effects on sow and litter performance.

Table 17.4. Mean voluntary feed intakes (kg/d) of lactating sows in five commercial herds. (Handley et al., 1996)

Herd	Primiparous sows	Multiparous sows
A	6.19 ± 0.20	6.66 ± 0.10
B	4.27 ± 0.20	5.53 ± 0.14
C	5.24 ± 0.10	6.36 ± 0.09
D	5.32 ± 0.11	5.84 ± 0.09
E	6.31 ± 0.27	6.52 ± 0.09
Overall	5.46± 0.07	6.19 ± 0.04

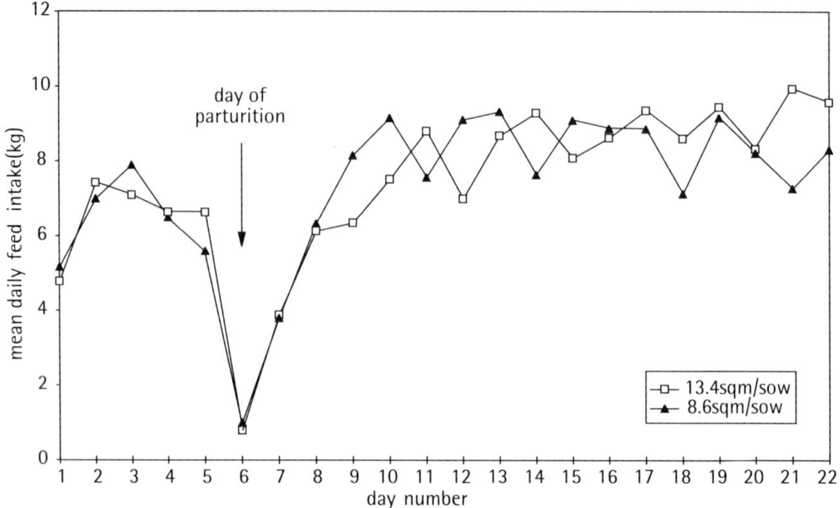

Figure 17.7. Mean daily feed intakes of ad libitum fed, group housed sows in two different space allocations providing 13.4m² and 8.6m² per sow from 5 days before parturition until day 17 of lactation (Burke, unpublished data)

Koketsu *et al.* (1996b) examined the records of 25,040 sows on 30 commercial farms and were able to characterise six distinct patterns of daily feed intake occurring during lactation. Average daily feed intake was 5.2 (SD 1.4) kg/d with the peak intake occurring at 12.6 (SD 4.6) kg/d days of lactation. Their data showed that sows having earlier peak feed intakes have higher average daily feed intakes and that average daily feed intake was highest for sows whose feed intake increased rapidly or gradually after farrowing with no drop in intake (Table 17.5). These sows also had the shortest weaning to conception intervals (Koketsu *et al.*, 1996a).

Although the major determinant of appetite is nutrient need, the wide variation in intakes reported in the literature reflect the moderating influence of a number of other variables.

It is well established that feeding levels in gestation affect sow feed intake during lactation (see review by Whittemore; Chapter 10). Several authors report increased overall lactation feed intakes when sows are fed *ad libitum* (Stahly *et al.*, 1979; Rudd *et al.*, 1994; Neil *et al.*, 1996b; Neil *et al.*, 1996a). The feeding of lactating sows *ad libitum* is also supported by Eastham *et al.* (1988) and Yang *et al.* (1989), who point out that even on this regimen, a degree of backfat loss is inevitable during lactation.

Increased feed intakes during lactation were reported in sows fed wet mash to appetite twice daily compared with those fed dry meal *ad libitum* (O'Grady *et al.*,

Table 17.5. Effect of pattern of feed intake in lactation on average daily feed intake, litter weaning weight and weaning to conception interval (After Koketsu et al., 1996a; Koketsu et al., 1996b)

Pattern of feed intake in lactation	Average daily feed intake (kg)	Litter weaning weight (kg)	Weaning to conception interval (d)
Feed intake increasing rapidly after weaning with no drop	$5.87 \pm .02^{2}$	$53.2 \pm .16^{2}$	6.6 ± 1.06^{2}
A major decrease of ≥ 1.8 kg/d observed relative to the previous peak level; intake remained low for ≥ 2d	$5.12 \pm .02^{2}$	$51.6 \pm .13^{3}$	6.9 ± 1.0^{2}
A minor decrease of < 1.8 kg/d observed relative to the previous peak feeding level	$5.42 \pm .02^{3}$	$53.3 \pm .14^{2}$	6.7 ± 1.01^{2}
Feed intake low throughout the lactation and did not exceed 4.5 kg/d	$3.24 \pm .08^{4}$	$51.3 \pm .66^{34}$	9.2 ± 1.07^{3}
Feed intake increased gradually during lactation with intake in the first week not exceeding 2.7 kg/d	$3.98 \pm .07^{5}$	$50.3 \pm .51^{4}$	7.9 ± 1.06^{3}
Feed intake increasing gradually with no drop. Peak at 10 d or later after farrowing	$5.91 \pm .03^{2}$	$53.6 \pm .20^{2}$	6.6 ± 1.02^{2}

^{234} Means in the same column lacking a common superscript letter differ ($P < 0.05$)

1985; Genest *et al.*, 1995) and in sows allowed to mix feed and water compared with those fed the same diet, dry (Pettigrew *et al.*, 1984). The feeding of high energy diets results in higher energy intake (Lynch, 1989), particularly when the energy is provided by fats or oils, which create less metabolic heat during digestion (Seerley, 1984; Whittemore, 1993).

17.4.3 Effects of Temperature

Increased metabolic heat production resulting from higher feed intake and the metabolic activity of milk production effectively reduces the lower critical temperature (LCT) of the sow. The zone of thermal comfort of the sow includes the range of temperatures between the LCT and the evaporative critical temperature (ECT), between which there are no extra demands for heat production and optimal feed intakes are achieved. The LCT varies widely according to sow body weight and condition and housing conditions and is considerably lower for lactating sows than for other classes of pigs. Lynch (1977) suggested that the LCT of sows in lactation ranged from 20°C to below 10°C depending on feeding levels. A more recent estimate of the lower limit to the zone of thermal comfort for the lactating sow was 12°C (Black *et al.*, 1993b). A number of authors have reported studies in which the relationship between ambient temperature and voluntary feed intake have been investigated. For example, Lynch (1977) demonstrated that for each 1°C increase in temperature between 21°C and 27°C, sows reduced feed intakes by 0.1kg/day. More recently, reductions in lactation feed intake of 0.2 kg/day per 1°C increase in environmental temperature from 18°C to 30°C were described by Stansbury *et al.* (1987). It is estimated that feed intake will be reduced by 1g for every 1°C above the LCT for every 1kg of body weight (Whittemore, 1993). Conversely, when ambient temperatures fall below the LCT homeothermy is maintained by reducing heat loss to the environment and increasing heat production through a rise in feed intake (Sorensen, 1961). Ambient temperatures above the evaporative cooling temperature (ECT) lead to a reduction in food intake, milk yield, reproductive performance and growth rate of piglets (Black *et al.*, 1993a).

17.4.4 Effects of season and photoperiod

The ancestral wild pig is a short daylength seasonal breeder with a period of anoestrous occurring during summer and autumn (Mauget 1982). The domestic pig appears to have remnants of this seasonality which is often manifested as 'summer infertility' (Love *et al.*, 1993). In many confinement management systems the sow is removed from seasonal photoperiod control as daylength is a function of the management regime. However, in less confined housing and 'outdoor' systems of sow management seasonal effects are significant (Love *et al.*, 1993). Summer infertility in pigs has been reviewed extensively by Claus *et al.*, (1985), Seren *et al* , (1987) and Love *et al.* (1993). Seasonal changes have a genetic component and the variability in expression of seasonality even in seasonally infertile sows suggests that local environmental factors such as boar presence (Bassett *et al.*, 1996) and nutrient status (Love *et al* , 1995) may be important modifiers.

For confinement systems a better understanding of the role of photoperiod and temperature on behaviour would enable controlled environments to be adjusted to optimise both sow and piglet performance. Reports on the effects of photoperiod duration on confined sows are equivocal. Both light intensity and light duration are important variables and no studies have considered both parameters in a systematic way. The most notable effect of photoperiod was reported by Stevenson *et al.*, (1983) who compared the lactation performance of sows given either <1 h or 16 h d-1 of supplemental light provided by cool white fluorescent light (32 to 266 lux). The only other light was from piglet heat lamps (<50 lux) which were on 24 hours per day. Sows given supplemental light weaned significantly heavier litters than controls (56.7 vs 53.4 kg $P<.05$) and significantly ($P<.01$) more treated sows (83%) than controls (68%) were remated by 5 d postweaning. As there were considerable differences in the light intensity at different positions in the farrowing house it was possible to regress litter weight at weaning against light intensity. Overall litter weight increased ($P<.05$) $141\pm$ 6 g for each 10 lux increase in light intensity.

Mabry *et al.* (1982b) compared the effects of a 16 h photoperiod with an 8 h photoperiod and found that piglets exposed to 16 h light suckled significantly ($P<.05$) more often than piglets exposed to 8 h light over the 24 h period. This was particularly noticeable during the 4 h periods 1600-2000 and 0800-1200 h. As a result litters exposed to a 16 h light pattern weaned significantly ($P<.05$) more pigs per litter with significantly ($P<.01$) heavier 21 d weights. Similar effects on piglet survival and growth were obtained in a second study (Mabry *et al.*, 1982a). In addition sow milk yield at day 15 of lactation was increased from 5.76 to 7.17 kg in sows subjected to the longer photoperiod. It seems likely that this effect may have resulted from sows having increased milk synthesis due to increased suckling stimulus.

In contrast, other workers have found no beneficial effect on lactation performance of extending the photoperiod (Greenberg *et al.*, 1982; Gooneratne *et al.*, 1990; Prunier *et al.*, 1994).

Few studies have investigated the hormonal status of sows subjected to different photoperiods. Neither prolactin (Cunningham *et al.*, 1981) nor FSH concentration (Prunier *et al.*, 1994) differed significantly in lactating sows subjected to an 8 or 16 h photoperiod. The latter workers found higher ($P<.001$) oestradiol -17β levels in sows on 8 h photoperiods in January but not in July.

Unfortunately, none of these studies reported on aspects of sow feeding behaviour or activity levels. Changes in either or both sow feeding behaviour and piglet suckling behaviour may be implicated in those studies where improved weaning weights were achieved. Similarly, studies of sow activity levels under different lighting conditions might provide some explanation for the reported differences in the survival rate of their piglets.

17.5 Drinking behaviour

Despite the importance of water intake for the maintenance of feed intake and milk production there is very little information available on the drinking behaviour of the sow. The onset of lactation in sows increases the demand for both water and feed immediately after farrowing (Friend, 1971). Milk contains around 80% water (range 74.2-82.9; Bowland (1966)) so a high yielding sow may need to consume up to 7 litres of water just to satisfy the demand for milk secretion. The factors affecting water demand have been reviewed by Brooks *et al.* (1990). Fraser *et al.* (1990) reviewed 12 studies of voluntary water consumption in sows. The lowest mean intake was 8.1 litres/day and the highest 25.1 litres/day with most of the studies having means in the range 13-19 litres per day. It is hardly surprising that large differences in mean values have been recorded in different experiments given the variability between animals within experiments. For example individual sow intakes ranged from 9.3 to 21.5 litres/day and 6.1 to 21.7 litres/day in the studies of Mahan (1969) and Fraser *et al.* (1989) respectively. Gill (1989) found that total water consumed (i.e. water mixed with the sow's feed plus water taken from drinkers) increased linearly up to farrowing and reached 12.2±1.1 litres on the day before parturition. On the day of farrowing water intake decreased sharply to 9.3±0.84 litres/sow. Thereafter, intake increased curvilinearly to reach a maximum of 24 litres/day 18 days post partum. The average daily water intake in this study was 18.9±0.27 litres/day. A similar pattern of water consumption has been described by Fraser *et al.* (1989).

Reduced water consumption results in increaced faecal dry matter and this in turn could predispose sows to mastitis metritis agalactia syndrome. Therefore, it is important to ensure that sows do not have restricted intakes around farrowing. Klopfenstein *et al.* (1995) investigated whether the time given to sows to adapt to a new environment and a different watering system affected water intake. In their study moving sows to farrowing accommodation 25 or 3 days prior to farrowing had no effect on water intake. However, they found that the average daily water consumption of most sows dropped drastically at farrowing and remained lower than the late gestation level for the first 3-4 days following parturition.

The study of Fraser *et al.* (1989) is interesting in that a very strong positive relationship was found between water intake of sows in the first three days after birth and piglet weight gain over the same period. Another interesting finding in this study was the relationship between the amount of time that the sow was active and water consumption (Table 17.6). This may imply that the time the newly farrowed sow allows for drinking is limited.

Table 17.6. Percentage of time spent active (standing and sitting) and water intake during the 24 h before and the 72 h after the start of farrowing (Fraser et al., 1989)

Time relative to farrowing	Percent time spent active (mean and range)	Water intake (l) (mean and range)	r^2
24 h before	30.5 (22.4-42.8)	12.8 (5.6-24.1)	0.63
1-24 h after	5.1 (1.5-14.9)	4.9 (0.0-15.7)	0.71
25-48 h after	6.5 (1.8-15.3)	8.4 (1.0-21.2)	0.92
49-72 h after	8.2 (2.7-15.3)	10.9 (3.2-20.0)	0.58

17.6 Sexual behaviour

17.6.1 Post partum oestrus

Oestrous cycling and sexual behaviour are normally suppressed in the lactating sow. Studies published in the 1950's indicated that a postpartum oestrus occurred in 50-99% of sows (Warnick *et al.*, 1950; Burger, 1952; Baker *et al.*, 1953; Self *et al.*, 1958) but that this was anovulatory except in the unusual circumstance that the piglets died or were removed at birth (Warnick *et al.*, 1950). However, no recent studies have made reference to the occurrence of postpartum oestrus in sows, even when the sows were group housed during lactation. Therefore, it must be questioned whether the sows reportedly showing postpartum oestrus in the 1950's were isolated cases or whether the tendency to show postpartum oestrus has been lost in modern genotypes.

17.6.2 Lactational oestrus

In theory, sow productivity could be increased if lactational anoestrous could be overcome and the sow successfully mated while still lactating. However, to be a viable alternative management strategy lactational oestrus would have to occur:

- in a high percentage of sows;
- at a predictable time after parturition;
- at an earlier time post partum than the normal post weaning oestrus.

In addition the survival rate and growth of the litter being suckled would have to be maintained and the size and viability of the succeeding litter would not have to be compromised.

As the process of lactation suppresses oestrus (Edwards, 1982) a number of workers have investigated the effect of reducing the suckling stimulus by 'partial weaning', that is removing the piglets from the sow for a portion of the day, and allowing pheromonal stimulation by providing daily contact with a mature boar (Smith, 1961; Cole *et al.*, 1972; Henderson *et al.*, 1984; Stevenson *et al.*, 1984; Newton *et al.*, 1987; Costa *et al.*, 1995) and additionally treatment with exogenous hormones (Crighton, 1970; Guthrie *et al.*, 1978; Hausler *et al.*, 1980; Cox *et al.*, 1982; Costa *et al.*, 1995). Although all these techniques have resulted in a limited number of animals ovulating during lactation they have not produced management practices that are worthy of commercial adoption.

Commercial herds have been observed in which sows did return to oestrus during long lactations (Table 17.7). Although a high incidence of lactational oestrus was recorded the sows that did conceive did so following a longer period post partum than would normally be expected for sows weaned at four weeks of age or less.

Table 17.7. Characteristics of sows showing lactational oestrus on two commercial farms

	(Rowlinson *et al.*, 1974)	(Petchey *et al.*, 1979)
Length of lactation (d)	46.3 ± 0.5	53.3 ± 0.7
Sows showing lactational oestrus (%)	49	100
Conception rate of sows mated during oestrus (%)	78	85
Farrowing to mating interval (d)	40.3 ± 1.81	35.5 ± 0.47

Three features of these farms appeared crucial to their success in stimulating oestrus in lactation. First, the sows were allowed to lactate for longer (45-55 days) than is allowed in most current commercial practice. Secondly, the sows were group housed during lactation with a mature boar present. Thirdly, they were provided with generous feeding which minimised weight loss.

Subsequent studies conducted under experimental conditions have confirmed that high incidences of lactational oestrus are only achieved if all three of these features are present. (Petchey *et al.*, 1980; Rowlinson *et al.*, 1981; Rowlinson *et al.*, 1982; Bryant *et al.*, 1983a). Although these techniques were capable of inducing lactational oestrus, there were a number of reasons why they did not find favour with producers. First, the costs involved and the management problems posed were too great. Secondly, they did not produce any increase in annual sow output compared with conventional management with weaning at 3-4 weeks of age. Thirdly, piglet growth performance was inferior and weaning weight was more variable than that of piglets reared in farrowing crates.

Some interest in lactational oestrus has been rekindled as a result of welfare concerns about restraining sows in farrowing crates for the duration of lactation. A desire to develop more welfare friendly housing systems has again led to sows being housed in more complex social environments with the result that some of the sows demonstrate oestrus (Henderson *et al.*, 1989; Stolba *et al.*, 1990; Hulten *et al.*, 1995a). However, in many cases this may reflect poor mothering and suckling behaviour on the part of the sow which reduces the suckling stimulus that she receives and hence removes the lactational inhibition of oestrus cyclicity.

Grouping sows during lactation seems to have little or no effect on sow feed intake (Bryant *et al.*, 1983b; Bryant *et al.*, 1984).

17.6.3 Interrelationships between suckling behaviour and lactational oestrus.

As indicated in the foregoing section lactational oestrus may be a consequence of reduced suckling stimulus. This may occur in one of three ways

- sows suckling small litters (as a result of post partum losses) may receive insufficient physiological stimulus to maintain lactation
- sows may abandon their piglets leaving other sows in the group to suckle them (in this situation the sow effectively weans herself early) (Boe, 1994)
- sows may reduce suckling stimulus by preventing access to their udders by sternal lying (Gotz, 1991) or by absenting themselves from their piglets (even though not abandoning them) in housing systems where the piglets are retained in nest areas by barriers (Boe, 1993; Hulten *et al.*, 1995b; Rantzer *et al.*, 1995b).

In the first of these situations there is no obvious behavioural component. In the other two the behaviour of the sow is instrumental in producing the effect. In both cases the sow may be motivated to the action as an escape from the constant attentions of her piglets (Jensen, 1988; De Passille *et al.*,1989). This behaviour parallels that of wild pigs where the sow increasingly absents herself from her piglets as lactation progresses (Mauget, 1982).

Grouping sows during lactation does result in some disruption of the normal suckling pattern. Bryant and Rowlinson (1984) found that true nursing was inhibited for a period after grouping ranging from 2.5 to 7.5 h in individual sows but that suckling frequency recovered thereafter to pregrouping levels. The incidence of false nursings increased following grouping and remained higher. In a comparison of group and individually housed sows it was found that nursing frequency was very similar as was the degree of synchronisation of suckling by sows sharing the same environment. However, the incidence of false nursings was much higher in the grouped sows (Bryant *et al.*, 1983b).

Group housing of lactating sows facilitates cross suckling by their piglets (Bryant *et al.*, 1983b; Bryant *et al.*, 1984; Algers, 1991; Wattanakul *et al.*, 1997). Algers (1991) found that about 30% of the piglets in the group housing system nursed sows other than their mother but only about 3% of the piglets totally abandoned their own mother for other sows. However, cross suckling could be seen as a mechanism by which less advantaged piglets could avail themselves of a better milk supply from a sow other than their dam. This would only be the case though, if the receiving sow had a spare teat, and this provided a superior milk supply to the teat abandoned on the natural mother. This is rarely the case. Furthermore, the alien pig still has to gain access to the teat of another sow and the more dominant piglets still outcompete the weaker pigs in the group (Braun *et al.*, 1988). This may help explain why the piglets of group housed sows have significantly poorer daily gain and higher consumption of creep feed prior to weaning (Rantzer *et al.*, 1995a). In addition the piglets of group housed sows in Rantzer's (1995a) study showed a dominance of haemolytic *E.coli* in rectal swabs at weaning indicating that the weaning process may already have begun. Thus although cross suckling may benefit some dominant individuals it may actually reduce the milk supply to the weaker pigs and result in reduced total milk output by the group of sows, as less productive teats are rejected, and atrophy due to the lack of stimulation of being suckled (Hulten *et al.*, 1995b).

Hulten (1997) studied the performance of sows and litters in commercial units where group housing was practised from about two weeks of lactation. Piglet mortality in the litters of multiparous sows was higher (6.5%) in the group housing period than for comparable litters of sows which were individually housed (1.4%). In primiparous sows housing system had no significant effect on mortality. Similarly, preweaning atrophy of mammary glands did not occur in primiparous sows (Hulten *et al.*, 1995b). These results suggest that the relationship between primiparous sows and their litters are not affected by group housing whereas the relationships between multiparous sows and their litters are.

17.7 Conclusions

This review has demonstrated that the success of the sow in rearing her litter to weaning is determined by a complex and interrelated series of behaviours. Many of these act through nutrition. Mothering and suckling behaviour in the perinatal period influence the success of the piglet in obtaining its first suckle, vital for the acquisition of both immunity and nutrients. Subsequently, the suckling behaviour of the sow affects the nutrient supply and thereby the growth of the piglet.

The feeding, drinking and sexual behaviour of lactating sows can have a significant effect on their nutrient intake, which in turn determines the quantity and quality of milk produced and hence the nutrients available to their piglets. The differences in behaviour of individuals and hence rearing success are considerable, even in systems of housing where sows are confined in farrowing crates. When sows are confined in farrowing crates sow temperament and mothering behaviour have less effect on the sow's success in rearing piglets and the interventions of the stockperson in the process assume greater importance. With consumer antagonism to confinement systems mounting, researchers and pig producers are actively seeking alternative forms of housing. There is renewed interest in loose and group housing of lactating sows. In such systems sow temperament and mothering behaviour are important components of success.

Our understanding of the reproductive physiology and nutrition of the sow has increased greatly in recent years and the housing systems that have been adopted have provided opportunities to exploit that knowledge. If, as seems likely, consumer concerns move the pig industry towards less confined systems of housing for lactating sows it will be essential to gain further insights into the contribution that different behaviours make to rearing success. Unless we can understand how lactation behaviour is, and can be influenced by the sow's environment, we will be unable to design housing systems and identify genetic selection criteria which will enable us to capitalise on our understanding of the sow's physiology and biochemistry. Future advances in sow management may depend less on the physiologist and the biochemist and more upon the research of the ethologist studying the sow and the psychologist studying the stockperson.

17.8 References

Algers, B. 1991., Group housing of farrowing sows. Health aspects on a new system. 7th International Congress on Animal Hygiene, Leipzig. 851-857.

Algers, B. & P. Jensen, 1985. Communication during suckling in the domestic pig. Effects of continuous noise. Appl. Anim. Behav. Sci. 14, 49-61.

Algers, B. & P. Jensen, 1990a. Thermal micro-climate in winter farrowing nests of free ranging domestic pigs. Livest. Prod. Sci. 25, 177-181.

Algers, B., S. Rojanasthien & K. Uvnas-Moberg, 1990b. The relationship between teat stimulation, oxytocin release and grunting rate in the sow during nursing. Appl. Anim. Behav. Sci. 26, 267-276.

Anderson, C.J.M., P.R. English, S.A. Edwards & O. MacPherson, 1990. Evaluation of different suckling strategies in lactation. Anim. Prod. 1990, 570-571 (Abstr.).

Arey, D.S. & E.S. Sancha, 1996. Behaviour and productivity of sows and piglets in a family system and in farrowing crates. Appl. Anim. Behav. Sci. 50, 135-145.

Auldist, D.E. & R.H. King, 1995. Piglets' role in determining milk production in the sow. 5th Biennial Conference of the Australasian Pig Science Association, Canberra, ACT, Australasian Pig Science Association, Werribee, Australia. 114-118.

Baker, L.N., H.L. Woehling, L.E. Casida & R.H. Grummer, 1953. Occurrence of oestrus in sows following parturition. J. Anim. Sci. 12, 33-38.

Barber, R.S., R. Braude & K.G. Mitchell, 1955. Studies on milk production of large white pigs. J. Agric. Sci. 46, 97-118.

Bassett, J.M., C.J. Bray & C.E. Sharpe, 1996. Summer infertility in outdoor sows: Lessons from studies on 'seasonally barren' sows. Pig J. 36, 65-85.

Baxter, M.R. 1980. The effect of restraint on parturition in the sow. International Pig Veterinary Society Congress, Copenhagen, Denmark. pp.84.

Black, J.L., B.P. Mullan, M.L. Lorschy & L.R. Giles, 1993a. Lactation in the sow during heat stress. Livest. Prod. Sci. 35, 153-170.

Black, J.L., B.P. Mullan, M.L. Lorschy & L.R. Giles, 1993b. Lactation in the sow during heat stress. Livest. Prod. Sci. 35, 153-170.

Blackshaw, J.K., A.W. Blackshaw, F.J. Thomas & F.W. Newman, 1994. Comparison of behaviour patterns of sows & litters in a farrowing crate and a farrowing pen. Appl. Anim. Behav. Sci. 39, 281-295.

Boe, K., 1993. Maternal behaviour of lactating sows in a loose housing system. Appl. Anim. Behav. Sci. 35, 327- 338.

Boe, K., 1994. Variation in maternal behavioural and production of sows in integrated loose housing systems in Norway. Appl. Anim. Behav. Sci. 41, 53-62.

Bowland, J.P., 1966. Swine-milk composition - a summary. In: Swine in biomedical research, Bustad, L.K., R.O. McClellan & M.P. Burns (eds.) Pacific Northwest laboratory, Richland, Washington. pp 97.
Braun, S. & P. Jensen, 1988. Cross-suckling in piglets in loose-housed sow groups or what makes a piglet become a cuckoo. International Congress on Applied Ethology in Farm Animals, Skara, Sweden.
Brooks, P.H., 1989. Opportunities for improving the survival rate of piglets by nutritional means. F.Hoffmann-La Roche, Basel, Switzerland. 27.
Brooks, P.H. & J.L. Carpenter, 1990. The water requirement of growing-finishing pigs - Theoretical and practical considerations. In: Recent advances in animnal nutrition - 1990, Haresign W. & D.J.A. Cole (eds). Butterworths, London. pp. 115-136.
Bryant, M.J. & P. Rowlinson, 1984. Nursing and suckling behaviour of sows and their litters before and after grouping in multi-accommodation pens. Anim. Prod. 38, 277-282.
Bryant, M.J., G. Palmer, D.J. Petherick & P. Rowlinson, 1983a. Lactational oestrus in the sow. 4. Variation in the incidence and timing of lactational oestrus in groups of sows. Anim. Prod. 36, 453-460.
Bryant, M.J., P. Rowlinson & H.A.M. Van der Steen, 1983b. A comparison of the nursing and suckling behaviour of group- and individually-housed sows and their litters. Anim. Prod. 36, 445-451.
Buchenauer, D., C. Luft & A. Grauvogl, 1982/83. Investigations on the Eliminative Behaviour of Piglets. Appl. Anim. Ethol. 9, 153-164.
Burger, J.F., 1952. Sex physiology of pigs. Onderstepoort J. Vet. Res. Supplement 2, 3-218.
Burke, J., P.H. Brooks, J.A. Kirk & J.C. Eddison, 1997. Feeding strategies and daily feed intakes of group housed sows fed ad libitum from 5 days before until 5 days after parturition. ISAE Winter Meeting 1997, London.
Castren, H., B. Algers, A.M. de Passille, J. Rushen, & K. Uvnas-Moberg, 1993. Early milk ejection, prolonged parturition and periparturient oxytocin release in the pig. Anim. Prod. 57, 465-471.
Castren, H., B. Algers, & P. Jensen, 1989a. Occurrence of unsuccessful sucklings in newborn piglets in a semi- natural environment. Appl. Anim. Behav. Sci. 23, 61-73.
Castren, H., B. Algers, P. Jensen, & H. Saloniemi, 1989b. Suckling behaviour and milk consumption in new born piglets as a response to sow grunting. Appl. Anim. Behav. Sci. 24, 227-238.
Claus, R. & U. Weiler, 1985. Influence of light and photoperiodicity on pig prolificacy. J. Reprod. Fert. (Supplement 33), 185-197.
Cole, D.J.A., P.H. Brooks & R.M. Kay, 1972. Lactational oestrus in the sow. Vet. Rec. 90, 681-683.
Costa, A.N. & M.A. Varley, 1995. The effects of altered suckling intensity, boar exposure in lactation and gonadotropins on endocrine changes, fertility and the incidence of lactational oestrus in multiparous sows. Anim. Sci. 60, 485-492.
Cox, N.M. & J.H. Britt, 1982. Pulsatile administration of gonadotrophin releasiong hormone to lactating sows: endocrine changes associated with the induction of fertile oestrus. Biol. Reprod. 27, 1126-1137.
Crighton, D.B. 1970, Induction of pregnancy during lactation in the sow. J. Reprod. Fert. 22, 223-231.
Cronin, G.M. & G. van Amerongen, 1991. The effects of modifying the farrowing environment on sow behaviour and survival and growth of piglets. Appl. Anim. Behav. Sci. 30, 287-298.
Csermely, D. & D.G.M. Wood-Gush, 1990. Agonistic behaviour in grouped sows, II. How social rank affects feeding and drinking behaviour. Boll. Zool. 57, 55-58.

Cunningham, F.L., R.R. Kraeling, G.B. Rampacek, J.W. Mabry & T.E. Kiser, 1981. The effect of photoperiod on serum prolactin concentrations in the lactating sow. J. Anim. Sci. 45 (Supplement 1), 21 (Abstr).
De Haer, L.M.C. & J.W.M. Merks, 1992. Patterns of daily food intake in growing pigs. Anim. Prod. 54, 95-104.
De Passille, A.M.B. & S. Robert, 1989a. Behaviour of lactating sows: Influence of stage of lactation and husbandry practices at weaning. Appl. Anim. Behav. Sci. 23, 315-329.
De Passille, A.M.B. & J. Rushen, 1989b. Suckling and teat disputes by neonatal piglets. Appl. Anim. Behav. Sci. 22, 23-38.
De Passille, A.M.B., J. Rushen & G. Pellether, 1988. Sucking behaviour and serum immunoglobulin levels in neonatal piglets. Anim. Prod. 47, 447-456.
Dividich, J. & J. Noblet, 1981. Colostrum intake and thermoregulation in the neonatal pig in relation to environmental temperature. Biol. Neonate 40, 167-174.
Dourmad, J.Y., 1993. Standing and feeding behaviour of the lactating sow: Effect of feeding level during pregnancy. Appl. Anim. Behav. Sci. 37, 311-319.
Eastham P., W.C. Smith & C.T. Whittemore, 1988. Responses of the lactating sow to food level. Anim. Prod. 46, 543-547.
Eddison, J.C. & N.E. Roberts, 1995. Variability in feeding behaviour of group housed sows using electronic feeders. Anim. Sci. 60, 307-314.
Edwards, S. 1982. The endocrinology of the post-partum sow. In: Control of pig reproduction. Cole, D.J.A.& G.R. Foxcroft (eds.).Butterworths, London. pp. 439-458.
Edwards, S.A. 1987. The effect of straw bedding on the behaviour of sows and their new born piglets. Appl. Anim. Behav. Sci. 17, 365-366.
Edwards, S.A. & S.J. Furniss, 1988. The effects of straw in crated farrowing systems on peripartal behaviour of sows and piglets. Br. Vet. J. 144, 139-146.
Edwards, S.A, W.J. Smith, C. Fordyce & F. MacMenemy, 1994. An analysis of the causes of piglet mortality in a breeding herd kept outdoors. Vet. Rec. 135, 324-327.
Ellendorf, F., M.L. Forsling & D.A. Poulain, 1982. The milk ejection reflex in the pig. J. Physiol. 333, 577-594.
England, D.C. 1986. Improving sow efficiency by management to enhance the opportunity for nutritional intake by neonatal piglets. J. Anim. Sci. 63, 1297-1306.
English, P.R. 1969. Mortality and variation in growth of piglets: A study of predisposing factors with particular reference to sow and piglet behaviour. PhD Thesis, University of Aberdeen.
English, P.R., W.J. Smith & A. MacLean 1982a. The sow: Improving her efficiency. Farming Press Ltd, Ipswich. 2nd, ed. pp. 354.
English, P.R. & V. Wilkinson, 1982b. Management of the sow and litter in late pregnancy and lactaion in relation to piglet survival and growth. In: Control of pig reproduction, Cole, D.J.A. & G.R. Foxcroft (eds.). Butterworths, London. pp. 479-506.
Fraser, D., 1980. A review of the behavioural mechanism of milk ejection of the domestic pig. Appl. Anim. Ethol. 6, 247-255.
Fraser, D., 1984. Some factors influencing the availability of colostrum to piglets. Anim. Prod. 39, 115-123.
Fraser, D., J.F. Patience, P.A. Phillips & J.M. McCleese, 1990. Water for piglets and lactating sows: quantity quality and quandries. In: Recent advances in animal nutrition 1990, Haresign W. & D.J.A. Cole (eds.). Butterwoths, London. pp. 137-160.
Fraser, D. & P.A. Phillips, 1989. Lethargy and low water intake by sows during early lactation: A cause of low piglet weight gains and survival? Appl. Anim. Behav. Sci. 24, 13-22.
Fraser, D. & B.K. Thompson, 1979a. The teat order of suckling pigs. III. Relation to competition within litters. J. Agric. Sci. 92, 257-261.
Fraser, D., B.K. Thompson, D.K. Ferguson & R.L. Darroch, 1979b. The 'teat order' of suckling pigs. J. Agric. Sci. 92, 257-261.

Friend, D.W., 1971. Self-selection of feeds and water by swine during pregnancy and lactation. J. Anim. Sci. 32, 658- 666

Genest, M. & S. D'Allaire, 1995. Feeding strategies during the lactation period for first parity sows. Can. J. Anim. Sci. 75, 461-467.

Gill, B.P., 1989. Water use by pigs managed under various conditions of housing feeding and management. PhD Thesis, University of Plymouth.

Gooneratne, A.D. & P.A. Thacker, 1990. Influence of an extended photoperiod on sow and letter performance. Livest. Prod. Sci. 24, 83-88.

Gotz, M., 1991. Changes in nursing and suckling behaviour of sows and their piglets in farrowing crates. Appl. Anim. Behav. Sci. 31, 271-275

Graves, H.B., 1984. Behaviour and ecology of wild and feral swine (Sus scrofa). J. Anim. Sci. 58, 482-492.

Greenberg, L.G. & J.P. Mahone, 1982. Failure of a 16h L: 8h D photoperiod to influence lactation or reproductive efficiency in sows. Can. J. Anim. Sci. 62, 141-145.

Gundlach, V.H., 1968. Brutfursorge, Brutpflege, Verhaltensontogenese und Tagesperiodik beim Europaischen Wildschwein (Sus scrofa L.). Zeit. Tierpsychol. 25, 955-995.

Guthrie, H.D., V.G. Pursel & L.T. Frobish, 1978. Attempts to induce conception in lactating sows. J. Anim. Sci. 47, 1145-1151.

Hansen, K.E. & S.E. Curtis, 1981. Prepartal activity of sows in stall or pen. J. Anim. Sci. 51, 456-460.

Handley, G., R.H. King & A.K. King, 1996. The voluntary food intake of lactating sows in five commercial herds. In: Manipulating pig production V. Hemery, D.P. & P.D Cranwell (eds.). Australasian Pig Science Association, Canberra. pp. 127 (Abstr).

Hartstock, T.G. & H.B. Graves, 1976. Neonatal behaviour and nutrition-related mortality in domestic swine. J. Anim. Sci. 42, 235-241.

Hartstock, T.G., H.B. Graves & B.R. Baumgardt, 1977. Agonistic behaviour and the nursing order in suckling piglets: relationships with survival, growth and body composition. J. Anim. Sci. 44, 320-330.

Hausler, C.L., H.H. Hodson, D.C. Kuo, T.J. Kinney, V.A. Rauwolf, & L.E. Strack, 1980. Induced ovulation and conception in lactating sows. J. Anim. Sci. 50, 773-778.

Henderson, R. & P.E. Hughes, 1984. The effects of partial weaning, movement and boar contact on the subsequent reproductive performance of lactating sows. Anim. Prod. 39, 131-135.

Henderson, R. & A. Stolba, 1989. Incidence of oestrus and oestrous trends in lacating sows housed in different social and physical environments. Appl. Anim. Behav. Sci. 22, 235-244.

Herskin, M.S., K.H. Jensen & K. Thodberg, 1997. Influence of environmental stimuli on maternal behaviour related to bonding, reactivity and crushing of piglets in domestic sows. 31st International Congress of the International Society for Applied Ethology, Prague.

Horrell, I. & J. Hodgson, 1992. The Basis of sow-piglet identification. 1. The identification by sows of their own piglets and the presence of intruders. Appl. Anim. Behav. Sci. 33, 319-327.

Houwers, H.W.J., R.G. Bure & P. Koomans, 1992. Behaviour of sows in a free acsess farrowing section. Farm. Build Prog. 109 (July), 9-11.

Hulten, F., A.M. Dalin, N. Lundheim & S. Einarsson, 1995a. Ovulation frequency among sows group-housed during late lactation. Anim. Reprod. Sci. 39, 223-233.

Hulten, F., A.M. Dalin, N. Lundheim & S. Einarsson, 1995b. A field study on group housing of lactating sows with special reference to sow health at weaning. Acta Vet. Scand. 36, 201-212.

Hulten, F., A.M. Dalin, N. Lundheim & S. Einarsson, 1997. Pre- and post-weaning piglet performance, sow food intake and change in backfat thickness in a group-housing system for lactating sows. Acta Vet. Scand. 38, 119-133.

Jensen, P., 1986a. Observations on the Maternal Behaviour of Free Ranging Domestic Pigs. Appl. Anim. Behav. Sci. 16, 131-142.
Jensen, P., 1988. Maternal behaviour and mother-young interactions during lactation in free ranging domestic pigs. Appl. Anim. Behav. Sci. 20, 297-308.
Jensen, P. & B. Algers, 1983/84. An ethogram of piglet vocalisations during suckling. Appl. Anim. Ethol. 11, 237- 248.
Jensen, P. & B. Recen, 1989. When to wean - Observations from free ranging domestic pigs. Appl. Anim. Behav. Sci. 23, 49-60.
Jensen, P. & I. Redbo, 1987. Behaviour during nest leaving in free ranging domestic pigs. Appl. Anim. Behav. Sci. 18, 355-362.
Jensen, P., G. Stangel & B. Algers, 1991. Nursing and suckling behaviour of semi-naturally kept pigs during the first 10 days postpartum. Appl. Anim. Behav. Sci. 31, 195-209.
King, R.H., B.P. Mullan, F.R. Dunshea & H. Dove, 1997. The influence of piglet body weight on milk production of sows. Livest. Prod. Sci. 47, 169-174.
Klopfenstein C., S. D'Allaire & G.P. Martineau, 1995. Effect of adaptation to the farrowing crate on water intake of sows. Livest. Prod. Sci. 43, 243-252.
Koketsu, Y., G.D. Dial, J.E. Pettigrew & V.L. King, 1996a. Feed intake pattern during lactation and subsequent reproductive performance of sows. J. Anim. Sci. 74, 2875-2884.
Koketsu, Y., G.D. Dial, J.E. Pettigrew, W.E. Marsh & V.L. King, 1996b. Characterization of feed intake patterns during lactation in commercial swine herds. J. Anim. Sci. 74, 1202-1210.
Lammers, G.J. & A. De Lange, 1986. Pre and post farrowing behaviour in primiparous domesticated pigs. Appl. Anim. Behav. Sci. 15, 31-43.
Lewis, N.J. & J.F. Hurnik, 1985. The development of nursing behaviour in swine. Appl. Anim. Behav. Sci. 14, 225-232.
Lewis, N.J. & J.F. Hurnik, 1986. An approach response of piglets to the sows nursing vocalisations. Can. J. Anim. Sci. 66, 537-539.
Love, R.J., G. Evans & C. Klupiec, 1993. Seasonal effects on fertility in gilts and sows. J. Reprod. Fert. Suppl. 48, 191-206.
Love, R.J., C. Klupiec, E.J. Thornton & G. Evans, 1995. An interaction between feeding rate and season affects fertility of sows. Anim. Reprod. Sci. 39, 275-284.
Lynch, P.B., 1977. Effect of environmental temperature on lactating sows and their litters. Ir. J. Agric. Res. 16, 2610- 2616.
Lynch, P.B. 1989. Voluntary food intake of sows and gilts. In: The voluntary food intake of pigs. Forbes, J.M., M.A. Varley & T.L.J. Lawrence (eds.). Br. Soc. of An. Prod., Edinburgh.
McBride, G., 1963. The 'teat order' and communication in young pigs. Anim. Behav. 11, 53-56.
Mabry, J.W., M.T. Coffey & R.W. Seerley, 1983. A comparison of an 8 vs 16 hour photoperiod during lactation on suckling frequency of the baby pig and maternal performance of the sow. J. Anim. Sci. 57, 292-295.
Mabry, J.W., F.L. Cunningham, R.R. Kraeling & G.B. Rampacek 1982. The effect of artificailly extended photoperiod during lactation on maternal performance of the sow. J. Anim. Sci. 54, 918-921.
Mahan D.C., 1969. Nitrogen and water metabolism in the lactating sow. PhD Thesis, University of Illinois, Urbana.
Martin, J.E. & S.A. Edwards, 1994. Feeding behaviour of outdoor sows: The effects of diet quality and type. Appl. Anim. Behav. Sci. 41, 63-74.
Mauget, R., 1981. Behavioural and reproductive strategies in wild forms of Sus scrofa (European wild boar and feral pigs). In: The welfare of pigs. Sybesma, W. (ed.). Martinus Nijhoff, The Hague.

Mauget, R., 1982. Seasonality of reproduction in the wild boar. In: Control of pig reproduction. Cole D.J.A. & G.R. Foxcroft (eds.). Butterworths, London. pp 509-526.
Moser, B.D. 1983. The use of fat in sow diets. In: Recent Advances in Animal Nutrition - 1983. Haresign, W. (ed.). Butterworths, London. pp.71-80.
Mullan, B.P., W.H. Close & D.J.A. Cole, 1990. Predicting nutrient responses of the lactating sow. In: Recent advances in animal nutrition, Haresign, W. & D.J.A. Cole (eds.). Butterworths, London. pp 332-346.
NCR-89 Committee on Confinement Management of Swine, 1990. Feeding frequency and the addition of sugar to the diet for the lacating sow. J. Anim. Sci. 68, 3498-3501.
Neil, M. & B. Ogle, 1996a. A two-diet system and ad libitum lactation feeding of the sow 1. Sow performance. Anim. Sci. 62, 337-347.
Neil, M. & B. Ogle, 1996b. A two-diet system and ad libitum lactation feeding of the sow 2. Litter size and piglet performance. Anim. Sci. 62, 349-354.
Newberry, R.C. & D.G.M. Wood-Gush, 1984. The Suckling Behaviour of Domestic Pigs in a Semi- Natural Environment. Behav. 95, 11-25.
Newton, E.A., J.S. Stevensonn & D.L. Davis, 1987. Influence of duration of litter separation and boar exposure on estrous expression of sows during and after lactation. J. Anim. Sci. 65, 1500-1506.
Nielsen, B.L., 1995. Feeding behaviour of growing pigs: effects of the social and physical environment. PhD Thesis, University of Edinburgh.
O'Grady, J.F., P.B. Lynch & P.A. Kearney, 1985. Voluntary feed intake by lactating sows. Livest. Prod. Sci. 12, 355- 365.
Petchey, A.M. & P.R. English, 1980. A note on the effects of of boar presence on the performance of sows and their litters when penned in groups in late lactation. Anim. Prod. 32, 107-109.
Petchey, A.M. & G.M. Jolly, 1979. Sow service in lactation: an analysis of data from one herd. Anim. Prod. 29, 183-191.
Petersen, V., 1994. The development of feeding and investigatory behaviour in free-ranging domestic pigs during their first 18 weeks of life. Appl. Anim. Behav. Sci. 42, 87-98.
Petersen, V., B. Recen & K. Vestergaard, 1990. Behaviour of sows and piglets during farrowing under free range conditions. Appl. Anim. Behav. Sci. 26, 169-179.
Petherick, J.C., 1982. A note on the space use for excretory behaviour of suckling piglets. Appl. Anim. Ethol. 9, 367-371.
Pettigrew, J.E., R.L. Moser, S.G. Cornelious & K.P. Miller, 1984. Feed consumption by lactating sows as affected by feeder design and corn particle size. J. Anim. Sci. 61 (Suppl 1), 107 (Abstr).
Prunier A., J.Y. Dourmad & M. Etienne, 1994. Effect of light regimen under various ambient temperatures on sow and litter performance. J. Anim. Sci. 72, 1461-1466.
Randall, G.C.B., 1972. Observations on Parturition in the sow. I.Factors associated with the delivery of the piglets and their subsequent behaviour. Vet. Rec. 90, 178-182.
Rantzer, D., J. Svendsen & B. Westrom, 1995a. Weaning of pigs raised in sow-controlled and in conventional housing systems. 1. Description of systems, production and bacteriology. Swed. J. Agric. Res. 25, 37-46.
Rantzer, D., J. Svendson & B. Westrom, 1995b. Weaning of pigs raised in sow-controlled and in conventional housing systems. 2. Behaviour studies and cortisol levels. Swed. J. Agric. Res. 25, 61-71.
Rohde Parfet, K.A. & H.W. Gonyou, 1991. Attraction of newborn piglets to auditory, visual, olfactory and tactile stimuli. J. Anim. Sci. 69, 125-133.
Rosillon-Warnier, A. & R. Paquay, 1984. Development and consequences of teat-order in piglets. Appl. Anim. Behav. Sci. 13, 47-58.
Rowlinson, P., M.J. Bryant & H.G. Boughton, 1974. Sows mated during lactation: observations from a commercial unit. Proc. Br. Soc. Anim. Prod. 3, 93 (Abst).

Rowlinson, P. & M.J. Bryant, 1981. Lactational oestrus in the sow. 1. The effect of interval between farrowing and grouping on the incidence and timing of lactational oestrus in sows. Anim. Prod. 32, 315-323.
Rowlinson, P. & M.J. Bryant, 1982. Lactational oestrus in the sow. 2. The influence of group-housing, boar presence and feeding level upon the occurrence of oestrus in lactating sows. Anim. Prod. 34, 283-290.
Rudd, A.R. & P.H. Simmins, 1994. Consequences of diet fed ad libitum to the farrowing and lactating crated sow. Anim. Prod. 58, 465-466 (Abst).
Schouten, W.G.P., 1986. Rearing conditions and behaviour of pigs. PhD Thesis, Landbouwhogeschool te Wageningen, NL.
Seerley, R.W., 1984. The best use of fats in sow diets. In: Fats in animal nutrition, Wiseman, J. (ed.) Butterworths, London. pp. 333-352.
Self, H.L. & R.H. Grummer, 1958. The rate and economy of pig gains and the reproductive behaviour in sows when litters are weaned at 10 days, 21 days or 56 days of age. J. Anim. Sci. 17, 862-868.
Seren, E. & M. Mattioli, 1987. Definition of the summer infertility problem in the pig. Commission of the European Communities, Brussels. pp.162.
Smith, D.M. 1961. The effect of daily separation of sows from their litters upon milk yields, creep intake and energetic efficiency. N. Z. J. Agric. Res. 4, 232-245.
Sorensen, P.H., 1961. Influence of climatic environment on pig performance. In: Nutrition of pigs and poultry. Morgan, J.T. & D. Lewis (eds.). Butterworths, London. pp. 88-103.
Spinka, M. & B. Algers, 1995. Functional view on udder massage after milk let-down in pigs. Appl. Anim. Behav. Sci. 43, 197-212.
Spinka, M., G. Illmann, B. Algers & Z. Stetkova, 1997. The role of nursing frequency in milk production in domestic pigs. J. Anim. Sci. 75, 1223-1228.
Stahly, T.S., G.L. Cromwell & W.S. Simpson, 1979. Effects of full vs restricted feeding of the sow immediately postpartum on lactation performance. J. Anim. Sci. 49, 50-54.
Stangel, G. & P. Jensen, 1991. Behaviour of semi-naturally kept sows and piglets (except suckling) during 10 days post partum. Appl. Anim. Behav. Sci. 31, 211-227.
Stansbury, W.F., J.J. McGlone & L.F. Tribble, 1987. Effects of season, floor type, air temperature and snout coolers on sow and litter performance. J. Anim. Sci. 65, 1507-1513.
Stephens, D.B., 1971. The metabolic rates of newborn pigs in relation to floor insulation and ambient temperature. Anim. Prod. 13, 303-313.
Stevenson, J.S. & D.L. Davis, 1984. Influence of reduced litter size and daily litter separation on fertility of sows at 2 to 5 weeks postpartum. J. Anim. Sci. 59, 284-293.
Stevenson, J.S., D.S. Pollman, D.L. Davis & J.P. Murphy, 1983. Influence of supplemental light on sow performance during and after lactation. J. Anim. Sci. 56, 1282-1286.
Stolba, A., R. Henderson & B. Wechsler, 1990. The influence of different social and physical environments on the incidence of lactational oestrus in sows. Appl. Anim. Behav. Sci. 27, 269-276.
Teilland, P., 1986. Strategies alimentaires et statu social chez le sanglier en capivite. Behavioural Processes 12, 327-347.
Warnick, A.C., L.E. Casida & R.H. Grummer, 1950. The occurence of estrus and ovulation in post partum sows. J. Anim. Sci. 9, 60-72.
Wattanakul, W., W. Sinclair, A.H. Stewart, S.A. Edwards & P.R. English, 1997. Performance and behaviour of lactating sows and piglets in crate and multisuckling systems: A study involving European White and Manor Meishan genotypes. Anim. Sci. 64, 339-349.
Weary, D.M. & D. Fraser, 1995. Calling by Domestic Piglets: Reliable Signs of Need? Anim. Behav. 50, 1047- 1055.
Weary, D.M., G.L. Lawson & B.K. Thompson, 1996. Sows show stronger responses to isolation calls of piglets associated with greater levels of piglet need. Anim. Behav. 52, 1247-1253.

Weary, D.M., S. Ross & D. Fraser, 1997. Vocalisations by isolated piglets: a reliable indicator of piglet need directed towards the sow. Appl. Anim. Behav. Sci. 53, 249-257.
Wechsler, B. & N. Brodmann, 1996. The synchronisation of nursing bouts in group housed sows. Appl. Anim. Behav. Sci. 47, 191-199.
Welch, A.R. & M.R. Baxter, 1986. Responses of newborn piglets to thermal and tactile properties of their environment. Appl. Anim. Behav. Sci. 15, 203-215.
Whatson, T.S. & J.M. Bertram, 1980. A comparison of incomplete nursing in the sow in two environments. Anim. Prod. 30, 105-114.
Whatson, T.S. & J.M. Bertram, 1982. Some observations on mother infant interactions in the pig (Sus scrofa). Appl. Anim. Ethol. 9, 253-261.
Whittemore, C.T., 1993. The science and practice of pig production. Longman Scientific and Technical, Harlow, Essex. 661.
Whittemore, C.T. & D. Fraser, 1974. The nursing and suckling behaviour of pigs. II. Vocalisation of the sow in relation to suckling behaviour and milk ejection. Br. Vet. J. 130, 346-356.
Whittemore, C.T. & C.A. Morgan, 1990. Model components for the determination of energy and protein requirements for breeding sows: a review. Livest. Prod. Sci. 26, 1-37.
Yang, H., P.R. Eastham, P. Phillips & C.T. Whittemore, 1989. Reproductive performance, body weight and body condition of breeding sows with differing body fatness at parturition, differing nutrition during lactation and differing litter size. Anim. Prod. 48, 181-201.

Subject index

F

G